Detox or Disease

Choosing Your Path To Better Health

William R. Kellas, PhD
Andrea S. Dworkin, ND, PhD

Disclaimer

The information presented in this book is for informational and educational purposes only, and is designed to help you make informed decisions about your health. Although benefits to specific illnesses are discussed, this book is not to be construed as patient-specific medical advice. If you have or suspect a serious medical condition, we strongly recommend that you consult with a knowledgeable healthcare practitioner prior to utilizing the information in this book. In addition, any questions or concerns, either general or specific to yourself, can be directed to the Center for Advanced Medicine, Encinitas CA, 888-244-4420 or 760-632-9042. Do not change any treatment or medication you are currently receiving without consulting with your physician. Having made these recommendations, the authors and publisher specifically disclaim responsibility for any adverse outcome resulting from the following of these procedures and protocols.

ISBN
Paperback 978-0-9636491-3-3
E-book 978-0-9636491-4-0

Published by Professional Preference, Carlsbad CA
Includes bibliographical reference and index

Keywords: Title, Authors, detox, detoxification diet, toxicity, sauna

Table of Contents

Table of Protocols and Summary Charts

About the Authors

Dr. William R. Kellas has a PhD in Nutritional Biochemistry. Over three decades ago he faced a severe hereditary arthritic condition and a wheelchair prognosis. He researched and tried progressive treatments, developed a deep understanding of how the body works, and over time has regained his health and vastly slowed the relentless advance of his disease. His desire to use his knowledge to help others led to his founding Comprehensive Health Centers in the 1980s and cofounding the Center for Advanced Medicine in the 1990s, in Encinitas, CA. This clinic integrates advanced medical, chiropractic, and other practices with biological dentistry, with a strong focus on detoxification. Dr. Kellas has also written the ***Toxic Immune Syndrome Cookbook*** and hosts the nationally syndicated radio program Health Talk: A Second Opinion. He has worked for several decades as a practitioner at the clinic.

Dr. Andrea S. Dworkin has a doctorate in Naturopathic Medicine (ND) and a PhD in Nutrition. She also has Bachelor's and Master's degrees in Chemistry, which gives her a strong background in toxicology and an understanding of how chemical toxins and nutrients affect the body. Like Dr. Kellas, Dr. Dworkin has overcome personal health challenges, utilizing the theories and protocols in this book. She has also worked as a practitioner at the Center for Advanced Medicine. Dr. Dworkin has coauthored, with Dr. Kellas, the Toxic Twins books ***Surviving the Toxic Crisis*** and ***Thriving in a Toxic World***, and is working to produce other books as well.

Part 1
Introduction and Basic Principles

Toxicity, Detoxification, and You

How are toxins and detoxification related to health?
Lately, news reports have given extensive recognition to the effects of toxins on our health. The environmental movement, and the resulting focus on green building products, has its roots, not only in increased awareness of our external environment, but in our health as we are exposed to such things as formaldehyde and paints in our homes, air pollution, water pollution, mold, food additives, and electromagnetic radiation.

Toxins can lead to disease in a number of ways. Chemicals and metals in excess often cause inflammation, which in turn can cause cardiovascular problems, pain, and other health issues. The clinic which inspired this book, the Center for Advanced Medicine in Encinitas, CA, has done decades of work with patients and found that toxicity is a major cause of illness and distressing symptoms. For over 25 years, Dr. Bill Kellas, the founder of the clinic, has addressed toxins as being the root cause of many health issues. The practitioners at the clinic have found that detoxification is usually the first step, and sometimes the only step, to a successful outcome.

Are there factors other than toxins and detoxification in the control of illness?
Although toxins are among the greatest factors in disease, there are certainly others. Structural imbalances, dental problems, nutritional deficiencies, genetic factors, electromagnetic radiation, energy imbalances, allergies and sensitivities…all these and more can contribute to illness. Most of these are covered more comprehensively in the Toxic Twins books, ***Surviving the Toxic Crisis*** and ***Thriving in a Toxic World***, written by the authors of this book. This book focuses on toxins – primarily chemicals, metals, dietary toxins, and the opportunistic microbes that accompany them – and detoxification, as well as dietary deficiencies, although other factors are mentioned where relevant.

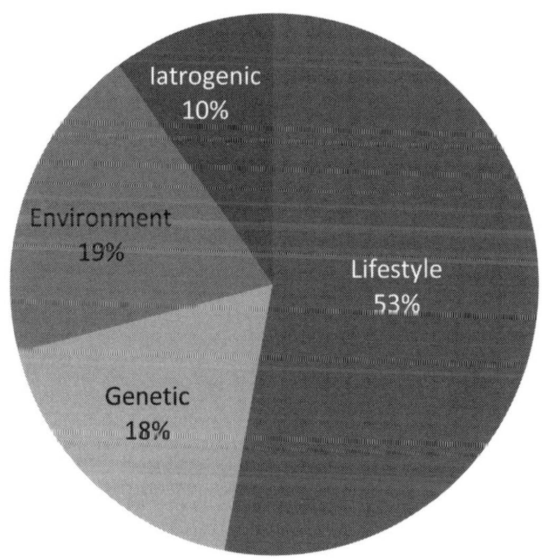

According to the CDC, 18% of illness is due to genetic factors, 53% lifestyle, 19% environmental, and 10% iatrogenic (caused by the medical profession). In other words, we can influence 82% of the factors. Where should we start?

Will detoxification help cure or prevent illness?

Detoxification can help to the extent that toxins are part of your health problems, and toxicity-related illhess is the case for many people. The importance of detoxification lies not only with detoxification in general, but with the selection and implementation of the type of detox that is right for your particular toxin overload. It can be said that there are three Rs of detox:

- Do the right thing
- in the right way
- in the right order

Although toxins may be a significant player in your health problems, they are not always the whole story, and other types of treatment may also be needed. Without detoxification, however, treatment for such things as opportunistic microbes may not be successful. This is one of the reasons why having your detoxification and overall health regimen monitored by a knowledgeable health professional is so important, although much of what is in this book is also suited to do-it-yourself evaluation and detoxification.

With this said, though, detoxification is so important, and is almost universally needed in today's world, that many progressive clinics and practitioners begin with toxin assessment and detoxification. Once toxins are cleared to a great extent, other causative factors can more effectively be identified and dealt with.

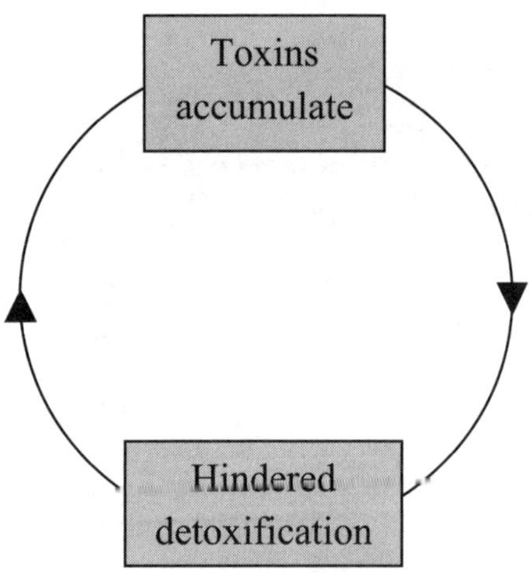

Aren't our bodies designed to eliminate toxins on their own?

A healthy body is designed to be able to eliminate toxins through such avenues as the cytochrome P450 system for chemicals and metallothionein for metals, but only up to a point. Most of us are exposed to more toxins than our bodies are capable of handling. Notice also that we said a *healthy* body, which so many of us no longer have. Ironically, the reason many of us have unhealthy bodies in the first place is due to toxins. So now we have a vicious cycle situation in which the toxins themselves are hindering our ability to detoxify them.

We clearly need to help our bodies along in our quest for detoxification, which is in turn the first step towards regaining our health. This book addresses both the necessity for detoxification, and, more importantly, how to detoxify.

Where does all of this knowledge come from?

The protocols in this book come in large part from protocols used successfully for decades at the Center for Advanced Medicine, in Encinitas, CA, just north of San Diego. Stories of the clinic's twenty-thousand-plus patients who have been helped by these protocols – in some cases getting their lives back after trying dozens of other doctors, clinics, and approaches – are interspersed throughout the book.

The story of how a clinic devoted to detoxification and other progressive treatments came to be is an interesting one. About three decades ago, Dr. Bill Kellas was told that he had a hereditary disease, ankylosing spondylitis, one of the most severe forms of arthritis. He was already starting to stiffen up in his 20s, and his doctors told him what was known about his disease at that time: almost nothing. No cure, no treatment, and the prognosis was that he would be in a wheelchair in a few years. Since he is not of the temperament to just accept the "expert" opinions and lie down and roll over and just give up on life, he thought outside the box and looked for anything that might work. His research led him to knowledge of the role of toxins and detoxification in his and other illnesses, and he was able to radically slow down the otherwise relentless progression of the disease.

After time he became so knowledgeable that other people started asking him for advice. He was able to help people with chronic and autoimmune diseases such as MS, lupus, arthritis and others that doctors had given up on. His postgraduate training of a sort was with masters in their field such as Dr. John Yiamouyiannis who fought fluoridation of water, and Dr. Hal Huggins who alerted the world to the dangers of mercury and other toxic dental work. After separating from his partner Dr. Robert Marshall in 1987, he founded the Comprehensive Health Centers in 1988, and in 1996 he and Mark Drucker, MD, co-founded the Center for Advanced Medicine, integrating the disciplines of detoxification of various types, biological dentistry, naturopathy, chiropractic, allergy treatment, osteopathy, nutritional guidance, chelation, and other healing modalities. More than twenty thousand people have been helped by their work and knowledge. That knowledge and record of success in the field of detoxification has been distilled and is presented here in this book.

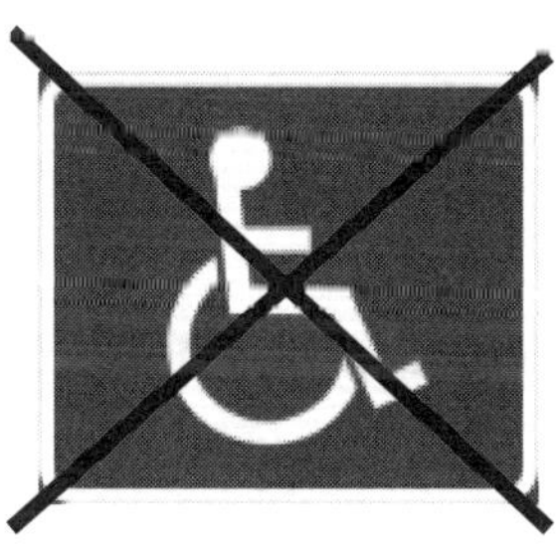

Dr. Kellas still works at the clinic; he was joined by Dr. Andrea S. Dworkin, who worked there as a practitioner and now focuses on writing and research. Oh, and more than thirty years since his devastating prognosis he still doesn't use a wheelchair.

About This Book

How is this book different from other detox books?
There are other detox books on the market, and most of them have a few things in common; this book takes a different approach.

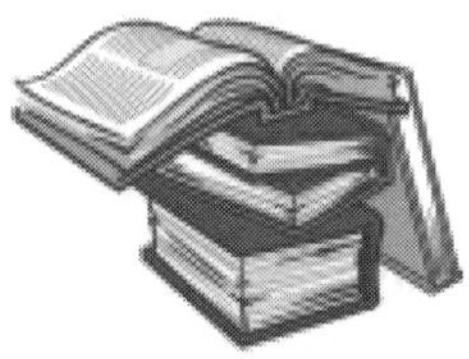

Most detox books focus on diet, both on dietary toxins and on a dietary solution. Although many toxins come from food sources, and while a detox diet is an important part of detoxification and is covered in detail in this book, other sources of and treatments for toxicity abound. You can be toxic even if your diet is impeccable, since toxins come from many sources other than food. In addition to dietary detoxification, detoxification for chemicals, metals, and parasites are included in this book.

Another important way this book differs from other books is in the way we address a complex subject. As is the case with diet books, many other detox book authors take the simplistic approach that their program is *the* right program for every reader. In the real world, different people have different exposures to toxins, and bodies are, to a certain extent, different in their reactions as well. This book, rather than presenting a single and simple one-size-fits-all solution, helps you to narrow down *your* particular toxin-related problems, and then helps you to find and implement the solutions that would best help *you*. Yes, a book that says "just do this" – to everyone – is the simplest to write and implement, just as producing clothing in just one size would be simpler, but in both cases it would be unlikely to find a good fit.

Another difference is that most detox books are geared towards the person who could use a cleansing tune-up, rather than one with serious toxin-related illness. This book is based on decades of experience helping people with serious and even life-threatening illnesses. Although a person with serious illness would be best served by working with a knowledgeable practitioner, the detoxification modalities in this book can be useful for nearly anyone, regardless of where they are on the spectrum of health and illness.

One size fits all? Not.
Plenty of books out there state, either definitively or by implication, that their program is *the* best and only program for anyone, regardless of each person's particular underlying problem or physical constitution. Such one-size-fits-all approaches sell books and appeal to those who want simplicity, who want one definitive expert approach that they can follow stepwise, who want to disengage their thinking processes and follow directions.

This book is different. It's about what is going on with *you*, how to figure that out, and what to do about it. We give the concepts and tools necessary to figure out and implement a detoxification and healing strategy tailored to you.

How should I use this book?

This book can be used in any of several ways, some of which may be more effective than others.

Pick and choose – One way is to go through the book and pick and choose detox modalities based on cost, appeal, availability, and other criteria that are not directly related to health. Will this be useful? Perhaps surprisingly, yes. Pretty much any detox will provide some benefit, especially in contrast to the way most of us live our lives. This is why there are a number of dietary and other detox books on the shelves, each of which have people saying how beneficial their program is. Did the program really help them? Probably yes. Is the program good for them in the long run? Unknown. Was the program the best one for them in particular? Possibly, but more due to coincidence than anything else. The pick-and-choose method definitely leaves something to be desired, but it's better than nothing.

Do everything – Another way is to do everything discussed in this book. This will certainly give great benefit and positive results. However, it is also likely to be a waste of resources. If, for example, you undergo chelation, a procedure that removes metals from the body but which can be expensive and somewhat invasive, and metals aren't a problem for you, then this is simply wasted time and money. You may think, after reading about sauna detox, that this is something you would like to or should do. However, if chemicals are a minor player in your particular health problems and your major issue is dietary, then sauna, while marginally useful for you, would be a waste of time and money better spent on diet.

Be selective – A third way – the most effective way – is to best utilize the structure of this book. Ready, aim, fire works a lot better than ready, fire, aim. This book, with its multitude of approaches, eliminates much of the chance and coincidence. There is considerable discussion about how you can narrow down what are likely to be *your* major toxic issues, and the detoxification approaches that can thus best benefit *you*. With the help of a knowledgeable practitioner, the best individualized approach is even more likely.

The best way to start using this book, therefore, is to read it carefully and thoroughly before actually doing anything. This will enable you to come up with a custom-tailored plan of action.

How is this book structured?

This book is laid out in five parts.

- **Why**: Part 1 is an introduction to a new way of looking at health and disease, as well as discussing the importance of toxicity and detoxification.
- **Who** is affected: Part 2, **Systems and Symptoms**, talks about the various ailments and their connection with toxicity, and how detoxification can help.
- **What** the problem is: Part 3, **Suppressors and Sources**, is about recognizing and eliminating sources of continuing toxicity; detoxification is of limited use by itself unless the sources are identified and eliminated. Detoxification is like draining the tub, but you won't make much headway unless you also turn off the tap, the influx of new toxins.
- **How** to do it: Part 4, **Solutions**, is the crux of the book, the detoxification modalities that, either with practitioner support or on your own, will allow you to detoxify. Ways in which to know what types of detoxification would likely be best for you are also covered.
- In addition: Part 5, **Support,** covers nutritional and other support to optimize detoxification.

Patient profiles throughout the book illustrate the principles discussed. Most of these profiles, and their outcomes, are of actual patients at the Center for Advanced Medicine.

For perspective

It is important to read the entire book before starting, since it is crucial to have an understanding of what is happening and why. While good results might well result from turning directly to Part 4 and starting to detoxify, it is most advantageous to know what is best for you, given your particular health manifestations, likely toxins, and resources.

A New Way of Looking at Health

Why is this book needed?

In the case of most chronic illnesses, there is no one cause, and therefore no one cure or treatment approach. Successful treatment lies in identifying the cause(s) of your particular case and addressing those. Silver bullets don't work – the one cause, one treatment approach. Nor does the symptoms = pill approach that so often characterizes allopathic (mainstream Western) medicine.

One cause can result in a number of health problems depending on the person's genetic weakest link. If, for example, ten people are exposed to pesticides, one may develop multiple chemical sensitivity (MCS), another chronic fatigue, another may develop cancer twenty years later, and another may appear to escape unscathed. On the other hand, one symptom or disease, for example chronic fatigue, MS, or heart disease, may have one or more causes that can differ from person to person depending on their genetic weakest link: chemical exposure, dental problems, structural imbalances, or nutritional deficiencies.

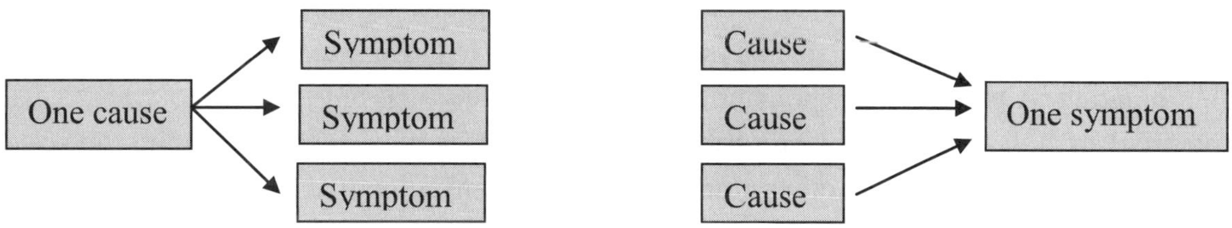

An approach that has met with considerable success is the naturopathic viewpoint, instead of identifying and treating the disease name or the blood test results. In this way of thinking, the body is designed correctly and will work as it should much of the time, but sometimes there is something that gets in the way of optimal function. In this case the body may need help. The key to giving this help lies in identifying the underlying problem, not in diagnosing the particular disease. Underlying problems fall into four basic categories:

- Too much of the bad stuff, or toxicity
- Too little of the good stuff, or nutrients
- Imbalance, as in structural or energetic imbalance
- The opportunistic microbes that take advantage of the weakness caused by the other three factors, much the way that flies, maggots, and vultures feed on decaying meat, or hyenas and jackals go after diseased and weak animals.

The focus of this book is on toxicity, identification and elimination of the source of toxins, and detoxifying the body. We are living in such a toxic world that many if not most people can benefit from detoxification.

Why we need to look upstream

In actually treating illness, instead of covering up the symptoms, it is important to identify and deal with the root cause. Let's look at an analogy.

If you wanted to clear up the water in the river that flows by your house, filtering the water that is right in front of you will not yield much in the way of results. It is crucial to look at what is happening upstream, such as a chemical plant discharging wastes into the water. The water in front of your house will not clear up until the chemical plant stops discharging toxins into the water upstream. Similarly, if one is treating a chronic illness, simply diagnosing and treating the presenting symptoms will have little efficacy; it is critical to look upstream to identify and eliminate the cause(s) of the symptoms.

In some cases, what appears to be the root cause has yet another cause farther upstream. For example, let's say the presenting problems are fatigue, brain fog, vaginal yeast infections, and abdominal bloating. A practitioner who is not looking upstream at all but is only looking at what is right in front of him or her might prescribe treatments for each of these symptoms separately. Looking upstream for a cause, another practitioner might determine that an overgrowth of candida yeast is the originating cause, and yeast control measures such as an antifungal medication and a strict anti-candida diet will have some limited success. However, one can look even farther upstream – since the body is designed to control the yeast appropriately, something else must be causing the yeast overgrowth. That something, in this case, might be the mercury in metal dental fillings that kills the beneficial bacteria in the intestines that would otherwise keep the yeast in check. Antibiotics, lack of breastfeeding in infancy, and whiplash are also upstream possibilities in this case.

The distinction between upstream, midstream, and downstream thinking can also be called source, system, and symptoms.

The three-legged stool

Getting well is a three-step process, and the three steps can be analogous to a three-legged stool – all three are necessary for the stool to stand, and all three, plus structure, are necessary for true healing to occur. The three legs are:

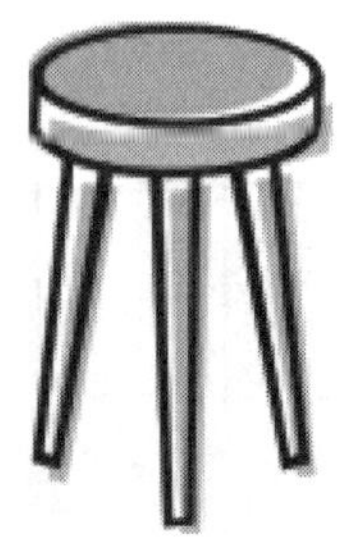

1. **Triggers** – Identifying the chemicals or other substances that trigger the problem and symptoms, and removing them from the immediate environment. Microorganisms are also triggers, secondary to the primary

triggers such as chemicals.

2. **Detoxification** – Removing these chemicals and other triggers from the body.
3. **Support** – The nutrients, foods, and supplements that can boost the healing power of the body in general as well as supporting the body's own detoxification efforts.

The body's skeletal structure, as well as other body systems, makes up the seat. Microbes sit on the seat.

What are the major triggers?

The usual primary triggers are chemicals and metals, as well as EMF and other types of radiation, which overload the body until it can no longer clear out the toxins, and the overwhelmed body can no longer function optimally. The result can be fatigue, pain, allergy, and disease. These are discussed in detail in Part 3 of this book, and in even greater detail in the book ***Surviving the Toxic Crisis***, written by the authors of this book.

What is Involved in Detoxification?

How is my health like a rain barrel?

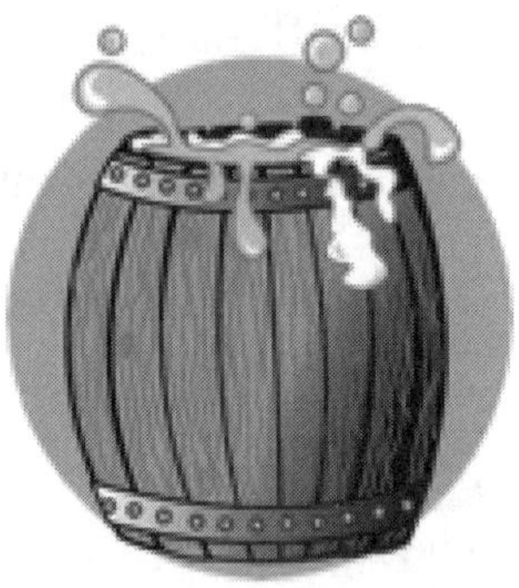

A rain barrel analogy can help you to see how toxins can affect you. In an admittedly simplistic analogy, imagine that your body is a rain barrel designed to hold and process toxins. Those who are genetically fortunate inherit a large rain barrel, while others get a medium-size or small one. The various toxic suppressors – chemicals, metals, structural problems, some kinds of dental work, microorganisms, electromagnetic radiation (EMF) and even emotional stresses – fill the barrel over time. Once the barrel is full and begins to overflow, symptoms start, and can worsen the more the barrel tries to hold. Imagine also that there is a spigot at the bottom of the barrel letting some of the contents out; this spigot is your detoxification systems. Some fortunate people have a large spigot, some have a smaller one, and some have a larger one that has gotten clogged with toxins; the size of this metaphorical spigot is the ability to detoxify and the speed at which one can do so.

Our approach to detoxification is threefold, keeping in mind the rain barrel image:

- Reduce the inflow of new toxins by identifying and avoiding them.
- Detoxify in order to reduce the level of toxins in the barrel, or body.
- Support and balance the systems and organs of detoxification as much as possible, analogous to unclogging and enlarging the spigot.

These three steps of detoxification follow the chapters of this book. One must first recognize and eliminate sources of continuing toxicity (Part 3), then detox the body (Part 4), during which time the body should be supported via nutrition in its detoxification efforts (Part 5).

What are the two stages of detoxification, and what are the implications?

Furthermore, detoxification occurs in two stages, once the influx of new toxins has been halted as much as possible.

- Stage One: The toxins, which have accumulated and have been stored in tissues, muscles, fat, liver, kidneys, the lymphatic system, and elsewhere, need to be pulled out of their storage places – especially fat – and into the bloodstream.
- Stage Two: The toxins in the bloodstream have to be eliminated via the body's usual channels: urine, stool, breath, and sweat, utilizing the kidneys, liver, digestive tract, lungs, and skin. This goes on to a certain extent anyway,

but when the body is so overloaded additional measures are needed. Liquid transports the toxins out.

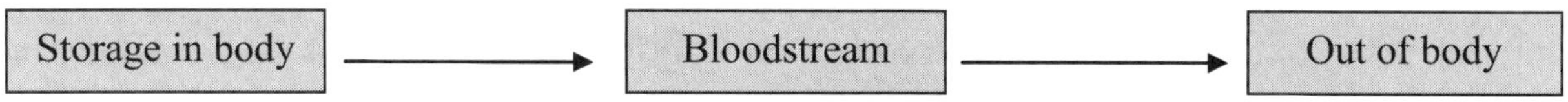

It is important to understand this. Quite often in detoxification of whatever type, as toxins are released from fat storage and enter the bloodstream, symptoms may worsen temporarily. This is why both heat and weight (fat) loss can cause symptoms to worsen – in both cases the toxins leave the fat and enter the bloodstream. The body doesn't differentiate between toxins from outside and toxins that enter the bloodstream from the various storage depots around the body. Thus during the early stages of detoxification your toxin-caused symptoms may temporarily worsen. Hang in there – this can actually be a good sign that the detox is working.

Assessment of Toxic Overload

How do you know whether toxins are a major player for you – and which toxins?
You can self-assess, or be assessed, for your toxin load in a number of ways. The resulting information will be of immense help in determining whether detoxification is likely to be of significant benefit. It is also crucial in determining what types of detoxification would most benefit you.

What is the first step in assessment?
The first step in assessment, both self-assessment and that done by a practitioner, involves looking at your symptoms and your personal history of exposure, and doing an overall physical assessment. Thinking about and talking or writing correlations down could come before doing any actual testing. Although, unlike the case in much of mainstream medicine, the disease diagnosis, if any, is not very important and is not what is treated. Instead, the symptoms and diseases are important clues as to what is going on at the root cause level. Symptoms other than the main one of concern can also be useful in diagnosis. Certain diseases or certain affected parts of the body tend to be due to particular causes; the next section on ailments, Part 2, discusses some of these.

Personal history of exposure to chemicals, once you know what to look for, is an important part of cause assessment. Some illnesses and symptoms come on rather abruptly, making it easier to see a cause and effect. For example, fibromyalgia or Parkinson-like symptoms such as tremors can come on soon after certain kinds of dental work due to the electrical charges generated, called the battery effect. In some cases, fatigue or chemical sensitivity can come on soon after spraying the house for ants or termites or having a new carpet put in. Thus there is a clear correlation between toxin exposure and the onset of symptoms, and this provides a good starting point. In the case of Dr. Andrea Dworkin, one of the authors of this book, her fatigue and severe chemical sensitivity followed years of working as a chemist and, before that, a chemistry student. In this case chemicals were the main cause, and chemical (sauna) detox was the way to go. Even in such a clear-cut case, however, additional approaches were needed.

Patient profile

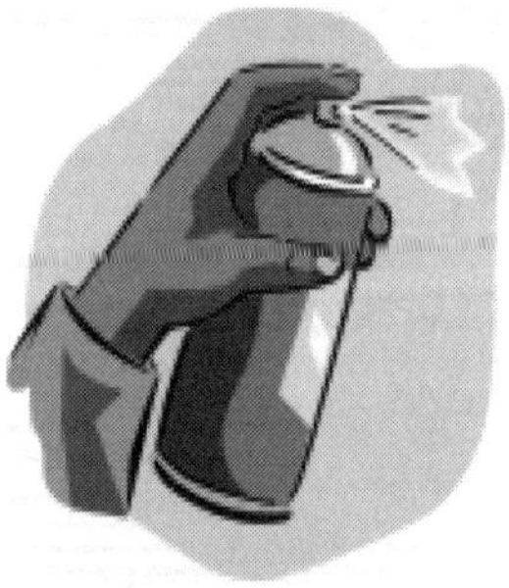

One patient had always had a trim figure, but suddenly she started putting on weight and couldn't lose it. Urged to search her mind for anything unusual that had happened just before the scale reading started to climb, she recalled that there had been an invasion of ants in her kitchen, and that she had grabbed the container of pesticide and just started spraying, breathing in a good bit of it in the process. As a result, her fat cells multiplied and grew to try to store the fat-soluble poison, since it was more than her body could handle all at once. She was also retaining water as her body, concerned more about survival than about her pants size, tried to dilute the toxin. The pesticide probably adversely affected her thyroid, the arbiter of metabolism and the rate at which calories are burned. Sauna detoxification helped to remedy the problem.

Be aware

Observe symptoms that correlate with exposure to a potential toxin; this can give valuable information. Take careful note of any change in the way you feel and try to correlate it with something you have been exposed to. For example:

- Itchy earlobes from wearing cheap earrings can be a sign of nickel allergy.
- Foggy thinking after pumping gas can indicate sensitivity to petrochemicals or to any of the components of gasoline.
- A flash of anger or irritability after smelling cologne on a passerby can indicate an allergy to artificially scented products, an allergy which is quite common and often unrecognized.
- Feeling poorly after a trip to the dentist can indicate increased mercury exposure, which can happen even when metal fillings are being removed if done improperly, or allergic reaction to any of a number of dental materials such as formaldehyde or latex.
- The "allergic salute" is the upwards rubbing of an itchy nose; see if this correlates to any particular inhalant exposure, especially pollen.
- Do sore, itchy, or red eyes occur during smog alert days, during pollen season, while wearing contact lenses, or when reading the newspaper? This can be a sign of allergy to these things.
- Fatigue can be a major allergic symptom. Take a look at what you did an hour to a day before.
- Aching may be correlated to a particular exposure.
- Mucus, throat clearing, stuffy or runny nose can be correlated with exposure.
- Higher pulse rate, discussed later in this chapter, can indicate allergy.
- A root canal or crown correlated with any resultant symptoms can indicate that the dental work is a problem.

As is the case with responses to an elimination diet, careful observation is more accurate than most tests because it measures actual responses. A written diary of exposure and symptoms may be helpful. Any of these responses can indicate a problem with a particular substance; the reaction can also indicate an overall toxic overload.

What are some kinds of testing I can do myself?

pH testing

Urine testing with a pH test strip is useful in helping to determine what broad category of toxins are the most likely players. Test strips are also valuable in helping to monitor your progress.

pH is the measure of acidity or alkalinity. 7 is neutral, neither acid nor alkaline; lower numbers are increasingly acid and higher numbers are increasingly alkaline. Water is, in theory, a 7, but due to added chemicals or acid rain, in actual practice water, including bottled water, tends to be slightly acidic. Optimal pH varies throughout the body; stomach acid should be about pH 2 to digest protein, the intestines should be slightly alkaline, and blood needs to be within a very narrow range of about 7.35-7.4. Urine, which is easy to test, should be around pH 6.0; urine pH is an indicator of the pH, and thus the condition, of the rest of the body.

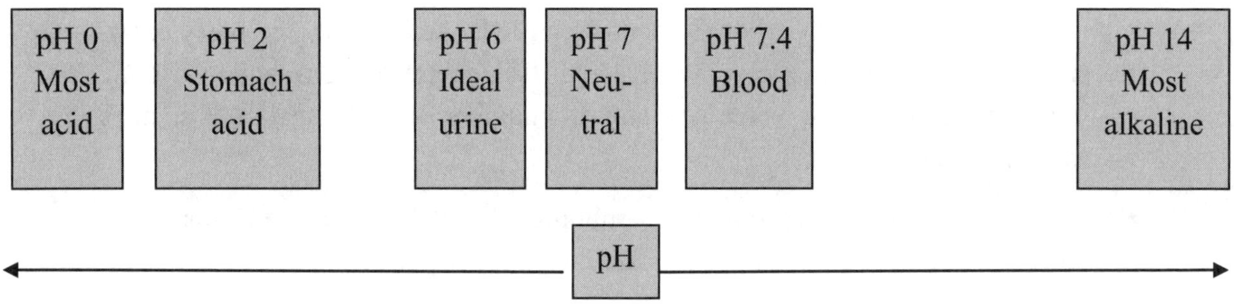

How is your body like a swimming pool?

In most of the body, including the blood, the optimal pH is around 7.4. Those readers with pools or hot tubs may recognize 7.4 as being the optimal pH of the pool water. This is not coincidental. In a pool, that pH is best for discouraging the growth of bacteria and fungus. This is true in the body as well.

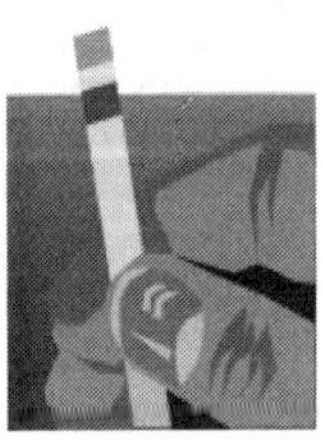

How is pH testing done?

pH test strips can be ordered from the Center for Advanced Medicine, 888-244-4420 or camhealthtalk.com, or bought at some drugstores. pH test strips come in different ranges depending on their purpose, so it is important to get a roll of strips with a range of pH 4.5-7.5. When exposed to the liquid that is being tested, the strip changes color to indicate pH, which is then compared with an enclosed color chart.

A sample of your first morning urine is tested. This is the first morning urination after the sun has risen; 3AM doesn't count, nor much after sunrise. Test around the end of the flow, not at the very beginning, since initial sediment can alter the actual pH. Tear off a 1" to 2" strip of pH paper and quickly dip it into the stream; don't hold it there or you may rinse off the testing chemical. After a few seconds, when the color change isn't still fluctuating, compare the color to the color chart to determine your urine pH. It is a good idea to keep a record of your diet and your urine pH on the following day to establish correlations.

How are the results interpreted?

The optimal urine pH should be between 5.8 and 6.2, and should be stable from day to day. If the pH is higher, around 7.0, this can indicate:

- Fermentation, which in turn can indicate a problem with sugar, yeast or bacteria.
- It can also indicate food allergies.

A pH of less than 5.5 is typically due to:

- Fermentation in a different stage – with fermentation, the pH can rise and then suddenly drop as a vinegar-like substance is made.
- Chemical or metal toxicity
- Low minerals

What about saliva pH testing?

Saliva pH testing is sometimes recommended, but it is not very useful. Salivary pH is more likely to reflect temporary and local conditions, such as what you have recently eaten. Urine, coming from the body itself, more accurately reflects what is going on systemically.

Detoxification diet

The detoxification diet, covered in detail in Part 4, has a diagnostic component. Your reaction to the diet – or lack of reaction – can provide valuable clues as to what is going on with you. With this diet, the protocol is both diagnosis and treatment.

Pulse testing

The pulse can be taken on the wrist at the base of the thumb, or at the temple. To take your pulse, put a finger (not the thumb, which has a pulse of its own) on the pulse point of the wrist just below the base of the thumb. Feel around until you find a definite beat. Count the number of beats in 30 seconds and multiply by two to get the beats per minute. First establish your baseline, or resting, pulse. This is your pulse rate when you haven't recently exercised or eaten, and is the rate to which your pulse will be compared under other circumstances. The resting pulse rate will probably be around 60-70 beats per minute.

Then test your pulse 15-20 minutes after eating a particular food or sooner after breathing something that you suspect is toxic. Don't change your basic posture (sitting, standing, lying) or activity level during these few minutes. Many times, although not always, the pulse rate will increase if the food eaten or the toxin breathed is one to which you are allergic or otherwise reactive. If the pulse is at least ten beats per minute higher than at baseline (before eating the food), this is a strong indicator of allergy to that food. Foods or other substances to which you are allergic are seen by the body as being toxic, and should be eliminated from the diet.

The accuracy of this method compared with the other methods is not known, but it has been shown repeatedly to have some validity. However, it costs nothing, involves no needles or discomfort, and can be done at any time without a doctor's assistance. After doing a detoxification diet (Part 4 of this book), pulse testing can be utilized as foods are added back.

Allergies to other foods ingested at the same time as the target food can confuse the results. Additives can also confuse the results; for example, if you eat a food preserved with sulfites and your pulse speeds up, this may be due to either the food itself or the sulfites, and the food may then be erroneously identified as an allergen. It is thus best to test pure foods by themselves whenever possible.

Other methods of determining food sensitivity

The following are also indicators of food sensitivity:

- Flushing after eating certain foods may be an indication of sensitivity to that food.
- A drop in energy a half hour to a couple of hours after eating may indicate food allergy or sensitivity. The midafternoon slump that comes on after eating a less than healthful lunch is common.
- Sublingual testing can be done; the food does not have to actually be eaten for the body to recognize the effect. Put a bit of the food under the tongue, and check your pulse; as is the case with food that has been eaten, the pulse rate will often rise if there is a problem with that food.
- Some foods, especially wheat and dairy, can cause mucus formation in sensitive individuals. See if you can correlate food intake with sniffling, throat clearing, or coughing.
- Body aches or headache after eating certain foods can indicate sensitivity.

What tests can professionals do to help determine toxic load?

If you have access to a knowledgeable professional or clinic, many more tests can be done. Some of these are screening tests, designed to give an idea of what might be going on with you; the results point the way toward more definitive testing. Screening tests give a bit of information on a lot of things, while more specific tests indicated by the screening tests give more information about one thing. Screening tests save time and money by narrowing down the testing possibilities.

Of course, many diagnostic tests other than those described here are available, such as X-rays or EKGs for heart rhythm. The ones discussed here are those that are most linked to the determination of toxicity.

Blood tests

The standard blood test, also called a CBC and chem panel, contains separate tests that can indicate toxicity. Elevated liver (SGPT, GGTP) or kidney (BUN/creatinine ratio) enzymes can indicate liver or kidney stress, or fungus in the case of high SGPT and GGTP; because both are organs of detoxification, such stress can indicate a high level of toxicity.

The levels of the different types of white blood cells are also measured, and an elevation of these can be a sign of microbial infection, which can be secondary to toxicity. Different types of white blood cells fight different types of microbes, such as bacteria (neutrophils) or viruses (lymphocytes, monocytes), and so the type of white blood cell involved can help narrow it down.

There is a caffeine clearance test, in which the person is given caffeine and then urine is tested at intervals for caffeine. The faster the caffeine is cleared out of the bloodstream, the better the organs of detoxification are doing their job. A slow clearance rate can mean that the liver and kidneys are overburdened with other toxins.

Preliminary blood tests, such as the CBC, are known as screening tests, since they give an overview of how the body is working. Abnormal results on these screening tests can lead to more detailed follow-up tests to determine the cause of the abnormal test results.

Live blood and dried layer analysis

Live Blood Analysis (LBA) is a simple testing technique that is rarely done in mainstream US medical venues but is more common in progressive clinics and in Europe and other parts of the world. If the technique seems a bit unfamiliar, consider that even the most mainstream doctors make use of blood tests to see how the liver, kidneys, and other systems are doing. The information about the entire body is in the blood, and these two microscopy blood tests are simply another way to access it.

In LBA, a drop of blood is taken from the finger and examined under the microscope. Among the large number of things that can be determined, there are some that relate directly to toxicity.

- Blood cells should float freely and separately. If they are clumped together like lozenges in a roll, this can indicate toxicity, as from chemicals or dietary toxins (coffee, fried foods, microwaved foods), or allergy.[1] Since blood cells carry oxygen, this clumping means there is less surface area on each cell for oxygen transport, and this can lead to fatigue, brain fog, and other symptoms.
- Spicules, or needle-like structures, can indicate liver stress, which can be caused by abuse or toxicity. However, if you are undergoing detoxification procedures of any kind at the time of the test, such as diet, sauna, colonics, or liver flush, the presence of spicules can be a positive indication that the liver is processing toxins for elimination[1].
- Cells can show a shiny grayish metallic outer surface if metals are present in the blood.

In dried layer analysis, also called Oxidative Stress Analysis (OSA), dried layers of a drop of blood are examined by microscope under a lower magnification than that used for OSA. Some of the toxicity-related indicators that can show up with OSA include[1]:

- Small white areas can indicate stress, emotional or physical, including allergy and chemical toxicity.
- A dark ring or dark spots around the outside of the blood drop usually indicate metals. The metals, heavier than other blood components, go to the outside of the drop by centrifugal action.
- Blood layers can actually show a shiny grayish metallic outer surface if metals are present in the blood, and black specks can be seen at the outer edges of the blood layer under magnification.
- Tan/grey areas can indicate yeast overgrowth, which is promoted by eating sugar or having mercury fillings. This is an *indication* of yeast (screening test), as compared with a *diagnosis* of yeast as obtained from a stool test, in which the actual yeast is seen.
- Dark areas within the drop may indicate parasites.

Hair testing

In hair testing, a sample of hair is taken, typically about an inch close to the scalp. Pubic hair, while less convenient, is good to test, since it is less exposed to environmental contamination or hair care products and thus more accurately reflects what is going on in the body. The sample is broken down chemically and analyzed for metals.

Why isn't hair testing useful for mercury and chemicals?

Because mercury is volatile – tends to evaporate – hair testing is less accurate for mercury than for other metals. Also, most mercury is in the kidneys bound to sulfur; like chemicals in fat, the mercury must be liberated from the kidneys to test for it. The best way to utilize hair testing for mercury is to use it indirectly: test for aluminum, which is cleared from the body using some of the same pathways (metallothionein) as the clearing of mercury. If aluminum levels are high, this is an indication that mercury levels are likely also high and the aluminum-clearing systems are busy dealing with the mercury overload. By the way, this correlation between mercury and aluminum may be why high levels of aluminum are found in the brains of those with Alzheimer's disease – this probably reflects high body levels of mercury, the more likely cause.

Hair testing is also not very useful for detecting chemicals. For one thing, hair tends to collect whatever is in the air so a hair test would not likely reflect what is going on in the body. Although a pre-testing shampoo could remedy that, there are other problems with hair testing for chemicals. For one, many chemicals are volatile and, like mercury, would evaporate during the preparation for testing. For another, chemicals are not typically eliminated into the hair follicle, so hair testing would not give an accurate indication of body chemical levels.

Urine testing

One of the best known uses of urine testing is to find various drugs or their metabolites. This is of limited use, if any, for our purposes, since you would likely know whether you have used any drugs. Most drugs of any type are potentially toxic, including street drugs, prescription drugs, over-the-counter (OTC) drugs, or the big three legal recreational drugs alcohol, tobacco, and caffeine – the body doesn't make distinctions based on legal status.

Another use of urine testing is testing for metals after provocative chelation. Chelation, discussed in Part 4, grabs hold of metal ions, and since the chelator-metal complex is now water-soluble, it is urinated out and can be collected during the eight hours immediately following chelation and tested. Since metals themselves are not water soluble, and metals in their unchelated form would not appear in the urine, testing for metals in urine without chelation is relatively useless.

The specific gravity of urine can be measured. Specific gravity is the measure of the density of a liquid; for example, syrup is denser than water, and oil is lighter, or less dense, than water. The specific gravity of pure water is defined as 1.0, and the preferred range for urine is 1.02, very close to that of water. If it is much denser than that, this can indicate something as simple and temporary as low water intake, or it can mean that chemicals and metals are thickening the urine enough to be measured. One way to distinguish between the two is to check the color – if the urine is dark in color, the problem can be simple dehydration, but if the urine is dense but light in color, the problem is more likely metals. A specific gravity that is too low can be an indication that minerals are low; when that is the case, water has a hard time entering the cells and is urinated out without the cells' waste products.

Urine pH, usually tested during a professional urine test, can be used by a knowledgeable practitioner as an indicator of metals, chemicals, fermentation, allergy, or low minerals, as described earlier in this chapter under do-it-yourself testing.

Urine testing can indicate an infection in the urinary tract, bladder, and/or kidneys by noting the presence of bacteria or white blood cells. However, urine testing won't pick up infection elsewhere in the body.

Muscle testing

Weak instead of strong? It may be an allergy

In muscle testing, also called kinesiology testing, the person being tested holds one arm out and resists the downward pressure on the arm applied by the tester. Once this baseline level of resistance is noted, the person holds some of the suspected allergen or toxin in the other hand, or smells it, and pressure is exerted on the arm again. The amount of substance tested can be small, and it can even be in a glass vial or other container. If the degree of resistance is about the same, the substance is not problem for that person. If the patient's arm lacks the strength to resist with certain substances, the patient is sensitive to them. This reaction, the weakening of muscles when exposed to toxins, helps to account for the muscle weakness and fatigue experienced by some toxin-laden people.

In an alternative method of do-it-yourself kinesiology testing, the person puts the thumb together with the first or second finger, and a second person tries to pull the thumb and finger apart. This is repeated with the test substance held in the other hand; a lack of strength indicates an allergy or unhealthy food or substance. However, this technique has its drawbacks when done by oneself, using one hand to test the other, since the testing hand will be weakened as much as the tested hand so often a meaningful conclusion can't be drawn.

There is a somewhat different type of muscle test that examines the particular detoxification pathways. The tester would have the subject smell a particular substance, such as ammonia or chlorine bleach, that is cleared by a certain detox pathway, and then use muscle testing to determine whether that pathway is weak. If, for example, the cytochrome P450 detoxification system is weak, and this system is used to detoxify chemicals, this can indicate an overload of chemicals. If the metallothionein system, used to detoxify metals, is weak, then metal overload is suspected.

Allergy testing

As mentioned, a substance to which the body is allergic or sensitive is one that the body senses as being toxic, and reacts accordingly. For some of our purposes, then, allergies can be treated in the same way as toxins.

What are the types of allergy tests?

Allergy tests can be provocative, noninvasive, or direct. Not all types of allergy testing give the same information.

Provocative testing involves trying to provoke a response by putting the substance in the body in some way – injection, ingestion (eating or drinking), inhalation, or on the skin. The immune system reacts to provide an unmistakable response. Severe reactions – even life-threatening anaphylaxis – or increased sensitization may result, even with homeopathic-level (tiny) doses. At worst, the deliberately induced allergic reactions are unpleasant. However, if allergies are ruining your quality of life, then the discomfort of testing is a small and worthwhile price to pay.

Noninvasive testing does not affect the body directly. Noninvasive tests include blood tests, in which the reaction is observed in the blood sample rather than in the body. Energy medicine tests such as EAV and kinesiology (muscle testing) – both of which are discussed in this chapter – are also noninvasive, and measure the body's energetic response to substances.

Direct testing is a subjective method that involves removing as many potential allergens and tox ins as possible, as through an elimination diet such as the detoxification diet in Part 4, and then carefully observing your reactions to individual substances. This is the best method, as it measures your body's reactions in real life situations.

EAV – The body electric

Electrodiagnosis makes use of the energetic pathways, sometimes called meridians, in the body. Electrodiagnosis is sometimes called EAV, for Electroacupuncture According to Voll, the researcher who developed it. When the device is used for allergy or toxicity testing, the patient holds a metal electrode in one hand and the tester places a metal probe against the acupressure points on the sides of the fingers or toes. After getting a baseline reading, the tester does a reading along with the test substance. If the wavelength, or frequency, of the substance causes a galvanic skin response reading – the basis of the lie detector test – significantly different from (usually higher than) the baseline reading, the substance is a probable allergen or toxin. A reading lower than baseline when nutrients are tested can indicate a deficiency of the nutrient. The procedure is harmless and little or no discomfort is involved. Many types of substances can be tested – foods, inhalants, liver toxins, chemicals, and metals. Verification with more expensive or invasive objective tests is sometimes done to follow up.

The concept of the frequency of a substance might be an unfamiliar one, and one that comes up again in Part 4, in the NAET chapter. By way of analogy, a scientific instrument called a spectrophotometer, or spectrometer, measures the precise color frequency of anything colored. Every paint chip in the paint department of the home improvement store has a different frequency, and your eye and mind together will judge any particular color to be pleasant, unpleasant, or neutral. Substances have a frequency as well, although most of them are not identified as a color. Your body may perceive that particular frequency – of a food, nutrient, or toxin – as helpful, harmful, or neutral, and precise instruments can measure your body's response to a particular substance frequency. Muscle testing makes use of the same type of reaction, although EAV is usually more objective.

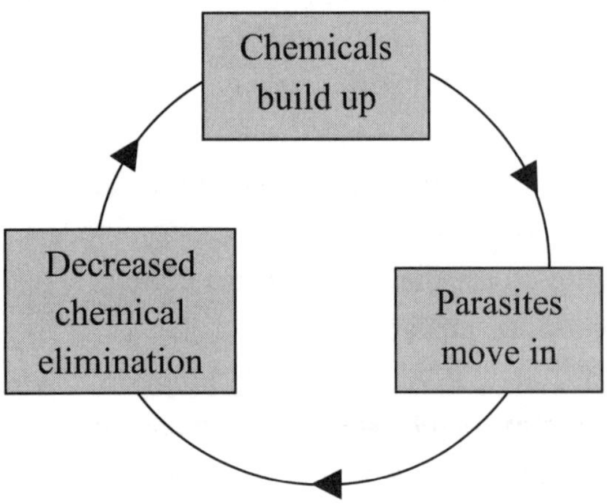

Stool testing

Stool testing is most typically used to determine the presence of parasites, such as microbes, yeast, bacteria, or worms, or their eggs. Their presence is an indication of possible toxicity, since parasites tend to be secondary suppressors that move in once the body is weakened, as by toxins. All of these parasites can affect the body's ability to digest oils that protect against toxic chemicals. Thus a vicious cycle can be set up in which chemicals set the stage for parasite invasion, which then interferes with the body's elimination of the chemicals.

Parasites tend to have a cycle which may be regulated by the moon, in which they come out to lay their eggs at a certain time of the month. This means that, if parasites are suspected but not detected, it might be necessary to test again in a few weeks to catch them at the time when they are most detectable. Unfortunately, a reliable correlation with a particular moon phase has not been found; if there were such a correlation, then testing could be done only at that particular time.

Chemicals do not show up reliably in the stool, unless the food eaten a couple of days previously had a high chemical content, so stool testing is not done for chemicals or metals directly.

Mercury vapor and voltage testing

In mercury vapor testing, a device similar to that used by OSHA to test air quality is utilized. The testing wand simply and painlessly samples the air inside the mouth, both before and after chewing gum, which mimics what happens when food is eaten. It is not uncommon to find mercury levels in the mouth far above what would cause OSHA or the EPA to evacuate a building or declare an alert.

Voltage testing can show whether a battery effect in the mouth is caused by dissimilar metals, such as mercury or nickel-containing stainless steel under metal crowns. Although voltage in the mouth is not, strictly speaking, a toxin, it can be an additional indicator that metal in the mouth may be a problem that should be addressed through removal.

Voltage in the mouth can affect the body's pathways, particularly the brain and heart, which have electrical signals of their own. In addition, high voltage can drive neurotoxins such as mercury into the body in increased amounts and at an increased rate, and can release more neurotoxic corrosion similar to that on car battery terminals.

Sputum testing

Sputum testing can be done to help diagnose the presence and cause of a respiratory infection. A sample of the sputum is sent to the laboratory and a culture is grown to determine whether there are pathogenic bacteria in the sample.

Saliva testing

Saliva testing, such as that done by Diagnos-Techs (diagnostechs.com), can test for adrenal function. Since a major cause of adrenal stress is an accumulation of chemical toxins, this can be a good screening test.

Saliva testing is not useful to evaluate chemical or metal toxicity, since chemicals are stored in fat and not released into the saliva.

Biopsy

Direct identification of toxins in body tissues can be made by taking a biopsy, or sample, of the body tissue, such as fat, muscle, or liver. This is one of the most invasive, as well as painful, types of tests, and should be done only as a last resort. However, fat biopsy is useful for chemical determination because chemicals are stored in fat, so it is worth weighing the risk vs. benefit in this case.

Other testing

A technique called gas chromatography can measure pesticides in a body fat sample. In addition, an IgG test can determine whether your blood cells are reacting to pesticides. This test determines reactivity rather than the direct presence of pesticides. Pesticides are rarely found in high levels in the blood or urine because they are stored in the fat.

Summary chart of testing procedures

Type of test	Type of toxin						
	Chemicals	Metals	Yeast	Microorganisms	Allergy	Low minerals	Liver stress
Urine pH	X	X	X	X	X	X	
Detox diet reaction			X		X	X	
Pulse testing					X		
Blood test (CBC)				X		X	X
Caffeine clearance	X						X
LBA/OSA	X	X	X	X		X	X
Hair testing		X					
Urine testing	X	X		X			
Provocative chelation		X					
Muscle testing				X	X	X	
Electrodiagnosis	X	X	X	X	X	X	X
Stool testing				X			
Mercury vapor testing		X					
Voltage testing		X					
Biopsy	X			X			

Part 2
Systems and Symptoms
Ailments That Can Be Related to Toxicity

Making the Best Use of This Section

How will I be affected by toxins?
Recall the discussion of the genetic weakest link in the previous chapter. You saw how the relationship of toxicity to illness depends in large part on the total toxin overload and your personal genetic propensity to a particular illness. However, certain illnesses are more likely to be associated with certain toxins.

What if I'm already sick?
The chapters in this section discuss some of the toxins associated with particular ailments. These are not necessarily *your* causes, but you might see a correlation between your symptoms and exposure to particular toxins. The causes discussed do not represent an exhaustive list of all possibilities; such a detailed listing could take up an entire book for one ailment. However, the correlations that you might see can point you in a direction towards your best type of detox.

What if I'm not sick but concerned about a particular disease?
You may not have any symptoms, but you might have a genetic predisposition to particular health problems. You may, for example, have a strong family history of cancer, neurological problems, or heart disease. You can take preemptive action to figure out what categories of toxins you most need to avoid, and to detoxify from what is likely to be a buildup of these toxins, even though you aren't having problems yet. Such detoxification can be very helpful in warding off your genetic legacy or even avoiding it altogether.

What if I'm just trying to stay healthy in general?
Even if you don't have any particular ailments in mind, this section is still a good one to read. Although it is organized by disease rather than by chemical, if you know that you've had a considerable exposure to a particular chemical or metal, you can see what that chemical can cause. Knowing this can provide good motivation to detoxify and to be the healthiest you can be.

In the next chapters in this section, we discuss the correlation of certain illnesses with certain toxins, as well as general problems and their causes common to that topic and specific ailments within each category.

What else is involved?

As discussed previously, many factors other than toxicity – such as allergens, stress, radiation, and structure – can contribute to any of the ailments; this section and this book focus on toxicity. Also, toxins other than those mentioned can be present; these are only some of them, in most cases the most likely ones.

Summary chart of ailments and causes

What is the chart about?

The chart on the following page summarizes the ailments and their primary causes. These are grouped by causes on the left by category (chemical, drug, food and nutritional, metal and dental, microorganisms, and structure) and body systems on the top (cardiovascular, nervous system, cancer, and others.).

These causes are marked as follows:

Most likely causes

Major causes

Minor causes

Not a likely cause

How can I best use this chart?

Take a look at your ailment(s) and, following the grid, their most likely causes. A transparent colored marker can help with this. You may very well find that certain causes, such as mercury or low minerals, show up for several of your health problems; these are a good place to start to address one or more root causes for your health problems in general.

What if I need more information?

This chart is intended as only a rough summary of ailments and their causes. This entire section, Part 2, goes into considerably more detail, and will tell you much more specifically which particular metals, microorganisms, or nutritional deficiencies might be causing your problems.

		Neurological	Cancer	Cardiovascular	Bones and joints	Gastrointestinal	Mental	Skin problems	Endocrine	Overweight	CFS, FMS, MCS
Chemicals	Chemicals, general										
	Pesticides										
	Chlorine										
	Fluoride										
	Silicone implants										
Drugs	Smoking										
	Alcohol										
	Drugs, medications										
Dietary	Food sensitivities										
	Food additives										
	Gluten										
	Sugar										
	Low minerals										
	Nutrient deficiencies										
Metal and dental	Mercury										
	Nickel										
	Root canals										
	Cadmium										
	Other metals										
Other	Microorganisms										
	Yeast										
	Structure										

Neurological Problems

The nervous system consists of the brain, spinal cord, and peripheral nerves.

Many neurological ailments are most closely associated with pesticides, solvents, and mercury, although almost any toxin overload can contribute to these ailments. Free radicals, the most damaging component produced by chemicals, can destroy brain cells, reduce immune responses, change neurotransmitter behavior, and modify the physical structure of brain cells.[1]

The brain is 60% fat, and most chemicals such as solvents and pesticides are oil-soluble, so it isn't surprising that a lot of toxins end up in the brain. While something called the blood-brain barrier protects the brain to a certain extent, a lot of poisons still enter the brain, causing various degrees of damage.

What is meningitis and what system is involved?
A three-layered covering of tissue, the meningeal system, covers the brain and spinal cord for additional protection. The meningeal system, or meninges, also acts as a shock absorber by providing a spring effect to counteract movement.

The ailment meningitis, the most familiar context of the meningeal system for many people, is an infectious inflammation of the meningeal system. Meningitis can cause stiffness as the muscles and meninges contract in response to the inflammation. Chemical toxicity, allergy, electrical charges produced by metals in the mouth, and even emotional stress can also cause meningeal inflammation, which in turn can lead to muscle contraction and pain as well as other neurological symptoms.

What are some of the chemicals that can cause general neurological symptoms?
Pesticides contain a penetrant which carries the poison into the insect's cells. Most pesticides affect the insect's nervous system; this means that pesticides can affect our nervous systems, too, especially when their action is aided by the use of a penetrant. The major difference between us and a bug in reactions to pesticides is the fat in our bodies that stores and dilutes the toxins, allowing us to experience chronic symptoms rather than sudden death.

Some of the effects of pesticides, especially nerve damage, are irreversible, and this has been known as early as 1958, as stated in a medical journal article at that time[2], yet the use of pesticides continues.

Solvents, whose purpose is to dissolve oils, can damage the fatty myelin sheath around the nerve cells and cause neurological symptoms and diseases such as multiple sclerosis. This condition is like the fraying of the insulation around an electrical wire, causing intermittent shorting out. Solvents can also cause the dissipation of the nerve impulse which can result in slowing of muscle response and shakiness. Other nervous system effects include both physical and behavioral symptoms such as:

- Memory loss
- Difficulty concentrating
- Impaired dexterity
- Reduced motor function
- Altered personality
- Multiple sclerosis (MS)

Trichloroethylene (TCE) is used as an industrial degreaser, dry cleaning fluid, and paint thinner. It is found in photocopy machines, correction fluid, carpet cleaning solution and floor polishes; therefore it is in many if not most office environments. It used to be used as a surgical anesthetic because it was so effective in causing loss of brain function[3]. Health effects of TCE pertaining to the nervous system include:[4]

- Headache
- CNS depression
- Burning eyes
- Tremors
- Fatigue
- Poor coordination
- Mental confusion
- Irritability
- Disturbed vision
- Loss of facial sensation
- Numbness and tingling in hands and feet

Fragrances – 95% of chemicals used in fragrances are synthetic compounds derived from petroleum – not harmless oils from aromatic flowers – including many toxins and sensitizers that are capable of causing central nervous system disorders.[5] And you thought they just smelled good. Actually, one of the signs of chemical overload is that colognes all start to smell like bug spray, a sign that you have been sensitized to the penetrant that is in both bug spray and cologne to make it stay on the skin and penetrate into the bloodstream.

Food additives can have neurotoxic (harmful to nerves) components. These additives and adulterants include[6]:

- Pesticides in commercial produce
- Food contaminants such as organochlorines, PCBs, and dioxin, which are especially concentrated in animal products
- Fried and high-fat foods, and processed foods with trans fats
- Seafood, especially large and predatory fish (any fish with teeth) such as swordfish and shark, which can contain methylmercury that goes up the food

chain and accumulates as larger fish eat smaller fish. Shellfish can contain cadmium.

- Neurotoxic food additives such as aspartame and other artificial sweeteners, and MSG, added to presumably improve the flavor.
- Some calcium supplements, especially those with bone meal, contain lead.
- Highly processed cheese, some OTC antacids, nondairy creamers, table salt, and baking soda can have high levels of aluminum.

Even some foods themselves can have a neurotoxic component:

- Potatoes, especially those left in sunlight that have developed green areas, contain glycoalkaloids such as solanine. If you eat potatoes, at least remove the green areas.
- Peanuts are sometimes contaminated with the potent neurotoxin aflatoxin.

Metals – General neurological symptoms can be caused by mercury exposure. These problems were documented decades ago.[7] Neurological damage was common in people who worked with mercury compounds in hat-making plants, explaining the origin of the phrase "mad as a hatter."

Central nervous system damage due to mercury includes:

- Light and sound sensitivity
- Headaches
- Convulsions, tremors, muscle twitches
- Numbness and tingling of extremities
- Dizziness
- Hearing or vision difficulty

Most of these are acute symptoms, with sudden onset following a single large exposure. Chronic symptoms can include these and more.

Dentists and dental assistants have been found to have neurological and behavioral impairments in direct proportion to their chelated and unchelated mercury excretion,[8,9] which in turn is related to their degree of unprotected exposure to mercury. In a study done in Norway, a group of dental assistants with a history of mercury exposure were compared to a group of non-exposed health personnel. The dental assistants reported a significant higher occurrence of neurological symptoms, psychosomatic symptoms, problems with memory and concentration, fatigue, and sleep disturbance[10].

Metals other than mercury can cause neurological problems. Lead poisoning can cause CNS (central nervous system) symptoms such as[3]:

- Seizures
- Learning disabilities, hyperactivity in children
- Headaches
- Tremors
- Muscular weakness and pain
- Sight loss
- Dizziness
- Fatigue, malaise (flu-like feelings)
- Nervousness
- Depression
- Disorientation

CNS symptoms of arsenic poisoning include dizziness, headache, weakness, and confusion.[3]

What microorganisms can cause or contribute to neurological problems?

Certain microorganisms and their toxins can cause or contribute to neurological problems when the microorganisms target nerve cells, the brain, or the spinal cord. Botulism's effect on the nervous system may be familiar to readers, since injections of the botulism toxin as Botox can temporarily paralyze the muscles, served by the nerves, where the toxin is injected.

Toxins and microorganisms from the bacteria in root canals are more neurotoxic than botulism. They can cause or contribute to many neurological symptoms and conditions, such as multiple sclerosis (MS).

Lyme disease, a bacterial infection carried by the deer tick, can affect various parts of the body, including the nervous system. An MS-like syndrome can result, with weakness, facial numbness, brain fog, and heavy fatigue.

What about specific neurological problems?

<u>Headaches</u>

Certain **foods and food additives** can cause or contribute to headaches. Artificial sweeteners, aspartame in particular, can contribute to headaches[11]. Chemicals in some foods lead to swelling of blood vessels that can lead to a headache. These foods include aged cheeses, which contain the amino acid tyramine; alcohol, especially red wine, brandy, and champagne; and nitrites in preserved meat products such as hot dogs and lunch meats.[12] A bologna and cheese sandwich washed down with a glass of wine would thus be a bad idea.

Heavy **caffeine** use (4-5 cups of coffee) can cause an increase in headache risk by 30% for males and 20% for females.[13] There is some irony in the fact that caffeine is an ingredient in some OTC medications for headache. Habitual caffeine use, when discontinued, can lead to a withdrawal headache. For caffeine withdrawal headache during detoxification, Epsom salt baths and an ice pack on the back of the head are recommended. Caffeinated drinks such as colas and energy drinks can give children headaches by affecting the expansion and contraction of blood vessels in the brain. However, since withdrawal from caffeine can also cause headaches, the child should be weaned off them gradually.[14]

Alcoholic beverages can lead to headache because alcohol dehydrates as part of its effect.[15] Alcoholic beverages can cause headaches more directly as part of their toxic effect – why do you think they call it in<u>toxic</u>ation?

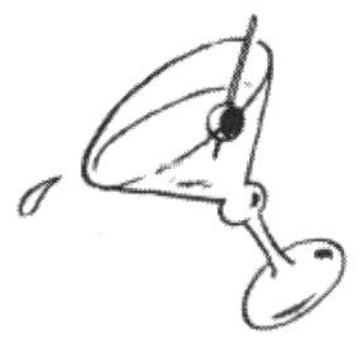

The morning-after headache that is part of the hangover is caused in large part by acetaldehyde, a neurotoxin produced from alcohol by the body as the body breaks down the alcohol for processing and excretion. During Prohibition, methanol, or wood alcohol, was consumed by some; methanol breaks down into formaldehyde (also known as embalming fluid), which is even more toxic than acetaldehyde, causing permanent nerve damage and blindness. Think this doesn't affect today's alcohol drinkers? Even today's alcoholic beverages can contain some methanol. Delirium tremens, an alcohol withdrawal symptom, is caused by the body's and brain's continued processing of aldehydes.

Ironically, **aspirin** and other painkillers and non-steroidal anti-inflammatory drugs (NSAIDs), frequently used to relieve headache and other pain, can cause rebound headaches once the body gets used to depending on them.

Other chemicals – Even short-term exposure to formaldehyde (found in many places, including carpets, cabinets, and building materials) can cause headache at levels as low as 0.8-1.0 parts per million (ppm) after only 10-30 minutes.[16] Toluene, found in cologne and some glues, can cause headaches[17], as can pesticides.

Metals can cause headaches:

- Mercury from dental fillings is a significant cause of headaches. Mercury poisoning can cause hangover-like headaches.[18] In a study of 233 patients with headaches, 222, or 95%, reported improvement in this symptom after removal of the fillings.[19]
- Copper, or foods such as citrus fruits that increase its availability, has been implicated in causing migraine headaches.[20] Excess copper combined with too little zinc can also cause migraines. Copper stimulates activity of vasoactive

amines, which influence the size of blood vessels; too much activity can trigger a migraine. Zinc supplementation can help keep the copper level down.[21]

Low oxygen, which can be secondary to carbon monoxide exposure, can cause headaches. If chronic headaches seem to come on or worsen at home or in a particular place, the furnace should be checked out. Low oxygen levels, as from carbon monoxide, can also have a different and less direct type of headache related effect. Depletion of oxygen can increase sensitivity to electromagnetic frequencies (EMF) such as those from fluorescent lights, microwaves, and radio waves, which can in turn lead to headaches.

Microorganisms such as helicobacter pylori, implicated in stomach ulcers, can also cause headaches.

Although not a toxicity issue, structural problems, such as when the head, neck, and/or bite are out of alignment, are major contributors to headache.

Multiple sclerosis

Solvents, made to dissolve oils, dissolve the fatty protective myelin sheath around the neurons (nerve cells). These include toluene (found in gasoline), and alcohol (in alcoholic beverages and in cologne and many personal care products). Synthetic musks, commonly used in fragrances, can break down nerve cells and their myelin sheaths, with MS-like symptoms.[22] Detergents, whose purpose is to dissolve oils, can have a similar effect; use rubber gloves when washing with detergents to prevent absorption through the skin on the hands. Alcohols and glycols such as those in antifreeze, paints and solvents, and aromatic (ring shaped and usually smelly) hydrocarbons, such as benzene and toluene, also dissolve the myelin.

Artificial sweeteners have been implicated in MS. Aspartic acid, an amino acid found in certain chelated mineral supplements and in the artificial sweetener aspartame, has a detergent (oil dissolving) effect on the myelin sheath. In particular, those who are low in body fat (although not necessarily underweight), such as athletes, would be advised to avoid aspartic acid, as it can take fat from the myelin sheath surrounding the nerves and use it for fuel. Although a necessary nutrient in small quantities, consistent doses of supplemental aspartic acid, sometimes listed as calcium (or potassium or any mineral) aspartate, can cause these nervous system problems.

Mercury, found primarily in dental fillings, is strongly correlated with MS. It is not necessary to have such fillings yourself; some evidence indicates that higher rates of MS are found in dentists and dental workers, due to their daily mercury exposure, than are found in the general population. Demyelinization, a significant cause of such diseases as MS, can be caused by mercury[23], primarily from dental fillings. In a study of 42 patients with MS[19], 33, or 78.5%, reported improvement in their MS symptoms after removal of all metal fillings.

Proper and safe mercury removal techniques are detailed in Part 4 of this book. A number of patients with MS have improved after chelation therapy, also discussed in Part 4. Not all patients will improve with chelation; as in other health cases the degree of improvement depends to a great extent on the degree to which mercury or other metals were a possible root cause of their health problems.

Patient Profile

One patient, Kathy, a nurse married to a doctor, had had symptoms since 1977, and was positively diagnosed with multiple sclerosis in 1992. Doctors could only recommend steroids for symptomatic relief. The steroids made her ill and were discontinued. By January 1995, she had facial paralysis on one side, trigeminal neuralgia (severe facial pain), extreme fatigue, vision problems in one eye, numbness in one leg, balance problems, pins-and-needles feeling in her hands and feet, and urinary problems. She used a walker to get around at home, and a wheelchair to cover longer distances.

Kathy came to Comprehensive Health Center, now called Center for Advanced Medicine, in March of 1995. Tests showed her level of mercury to be 81 – normal or optimal should be below 1, and 81 is higher than that of most dentists. She had her mercury fillings safely removed and replaced with non-toxic dental composite material, and had chelation to remove the mercury from her body. She went on an eight-day detoxification diet and felt much better after three days, with the numbness and tingling subsiding.

Other than this, however, the changes were at first slow. Typically with MS, some days are better and some are worse, without any apparent pattern. Over several months she noticed more good days and fewer bad days, she could walk farther, and she no longer needed an afternoon nap. By June 1995 she was able to walk around EPCOT Center in Florida, and she was previously barely able to shop for a few groceries without leg pain. Her MS tests used to be positive, and are now negative. No brain lesions show on the MRI test, and her spinal tap is negative.[3]

Kathy's story has been repeated many hundreds of times using a similar approach at Center for Advanced Medicine (CAM), with over 90% success. In fact, about 20% of patients at CAM are now MS patients, such is CAM's reputation of success with the illness.

Mercury contributes to MS indirectly as well as directly. Yeast overgrowth is often found in MS patients, often secondary to mercury overload, which kills the protective bacteria that should be keeping the yeast under control. A strict yeast-free diet (described in the Detox diet chapter in Part 4) is typically part of the protocol to alleviate MS symptoms. Yeast can cause MS problems in part because of its conversion to aldehydes in the body.

Mercury allergy, not just mercury toxicity, can be a causative factor in MS. With an allergy, even less mercury is needed to bring on symptoms. Treatment for the allergy as well as the removal of mercury from the mouth and from the bloodstream via chelation may be necessary.

However, mercury is not the only implicated metal. There is a possible correlation between aluminum or nickel (toxicity or allergy) and multiple sclerosis; nickel is found in root canal posts, some crowns, bridges, and other dental work. The battery effect that is set up when there are different metals in the mouth, root canal bacteria, and allergy to nickel and other dental materials can cause problems in themselves and also cause mercury to be released from the teeth into the body faster.

Viruses can be a contributory cause of MS.[24] Lyme disease, which is bacterial, can cause, in its later stages, MS-like symptoms.

MS patients tend to be thin, with low body fat. Chemicals are stored in fat, and if there isn't enough fat to store the chemical overload, the chemicals can end up in the bloodstream, causing neurological symptoms. The thinness may be genetic, or the result of strenuous dieting; in some cases the low body fat is due to a problem with assimilation of nutrients. Gluten intolerance, common in those with MS, flattens out the villi in the intestine through which nutrients are absorbed, resulting in less nutrition reaching the cells regardless of diet. A low or non-gluten diet, described in the Detox diet chapter, can help with this.

Amyotrophic lateral sclerosis (ALS), or Lou Gehrig's disease

Mercury has been implicated as a major factor in the development of ALS.[25] Some patients with ALS have improved or even recovered following properly done mercury amalgam removal.[26] ALS can also be caused by parasites, which can themselves be secondary to mercury, as mercury kills the beneficial bacteria that help keep parasites in check.

Hair lead levels were found to be elevated in ALS patients compared with controls, so lead may be causative for ALS.[27]

A number of patients with ALS have improved after chelation therapy, which removes metals from the body. Not all patients will improve with chelation – the degree of improvement depends to a great extent on the degree to which mercury or other metals were a possible root cause of their health problems.

Gulf War Syndrome – In a study of 2.5 million veterans, it was found that Persian Gulf War (1991) veterans are twice as likely (6.7 cases per million persons) to develop ALS than veterans who served elsewhere (3.5 per million).[28] This study, along with studies of the pro athletes affected, strengthens the likelihood of the illness being related to chemical exposure in many of those with the disease.

A particular **body type** is typically found along with ALS. As is the case with MS and other neurological diseases, ALS disproportionately affects those with a wiry, athletic, low-body-fat build, usually but not always men. Since ALS is known to affect athletes – it is not coincidental that ALS is also called Lou Gehrig's disease after the well-known ballplayer who died from it – there are a couple of possible correlations. Fat stores neurotoxic chemicals so they are less likely to affect the brain; a person with low body fat is less able to store chemicals, which then end up in the bloodstream and from there, the brain. In addition, many athletes typically spend a lot of time playing their sport on a heavily pesticided grassy field, increasing their exposure to these neurotoxic chemicals.

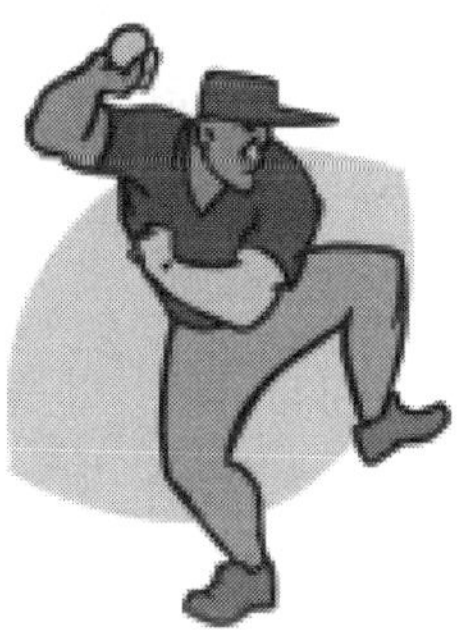

Catfish Hunter, a major league baseball player who spent years playing on grassy fields, was another professional athlete who succumbed to ALS in 1999.

Dizziness, vertigo, and disorientation

Dizziness is a term sometimes used interchangeably with vertigo. The typical symptom is a feeling that the room is spinning and it is difficult to walk straight.

Acetone, a common solvent used in nail polish remover and in cellulose production, can cause vertigo and weakness.[3] Other chemical and metal causes of dizziness or vertigo include excess silver, arsenic, iron, potassium, mercury, manganese, sodium, nickel, lead, selenium, pesticides, aspartame, inhaled chemicals, h.pylori bacteria, and giardia.[29]

Even short-term exposure to formaldehyde (found in many places, including carpets and building materials) can cause disorientation at levels as low as 0.8-1.0 parts per million (ppm) after only 10-30 minutes.[30]

Numbness and tingling in hands and feet

Solvents, especially topical contact with them, is a common cause of numbness and tingling in the hands and feet. Trichloroethylene is a particular solvent associated with this condition[29], but other solvents can also be triggers.

> **Patient profile**
> A type of skin effect was experienced by a patient, Rick, who used to work on cars and would clean his hands with whatever solvent was available such as gasoline or transmission fluid. Years later his hands are still slightly numb, as if he were wearing gloves. It is possible that the fatty myelin sheaths of the nerves in his hands were damaged by the solvents that were absorbed through his skin, resulting in a garbled message when sensations such as touch are relayed from the hands to the brain.[3]

The toxic water additive **fluoride** can cause neurological symptoms. A fluoride pump malfunction in Hooper's Bay, Alaska, caused too much fluoride to enter the water. One death and over thirty cases of illness resulted, including neurological symptoms such as tingling hands and arms, as well as nausea and vomiting and fatigue.[31] Since most municipal water is now fluoridated, it is possible that lower but cumulative exposure over time can cause the same types of problems.

Mercury is implicated in this symptom. One patient with an abscessed tooth had numb hands and feet. He subsequently had the tooth extracted, then had his mercury fillings removed, had chelation to remove the mercury from his body, and started getting better.[3]

Parkinson's disease, tremors, shaking, muscle twitches

Pesticides – A study published in the respected medical journal ***Journal of the American Medical Association (JAMA)*** claimed that environmental chemicals, including pesticide exposure, cause most cases of Parkinson's disease.[6] An analysis of data in California showed that there was an increased mortality rate from Parkinson's disease in counties that used agricultural pesticides.[32] In one study, Dieldrin, a pesticide, was found in the brains of 6 out of 20 Parkinson's disease victims, but in none of the fourteen control samples.[33] This implicates Dieldrin and possibly other pesticides in the causation of, or at least contribution to, Parkinson's disease. Another study links pesticides to young-onset Parkinson's disease, which more typically affects the elderly.[34]

Heavy metals such as mercury, iron, manganese, and aluminum have been shown to increase the risk of Parkinson's disease.[6]

Mercury, in addition to being toxic in itself, contributes to the battery effect. The battery effect is what occurs when dissimilar metals are placed in an electrolyte solution; this is in fact how a battery is constructed. A mouth with electrolyte-containing saliva in which two or more different metals are placed thus becomes a battery, which generates measureable current. This current in turn can upset the normal electrical impulses in the brain, leading to Parkinson's-like symptoms, much the way connecting a battery to your TV set or household appliance is likely to lead to poorer function.

If Parkinson's symptoms abruptly come on or worsen just after crowns or other metal dental work has been done, this is an indication that dental work is a cause. Confirmatory testing can be done using a special ammeter /voltmeter for this purpose. If voltage is high, try having your dentist remove, but retain, the crown and replace it with a plastic temporary crown to see whether symptoms improve. In some cases, the symptoms cease almost immediately, as if an electrical switch had been turned off – which is almost literally the case – but more often it takes some time for the body to adjust to the change and to heal enough for the symptoms to ease.

Medications such as chlorpromazine and haloperidol, prescribed for psychiatric disorders, can cause Parkinson's symptoms, as can metoclopramide for stomach problems and reserpine for hypertension.[6] Movement disorders such as tardive dyskinesia, which can mimic Parkinson's disease, can be a result of taking psychiatric medications.[35]

The use of statin drugs, used for lowering cholesterol, has been correlated with the development of Parkinson's symptoms. Cholesterol, unfairly reviled in the health press, is necessary for the support and protection of the central nervous system. Drugs that suppress the formation of cholesterol would thus deprive the nervous system of this protection. This correlation was made after a number of patients were observed to have Parkinson's symptoms come on soon after starting a regimen of these statin drugs.

Vitamin B6 supplements should not be taken by Parkinson's disease patients who are taking l-dopa, because B6 will counteract l-dopa and can increase Parkinson's symptoms.[29] This is an example of a normally beneficial vitamin that can act as a toxin under certain circumstances.

Seizures, epilepsy, convulsions

Cologne – A number of patients have been known to go into seizures as soon as they were exposed to cologne. Seizures can be triggered by toluene, found in cologne as well as in gasoline and oil degreasers.[17]

One of the most common **insect repellents** is N,N-diethyltoluamide, better known as Deet. It can be absorbed into the bloodstream through the skin, causing allergic reactions and nerve damage. Seizures have been linked to this compound.[36]

The Seeds of Cancer

Cancer is on the rise

In 1900, about one out of thirty people got cancer; today the rate of cancer is more like one out of three who will develop the disease at some time in their lives. Cancer is typically a disease of older people, in large part because the older you get, the more cumulative toxins you have amassed. However, cancer is touching people at younger and younger ages. Sadly, cancer incidence in children and adolescents rose at a rate of 1-1.5% per year from 1969-1999, according to a 2009 article.[1]

Cancer is due to...

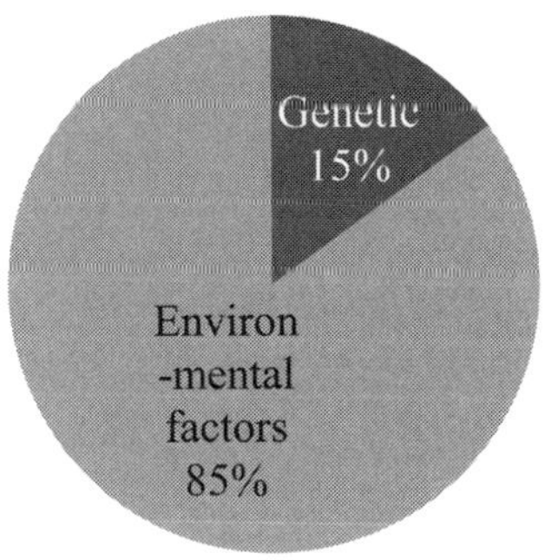

Is cancer due more to genetics or to environment?

Genetics is only a small part of the cancer story. A study conducted at the University of Copenhagen and published in the ***New England Journal of Medicine*** found that people adopted at birth had a cancer risk much more related to that of their adoptive parents than of their biological parents. In other words, environmental factors, including diet, had much more of an effect on cancer risk than genetic propensity. Genetic factors contribute 15%, at most, to one's risk of cancer[1], meaning that 85% is environmental and thus within our control.

Chemicals are a major player in the development of cancer; it is considered to be 75-90% environmentally caused.[2,3] Thus if chemical exposure is identified and limited, cancer can be prevented, or at least the risk can be substantially reduced.

A couple of things that foster the growth of cancer are a weakened immune system that is less capable of detecting and destroying cancer cells, and low-grade chronic inflammation that allows cancer cells to take hold in the weakened tissue.[1]

Find the arsonist

As with all ailments, the approach taken in this book is to figure out the cause of the problem, cancer in this case, and remove the causative factors to the greatest extent possible. Mainstream medicine often takes the approach, "It doesn't matter what caused your cancer – or any disease – the important thing is that you've got it now and so let's treat the disease itself." This approach is like putting out a series of arson fires, endlessly, without attempting to find and stop the arsonist.

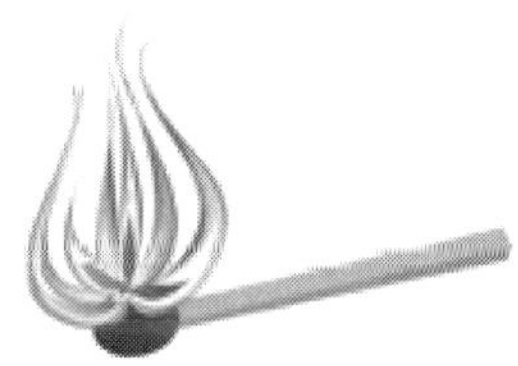

What are some of the toxins that can lead to cancer in general?

Many **solvents** are linked to the development of cancer, since they can penetrate the lipid (fat) membrane around the cells and damage the DNA (blueprint for reproduction). Vinyl chloride from plastics[4] and benzene from gasoline and other sources can cause DNA damage.

Acrylamide, found in tobacco smoke, is also found in lower concentrations in fried and starch-based foods. Acrylamide can lead to potentially carcinogenic DNA changes.[5]

Pesticides – The cancer causing potential of pesticides is further discussed in the chapter on Carcinogens in ***Surviving the Toxic Crisis***[6]. A study of farmers in Italy who were licensed to use pesticides showed a significant increase in cancer, especially that of the stomach, kidney, rectum and pancreas[7]. Women working in the agricultural field have higher rates of cancer of the breast, ovary, and cervix as well as of the lung and bladder, and lymphoma and leukemia, as compared with women overall.[8] Pesticide exposure is the most likely risk factor. Independent research has found a link between elevated pesticide concentrations in fatty tissue and the incidence of cancer as far back as 1968.[9]

Personal care products – You might never think that all the pretty perfumes and potions on your dressing table or in your bathroom can have cancer-causing potential, but that is indeed the case. 95% of chemicals used in fragrances are synthetic compounds derived from petroleum, including many toxins and sensitizers that are capable of causing cancer as well as other health problems.[10] Toluene (found in cologne as well as other places) has been linked to cancer development.

Several ingredients found in a number of cosmetic products are known to be carcinogenic. These include:

- Talc found in powders
- Coal tars found in eye makeup
- Mineral oil found in lipstick
- Saccharin found in toothpaste

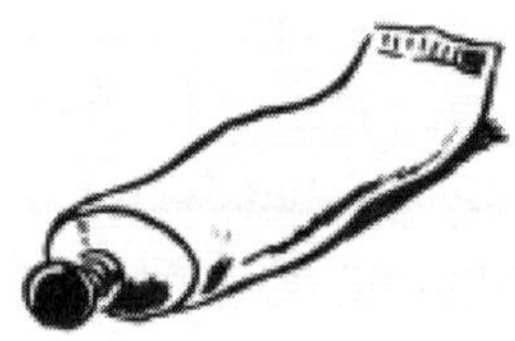

These ingredients may be found in other products as well. Read the labels.

Hair dye, as well as mascara, contains coal-tar dyes and metals. They may also contain aniline dyes, known to cause cancer in animals. Women who used synthetic hair dyes had a 50% greater chance of developing non-Hodgkin's lymphoma, a cancer of the lymph system, than women who never dyed their hair. Hair dyes were also implicated in leukemia and multiple myeloma.[11]

Fluoride – Cellular mutations occur more or less regularly in even a healthy body. DNA is the genetic component of the cell that is the blueprint for the development of new cells, and the cell has a built-in repair system to repair genetic damage so that mutations are not passed on. Researchers have found that 1 ppm of fluoride inhibits DNA repair enzyme activity by 50%. Both genetic abnormalities such as birth defects and cancer would be expected to increase as a result of fluoride ingestion. A number of experiments on animals, insects, and plants[12] have demonstrated this to be the case. High fluoride exposure has been linked to osteosarcoma[13] and possibly other cancers as well.

Fluoridation of water, especially in municipal areas, is becoming increasingly common, due to faulty studies, politics, and the votes of misinformed people. In a study done in 1975 by Drs. John Yiamouyiannis and Dean Burk, the cancer death rate of the ten largest fluoridated cities was compared with the cancer death rate of the ten largest nonfluoridated cities. The cancer death rates were comparable up to the period from 1940-1952, before artificial fluoridation was introduced. By 1969, the nonfluoridated cities averaged 195-200 cancer deaths per 100,000 people, while the fluoridated cities averaged 220-225. There was no other difference between the cities that could account for this 10% difference in only one generation.[6] In the decades since then, even more cities have their water fluoridated. Are you comfortable with having a chemical added to the water supply that could increase your chances of developing cancer by 10%?

Another study found that the bone cancer rate among 10- to 19-year-old males was 6.9 times higher in fluoridated than in nonfluoridated areas of New Jersey.[14] Fluoride in drinking water at the 0.5 to 1 ppm level increased tumor growth rate in cancer-prone mice by 15-25%, most likely by inhibiting the immune system's effectiveness.[15]

How does diet affect cancer development?

Diet is a major player; according to the American Cancer Society, 30% of all cancer deaths are attributed to dietary factors[16], although the numbers may be even higher. "The National Academy of Sciences found that 60% of all cancers in women and 40% of all cancers in men may be due to dietary and nutritional factors[9]."

Trans fatty acids, which hold chemicals as well as being toxic in themselves, have been implicated in degenerative diseases such as cancer, especially breast, prostate, and colorectal cancers.[17]

Sugar intake increases the glucose in the blood. Cancer cells use much more glucose than normal cells, so eating a lot of sugar feeds cancer cells, which depend on a fermentative environment for their growth. Refined white flour quickly turns to sugar in the body and is thus similarly harmful.

When sugar is eaten, the cancer cells convert glucose to lactic acid anaerobically, leading to, among other things, fatigue. This inefficient anaerobic energy metabolism pathway yields only 5% of the ATP energy available in food, leading to malnutrition, which kills 40% of cancer patients.[18] Sugar feeds cancer cells, decreases immune system effectiveness, and contributes directly and indirectly to malnutrition, a triple negative effect.

Fructose (fruit sugar), although it is promoted as a healthy alternative to sucrose (table sugar), can actually enhance the growth of some tumors by stimulating excess insulin production.[19] Fructose is a major part of high fructose corn syrup, said by some to be worse than sugar.

Meats contain arachidonic acid, linked to cancer development. Meats that have been grilled, charcoal-broiled, cured, or smoked are especially carcinogenic.[17]

What about the legal recreational drugs?

Alcohol intake is strongly correlated with the development of cancer, in particular its metabolite, acetaldehyde.[20] Beer, especially, is linked to higher cancer rates.[21] This is likely due to the fermenting yeast in beer being similar to fermenting cancer cells.

Laboratory data suggest that **caffeine** or some components of coffee may cause DNA mutations and inhibit tumor suppression mechanisms, leading to neoplastic (cancer) growth.[22] This is most likely with high consumption of caffeine. Caffeine also sets up a fermenting environment, preferred by cancer cells.

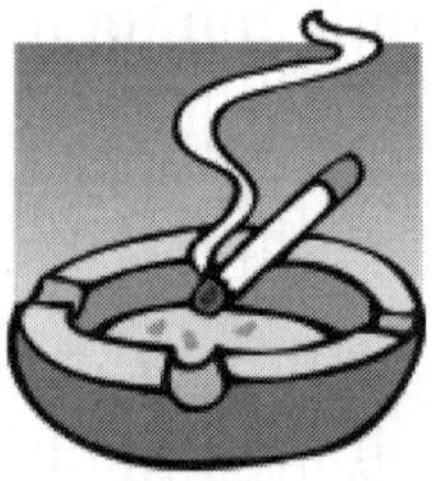

Smoking is well-known to be implicated in the development of cancer. Lung cancer is the best known smoking-caused cancer, but smoking and the use of chewable tobacco products have been shown to be a factor in the development of cancer in general.

How can metals cause cancer?

Cadmium, found in tobacco and in the dust from car tires and brakes, is a major player in the development of cancer. It has been classified as a human carcinogen by the International Agency for Research on Cancer (IARC). Administration of cadmium to animals results in tumors of multiple organs and tissues.[23] Since cadmium is found in sources other than tobacco, even nonsmokers face a cancer risk from cadmium.

Nickel, found in root canal posts, crowns, and other dental work, as well as stainless steel pans and earrings, is a major carcinogen. In fact, when laboratory researchers want to give lab animals cancer, nickel is such a reliable developer of cancer that it is frequently used for this purpose. Nickel is especially implicated in cancer of the breast, urinary tract, and esophagus.

What are some of the causes of specific cancers?

Bladder and urinary tract cancer

Although bladder cancer doesn't get as much press as some other cancers, bladder cancer is the fourth leading type of cancer among men in the US.[24] Early symptoms of bladder cancer are blood in urine and increased urinary frequency.

Chlorine – The consumption of chlorinated water accounts for 9% of all bladder cancers in the U.S. People drinking chlorinated water over a long period of time have a 21% increase in bladder cancer risk.[25] Chlorinated water, in conjunction with fluoride and chemicals such as ammonia, forms chloramines, which are highly toxic and carcinogenic.

Dyes are used in industry, foods, and hair coloring. They can lead to bladder and urinary tract cancers. Unlike many other toxins that are collected and eliminated by the lymph glands, dyes do not leave the lymph glands but instead simply collect there. Eating or drinking highly and artificially colored foods such as soft drinks does not change the color of the urine, indicating that these dyes are not excreted.

Tobacco smokers have an incidence of bladder cancer two to three times that of the nonsmoking population.[26] 50% of bladder cancers are in smokers.[27]

Brain cancer

Chemicals – Chlordane and Heptachlor, used mostly for termites, can cause brain tumors[6], as can other pesticides. Formaldehyde (found in carpets and particle board, and elsewhere) is linked to brain cancer.[28]

Childhood brain tumors are linked to parental occupation. Women and men who worked in the chemical industry in the five years prior to a child's birth were 3.3 and 2.1 times more likely, respectively, to have a child with an astroglial brain tumor.[29]

Metals such as mercury, nickel, and lead are also associated with brain cancer.[30]

Breast cancer

Breast cancer is the second leading cause of cancer death among women. Breast cancer afflicts one out of every eight women. Men have breast tissue too, so they are not immune; men account for 1% of breast cancer cases, and breast cancer is 0.2% (1 in 500) of all malignancies in men.[31] In both genders, there is lymph tissue in the breast area, and toxins are stored in the lymph. Bras, especially underwire bras, constrict the lymph channels and allow toxins to accumulate in that area, which may account in part for the much higher breast cancer rate in women, or at least women in developed countries where all-day bra-wearing is customary.

Pesticides such as DDT, DDE, and PCBs affect the body the way too much estrogen does, and in this way can contribute to the development of estrogen-dependent breast cancer. A Connecticut study cited in ***Archives of Environmental Health*** found 50-60% more DDE, DDT, and PCBs in women with breast cancer than in women without cancer.[32] Three carcinogenic pesticides were banned in Israel, which may be linked to a 30% drop in breast cancer cases in that country between 1976 and 1986.[32] Xenoestrogens such as those found in pesticides stimulate the growth of estrogen-dependent cancers even in men.

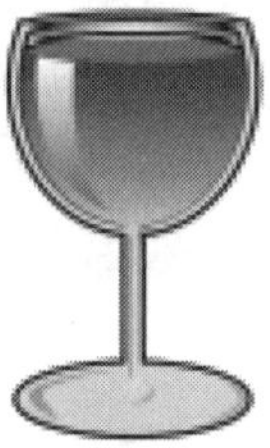

Alcohol – A number of studies show the link between alcohol consumption and breast cancer. Breast cancer risk is shown to be increased by 39% with one alcoholic drink per day average lifetime consumption, by 69% with two drinks per day, and by 130% (more than double) with three drinks per day, as compared with nondrinking controls.[33] Even more dire statistics show that, as reported in the ***New England Journal of Medicine***, drinking as few as three alcoholic drinks a week increases breast cancer risk by 50%.[34]

Smoking –A Canadian study of almost 3000 women found that premenopausal women with a long-term exposure to secondhand smoke had more than twice the risk of developing breast cancer compared with those with little or no such exposure. For postmenopausal women the risk goes up 30% with exposure.[35]

Other chemicals and drugs –A clear correlation between chemicals and breast cancer has been made. US counties with toxic waste sites were 6.5 times more likely to have elevated breast cancer rates.[32] A 2001 study looking at residential toxin exposure detected the presence of 33 different carcinogens in house dust implicated in breast cancer, and 24 different compounds in air.[36]

Even substances considered to be harmless cosmetics can be problematic. One study suggests that women over the age of fifty who have used hair dyes for ten or more years have an increased risk of breast cancer.[37]

Metals – Nickel from root canals, especially in the lower front teeth, can be a contributing factor in breast cancer. The nickel drains through the lymph channels into the main collector lymph node in the chest, close to the breasts.

Iron supplements should be avoided by women with breast cancer because iron can feed the cancer and promote its growth.[34]

A report in the ***Journal of the National Cancer Institute*** links high cadmium levels to increased breast cancer risk.[38] Cadmium also suppresses zinc, which is in the same column of the periodic table and so binds similarly to cells; zinc is necessary for a healthy immune response. A metallic taste can be a sign of a high cadmium level.

Root canals – A study done by Dr. Thomas Rau, who runs the Paracelsus Clinic in Switzerland, checked the records of the 150 most recent (at the time of the study) breast cancer patients treated there. He found that 147 of them, 98%, had one or more root canalled teeth on the same pathway as the original breast cancer tumor.[39]

Dietary causes – Dietary fat has been implicated in the formation of some cancers, especially breast cancer. It is likely that PCBs (polychlorinated biphenyls, a type of plastic) and other fat soluble chemicals stored in both dietary fat and breast and body fat are at least partially to blame, rather than the fat itself. Tissues of women with breast cancer had PCBs and certain pesticides at levels 50-60% higher than in women without breast cancer.[40]

High stool pH can be due to putrefaction, fermentation and allergy, which are in turn linked to a diet high in animal foods and fats. Decrease intake of these foods, increase fiber, and take bifidus and acidophilus.

Polyunsaturated fats such as those in vegetable oils, sometimes advertised as being heart-healthy, can increase a woman's risk of breast cancer.[41] However, monounsaturated fats such as those in olive oil can absorb and dilute chemical toxins and reduce the breast cancer risk.

Women who eat sugar-laden foods more than three times a week have a higher risk of developing premenopausal breast cancer, according to preliminary research from the National Cancer Institute. The proposed connection is that sugar increases insulin levels, which could promote cancer cell growth[42], as well as feeding the cancer cells and lowering immune response.

Colon and rectal cancer

Chlorine – The consumption of chlorinated water accounts for 15% of all rectal cancers in the U.S. People drinking chlorinated water over a long period of time have a 38% increase in rectal cancer risk.[43] Chlorination byproducts such as chlorinated hydrocarbons are linked to increased risk of colon cancer and total combined cancer. It is wise not to drink or cook with tap water and to use a filter for showering.[44]

Diet – Sugar, salt, alcohol, animal protein and fat, and obesity increase the risk of colon cancer.[45] High stool pH, due to putrefaction, fermentation and allergy is linked to colon cancer.

Alcohol – Even one or two alcoholic drinks per day can increase the chance of developing colon cancer, as it irritates the intestinal tract.

Kidney cancer

Cigarette smoking is the single most important cause of kidney cancer. Smokers are twice as likely to develop it as nonsmokers.[46]

Formaldehyde, found in carpets and particle board, and elsewhere, can contribute to kidney cancer.[47]

Regular users of the painkiller **acetaminophen** (Tylenol) may be doubling their risk of kidney cancer.[48] Phenacetin, also a painkiller, was banned due to its severe kidney toxicity; acetaminophen is the major metabolite of phenacetin.[49]

Lead – Rats inhaled so much lead from discarded batteries burning in dumps that they developed kidney tumors.[50] Lead that enters the air from burning and that enters the water table from discarded material in landfills is probably doing us similar harm.

Leukemia

Benzene is linked especially to leukemia; workers exposed to it for over ten years have 33 times the leukemia risk of the general population. Most people have been exposed to benzene for several decades since catalytic converters and benzene have replaced lead in gasoline.

Indoor **pesticide** use has been found to result in a fourfold increase in the risk for childhood leukemia, and the risk climbed to sevenfold for children of parents who used garden pesticides.[9,51] Chlordane and Heptachlor, used mostly for termites, can cause leukemia, as can other chlorinated pesticides.[6]

Fiberglass, a fibrous material like asbestos, is used as a construction and insulating material. Exposure leads to higher rates of leukemia.

Mercury – Hal Huggins found that both low white blood cell counts and high counts (leukemia) were normalized following dental metal (mercury) removal[52], indicating a causal relationship.

Liver cancer

Alcohol and tobacco – 60-90% of liver cancer cases occur when the liver is already damaged by cirrhosis, alcoholism, or hepatitis B.[46] 90% of cancers of the liver are in those who both smoke and drink alcohol, and these two drugs are often used together.

Trichloroethylene, used as a dry cleaning agent, is one of many chlorinated solvents; many glues and plastics fall into the same category. Their carcinogenic effects focus mostly on liver cancer, with the lungs a secondary target.

Vinyl chloride, primarily from occupational exposure, is a known risk factor for liver cancer.[4]

Lung cancer

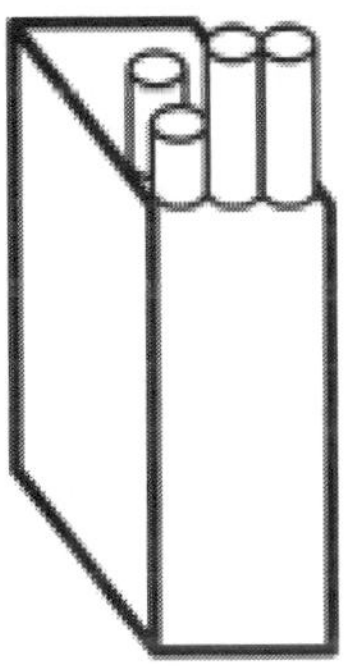

Smoking – The biggest correlation for lung cancer is smoking, although it can be found, though rarely, in those who have never smoked. Dana Reeve, wife of actor Christopher Reeve, is one high profile nonsmoker who died of lung cancer in 2006. Lung cancer is the most frequent cause of death in smokers after heart attacks and strokes. The connection between smoking and lung cancer was noted in a 1950 ***Journal of the American Medical Association*** article[53], if not before, so the association is nothing new. About 85-90% of lung cancers are caused by smoking, for a total of about 100,000 deaths a year in the United States.[26] These deaths are among the most preventable, since smoking, or at least the starting of the smoking habit, is in almost all cases a choice; the exceptions would be children exposed to secondhand smoke.

Passive smoking is a danger. The term refers to the secondhand smoke inhaled by a nonsmoker who is in the vicinity of a smoker. The EPA officially linked passive smoking and increased risk of lung cancer.

Many components in tobacco smoke can contribute to lung and other cancers. Carbon monoxide, produced by a burning cigarette, may be partially responsible for cancers caused by smoking. Tar, the brownish-yellow stuff that can be seen on the cigarette filter and that is a relative of black sticky road tar, clogs the alveoli in the lungs and is carcinogenic. Sticky blackish deposits on the lungs, like road tar, can be seen at autopsy. The tar, nickel, and some other compounds in cigarettes are carcinogens, and cadmium, a metal element found in cigarettes, suppresses the immune system thus allowing the cancer to gain a foothold.

Formaldehyde, found in carpets and particleboard and a number of other building materials and furniture, is a contributor to lung cancer[47]

Soot, coal tar products, road tar, waxes, benzene (a coal tar byproduct), and creosote (a wood preservative used on telephone poles) are linked to cancers of the lungs.[6]

Asbestos is a fibrous, naturally occurring mineral widely used until recently in construction and other applications due to its fire retardant and insulating qualities. Fine asbestos dust contains needle-like crystals which look like burs or stickers from a plant. The crystals lodge in the lungs, attaching like a plant bur, causing scarring of the lungs and lung cancer. These fine crystals can puncture cell walls, letting in other carcinogens. Asbestos workers are ten times as likely as the general population to develop lung cancer. If they smoke, the risk becomes 90 times greater.[6] Fiberglass, a fibrous material like asbestos, is used as a construction and insulating material; exposure leads to higher rates of lung cancer.

Metals – Lung cancer can develop when nickel dust is inhaled. Nickel dust is a known carcinogen with an incubation period of 25-30 years, similar to that of cigarettes.[54] Exposure to chromium can lead to a thirty- to forty-fold increase in the risk of lung cancer 10-20 years after exposure.[6] Cadmium can contribute to the development of lung cancer.[55]

Radon – The National Cancer Institute states that radon may be responsible for at least 30,000 lung cancer deaths each year,[56,57] and is second only to tobacco as a lung cancer cause. Radon is found in the ground in certain parts of the country and the world. The radon, which is radioactive, can enter the house, especially through the basement if there is one. There are maps online that show areas of greatest radon exposure, and testing can be done if radon exposure is suspected. Several methods of sealing the basement can be used to prevent radon from entering the home.

Lymphoma

Pesticides – A Southern California study found that children whose parents use pesticides in the home are seven times more likely to develop non-Hodgkin's lymphoma compared with children whose parents never use them.[58] Non-Hodgkin's lymphoma is on the rise in three predominantly agricultural counties in Ireland, suggesting the strong effect of agricultural chemicals.[59]

Pasteurized **milk** consumption has been associated with greater frequency of lymph system cancer.[60]

Mouth cancer, oral cancer

A chronic ulcer in the mouth is a warning sign of oral cancer.

Smoking and tobacco – Cancer of the mouth is five times more prevalent in smokers than in nonsmokers, and cancer of the larynx is 6 to 9 times more prevalent.[26] Tobacco and alcohol are considered the main risk factors for oral cancer, due in large part to local tissue irritation, which can cause cell mutation. Smokeless (chewing) tobacco, the use of which is on the rise, is associated with a high incidence of mouth and throat cancers. 90% of cancers of the mouth, larynx, and esophagus are in those who both smoke and drink alcohol.

Tobacco isn't the only kind of smoking that can cause problems. Cancers of the mouth, jaw and tongue are linked to the frequent and/or heavy use of marijuana.[61]

Oral leukoplakia, a precancerous mouth lesion, is frequently found in those who smoke or chew tobacco or drink alcohol, both of which irritate the tender mucous membranes in the mouth as well as exposing these tissues to carcinogens.

Nickel is such a potent carcinogen that scientists desiring to give laboratory rats cancer will often inject them with a nickel solution.

> **Patient profile**
> A 26-year-old nurse had dental braces with a loose bit of nickel-containing stainless steel wire that kept poking and irritating the inside of her mouth. Her orthodontist said not to worry about it, that it was no big deal and that it happens to many patients. She developed cancer right where the wire was poking her and essentially injecting nickel, a growth that was half the size of her head when she finally came to a clinic for treatment.[6]

Those with **celiac disease** or gluten intolerance have a greater risk of cancer, particularly of the mouth, pharynx and esophagus, as well as other autoimmune diseases. Studies have shown that even asymptomatic celiac patients should avoid gluten for life to reduce their cancer risk to that of the general population.[62] A conclusion that can be drawn from this is that even those with no particular gluten sensitivity should avoid gluten, since it appears to promote cancer to a certain extent.

Women who use **mouthwash** daily have an increased risk of oral cancer[46], probably due to the alcohol content and its irritation of mouth tissues.

Nasal and sinus cancer

Formaldehyde has been associated with cancers of the pharynx, sinus and nasal cavity.[47] **Soot**, coal tar products, road tar, waxes, benzene (a coal tar byproduct), and creosote (a wood preservative used on telephone poles) are linked to cancers of the sinuses.[6]

Metals – Nasal cancers can develop when nickel dust, a well-known carcinogen, is inhaled. Exposure to chromium can lead to a thirty- to forty-fold increase in the risk of nasal carcinoma (cancer) 10-20 years after exposure.[6]

Prostate cancer

Chlorine in water is major cause of prostate cancer.

Smoking doubles a man's risk of developing prostate cancer.[63]

Diet – Free radicals produced when fat is cooked may play a role in the development of prostate cancer.[63] One study reported that eating five or more servings of red meat weekly could be increasing their prostate cancer risk by almost 80%.[64]

Nickel – Several epidemiological studies have suggested an association between nickel exposure and prostate cancer risk.[65,66]

Cadmium is linked to the development of prostate cancer, and metallothionein, the body's own metal detoxification system, has a protective effect against cadmium and other metals.[67]

Skin cancer

Soot, coal tar products, road tar, waxes, benzene (a coal tar byproduct), and creosote (a wood preservative used on telephone poles) are linked to cancers of the skin. Formaldehyde is linked to skin cancers, especially squamous cell carcinoma.

Coffee – Basal cell carcinoma patients were studied, and it was found that caffeine consumption was higher in cancer patients than in controls.[68]

Personal care products

> **Patient profile**
> A woman in her fifties had skin cancer, which was very likely caused by the cosmetics she used and/or her sunblock/tanning lotion. She stopped using them, and did sauna and chemical detoxification and took flax oil as part of her treatment. She regained her health. She switched to only CA Botana natural cosmetic products.[6]

Stomach and esophageal cancer

Nickel, found in some dental work such as root canal posts, is implicated in the development of esophageal cancer. Nickel is an RNA modifier which can change the genetic expression of cells, including the development of cancer cells.

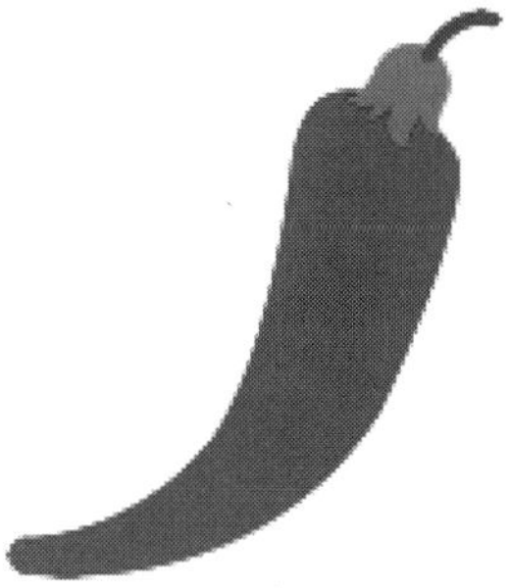

Hot chili peppers may cause stomach cancer when eaten regularly due to the irritation of the stomach lining. Mexicans eat an average of one chili pepper per day, and 10% of all cancer deaths in Mexico are from stomach cancer. Scientists surveyed hundreds of people with and without stomach cancer and concluded that the incidence of stomach cancer increased with chili pepper intake, and those who had the highest intake of the peppers had a huge 17-fold greater risk of stomach cancer compared with those who didn't eat the peppers. The scientists concluded that 76% of stomach cancer cases in Mexico City could be attributed to eating chili peppers.[69]

Cardiovascular Problems

Heart health in general

Much cardiovascular damage is caused by acute chemical exposure; some means are cocaine or overdoses of cardiac drugs such as digitalis, a synthetic derivative of the herb foxglove.

Caffeine use can cause fungus growth, constricted arteries, constipation, and faster blood clotting which can in turn lead to stroke, heart attack, or phlebitis. The faster clotting time is visible under the microscope during the Live Blood Analysis (LBA) test, discussed in the Assessment chapter.

Cardiovascular problems caused by **mercury** include abnormal heartbeat, pressure and pain in chest, high or low blood pressure, and anemia.[1,2] Mercury can damage blood vessels, reducing blood supply to the tissues.[3] Heart problems have been traced to metal toxicity.[4]

Trans fatty acids in general and margarine in particular have been linked to heart disease and heart attacks[5], although some margarines have recently been reformulated so as not to contain trans fats. Corn oil, egg substitutes and even some "healthy" breads are made with hydrogenated oils. Ironically, margarine and egg substitutes have been and sometimes still are recommended by cardiologists, the (incorrect) theory being that such products will reduce cholesterol. By saturating oils to make margarine, manufacturers are selling you the very saturated fats they claim to be helping you avoid. In one study, researchers found that eating margarine causes trans fatty acids to be deposited in the heart itself, which blocks the protective oils from the heart muscle.

Arrhythmias, palpitations, rapid heartbeat

Fluorocarbons and other halogenated (containing halogen) elements such as chlorine or bromine) alkanes (straight-chain molecules) can cause cardiac arrhythmias (irregular heartbeat). These arrhythmias can be brought on simply by wearing a newly dry-cleaned suit.[6]

Aspartame, a sweetener found in some sodas and sugarless gum, can cause rapid heartbeat.[7]

Certain **drugs** can cause or contribute to heart arrhythmias:

- Heart arrhythmias can result from the use of stimulant drugs such as phenylpropanolamine in diet aids as well as herbs such as Ma Huang.
- The cause of heart palpitations can be as simple as caffeine. Eliminate caffeinated beverages to see if this helps to reduce palpitations.
- Alcohol is also a major contributor to the incidence of heart arrhythmias.[8]

- Heart palpitations can be caused by antihistamine drugs.[9]
- Smoking can cause or worsen palpitations.[10]

Nickel can block calcium channels in the heart, lowering magnesium levels and leading to heart arrhythmias.[11]

Mineral deficiencies can cause heart rhythm problems. A deficiency of magnesium or excess of calcium can cause arrhythmia, and a deficiency of potassium can cause a rapid heart rate. Taking the indicated mineral, typically 1-2 tablets or capsules, can restore the heart rate or rhythm to normal in as little as a half hour if a deficiency of that mineral was the cause.

Lyme disease has a number of puzzling symptoms, one of which, especially in the later stages, is heart arrhythmia, possibly due to the spirochete bacteria burrowing into the heart muscle.

Heart attack

Drugs, both prescription and recreational – even, and especially, the legal ones are linked to heart attack incidence.

- Heavy coffee consumption (5 or more cups per day) has been shown to increase the risk of heart attack in a study done on women.[12]
- The anti-impotence drug Viagra is linked to acute myocardial infarction, even in men with no known risk factors or pre-existing disease. The FDA has reported 69 deaths, mostly from heart attack, associated with Viagra, in addition to 54 unconfirmed cases.[13]
- Aspirin was tested and found to be effective for the prevention of myocardial infarction (MI), or heart attack, in this country. Aspirin studies in England showed very little effect. The difference? Buffered aspirin containing magnesium was used only in the U.S. study, so it was very likely the magnesium and not the aspirin which had the protective effect.

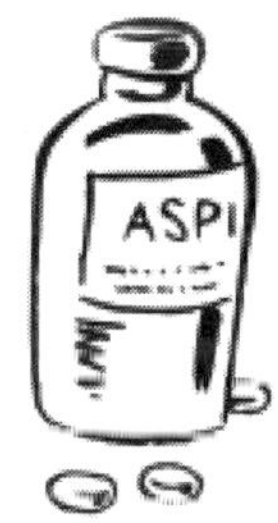

Smoking has been proven to be strongly linked to the incidence of heart attack. Smokers under age 40 are five times as likely to have a heart attack as nonsmokers, according to analysis of World Health Organization data from 21 countries. About 80% of people age 35-39 who had heart attacks were smokers.[14] Women smokers risk a heart attack 19 years earlier than nonsmokers.[15] Stopping smoking can reduce heart attack risk 50-70%.[16]

Secondhand smoke may be an even more powerful factor in heart attacks than previously believed. When the city of Helena, MT, prohibited smoking in public buildings, heart attack rates immediately dropped about 60%. Researchers tracked cases of heart attacks at the major medical center in Helena for four years prior to the ban and then during the six months of the ban, which did not survive a court challenge. Heart attack rates in Helena have risen again since the ban was lifted. The average heart attack rate before the ban was 6.8 per month, which dropped dramatically to 3 per month during the ban. Secondhand smoke causes about 240,000 heart attacks annually in the US, 60,000 of them fatal.[17]

Iron, usually considered to be a beneficial mineral, can actually increase heart attack risk. Men over age 60 were 1.4 times as likely to have a heart attack for every 50 mg of iron they take.[18] Too much iron can lead to free radical damage, which includes heart attack due to damage to the heart muscle lining. Men, by the age of 45, have 300% more stored iron than women, and 300% more risk of having a heart attack. After menopause, women's iron stores go up, and so does their risk of heart attack. Chelation, discussed in Part 4, is quite useful in removing excess iron from the blood.

Calcium may crystallize out of the blood, plaquing on the blood vessels. This leads to the narrowing of the interior blood vessel diameter which can eventually result in heart attack or stroke. This excess calcium is removable by chelation, discussed in Part 4.

Heart disease

Heart disease is the number one cause of death in the US, responsible for over 700,000 deaths annually.[19]

Calcium channel blockers, ironically prescribed for heart health, may increase the risk of cardiovascular disease and/or incidence of mortality.[20] Calcium channel blockers allow more beneficial magnesium into the heart cells; simply taking magnesium supplements can provide the benefits without the risk, as long as they are not taken to excess. Magnesium can cause loose stools and a large excess can cause heart rhythm problems. See recommendations on the supplement bottle or consult your practitioner.

Coffee drinking has been shown to elevate homocysteine levels, a risk factor in cardiovascular disease. Although coffee drinking is associated with higher levels of tobacco smoking and lower intake of supplements and fresh fruits and vegetables, which also raise homocysteine levels, coffee drinking alone was shown to raise homocysteine levels even after these other variables were corrected for.[21]

Smoking – In one study, the death rate from heart disease in male smokers under age 65 was 427 per 100,000 compared with 166 per 100,000 for those who never smoked[16], or nearly three times as high. The CDC estimates that secondhand smoke causes 35,000 deaths a year from heart disease in the US.[22] Acetaldehyde, found in both cigarette smoke and smog, is a strong cross-linking agent. Cross-linked arterial tissue toughens and leads to cardiovascular disease.

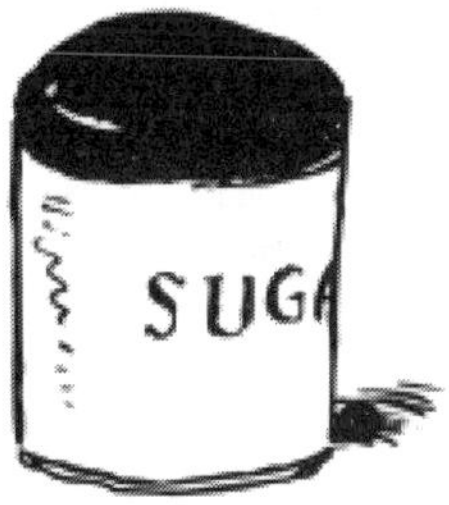

Sugars, especially sucrose (table sugar), fructose (fruit sugar) and lactose (milk sugar) are associated with a higher rate of ischemic heart disease. [23] In the 1960s, John Yudkin, MD and researcher, noticed the relationship between sugar intake and heart disease risk. Sugar increases levels of blood fats such as triglycerides. In addition, sugar makes blood platelet cells stickier and more likely to clump together; these clots can cause heart disease, heart attack, and stroke. This is why diabetics, who by definition tend to have high blood sugar, also tend to have higher rates of cardiovascular disease. Both high glucose and high insulin levels increase the formation of thromboxane, which in turn triggers blood clot formation. On top of all of this, elevated glucose generates free radicals, which also contribute to cardiovascular problems.[24]

People with high **mercury** levels are much more likely to experience heart failure.[25]

High blood pressure

Over 70% of American women and 50% of American men over age 70 have high blood pressure[26], although it is also a problem for many younger people.

Inflamed arteries provide rough surfaces inside them upon which calcium-containing plaque can build up just as mineral deposits build up in household plumbing or in showerheads. The openings in the blood vessels get smaller and the blood pressure rises. Chelation, discussed in Part 4, can help reduce these calcium deposits.

People with a blood pressure over 140/90 have four times the risk of heart disease.[27] It is not definitely known, however, whether high blood pressure is responsible for the higher risk, the usual interpretation, or if the hypertension is caused by the heart disease in any way such as narrowing the blood vessels, or if some other factor contributes to both conditions.

Certain **drugs**, including the Big Three legal recreational drugs (alcohol, caffeine, smoking), can increase blood pressure:

- Studies show a direct correlation between the amount of coffee or caffeine consumed and the raising of blood pressure. High blood pressure can also result from the use of stimulant drugs such as diet aids as well as herbs such as Ma Huang.
- Nicotine constricts blood vessels and raises blood pressure.

- NSAIDs (non-steroidal anti-inflammatory drugs used for headaches and other pain) such as aspirin, ibuprofen, and naproxen have been shown to raise blood pressure in those who take them regularly.
- Having three or more alcoholic drinks a day doubles the number of people who have blood pressure of over 160/95. However, cutting down on alcohol consumption can reverse high blood pressure for which this is the main cause.[28]

One of the first symptoms of **cadmium** overexposure is high blood pressure. Cadmium is found in cigarettes, and is shed by brake linings and tires, and thus can be found in higher concentrations in those who live close to major highways. Those with high blood pressure have been shown to have blood cadmium levels 3-4 times higher than those with normal blood pressure.[29] With higher exposure, the kidneys and liver are damaged and the blood pressure then falls. This may be due to cadmium's effect on aldosterone, a hormone produced by the kidneys which affects blood pressure.

The supplement Cardio-Health (Integris) is recommended for high blood pressure and overall heart health. It can normalize blood pressure through normalizing systems' stress levels, and can raise HDL (beneficial cholesterol) and lowers LDL cholesterol.

Low blood pressure

Yes, there is such a thing as too-low blood pressure, which is more likely to be a problem in women. Chemical and metal causes include:

- **Poisons** that exaggerate the effects produced by acetylcholine release are called cholinergics. These compounds slow the heart and lower blood pressure. Toxic doses may lead to death by circulatory failure. These compounds include pilocarpine, found in glaucoma medications.[30]
- Men who are taking nitroglycerine as sublingual tablets or patches are warned against taking **Viagra**, as the combination may cause a dangerous lowering of blood pressure.[31]
- Low blood pressure, with accompanying dizziness on arising and lack of energy, can be caused by **nickel**.[32]

An abrupt drop in blood pressure, leading to dizziness and a prickling feeling in the face, can be one of the symptoms of acute chemical sensitivity for some people.

High cholesterol and triglycerides

Carbohydrates – Although the eating of foods containing cholesterol has been promoted – and more recently debunked – as a cause of high blood cholesterol, sugar and refined carbohydrates are contributors to the condition. Refined sugars are more likely to become sticky harmful triglycerides, which can cause weight gain from the deposit of fat, insulin swings, and eventually blockage of arteries. Eating refined carbohydrates causes an outpouring of insulin, which raises the triglyceride level.[25,33] Insulin converts blood sugar, glucose, to glycogen, which is an essential stored body fuel. However, excess glycogen is stored as triglycerides[25], and high triglycerides are often the precursor to heart disease. This explains why diabetics are more prone to heart disease than is the general population. The diabetes does not cause the heart disease; rather, they are both manifestations of insulin resistance. The detoxification diet in Part 4 removes all sugars and refined carbohydrates from the diet, and a beneficial side effect of this may be the lowering of cholesterol and triglyceride levels.

Smoking is another thing that raises triglyceride levels[34]. This may also apply to passive smoking.

Arteriosclerosis and atherosclerosis, plaque on blood vessels

Inflammation is the body's natural response to an injury. It can occur inside the blood vessel walls in response to chemical and other irritation, and the resulting free radical damage. Plaque is the body's response to this inflammation, and in time plaque can build up to a point of blocking the blood vessel.

Arteriosclerosis and atherosclerosis, although not the same thing, are similar, and they often occur together. Arteriosclerosis is the progressive hardening and thickening of the arterial walls, while atherosclerosis is the narrowing of the arteries from plaque deposits.

Chemicals – The body, in its desperation to find somewhere to store toxins until it can deal with them, may deposit them in blood vessels as plaque. Analysis of coronary artery plaque has shown that it can contain pesticides, BHT, toluene, aromatic hydrocarbons and other toxic organic chemical compounds.[35] In addition to the direct contribution of chemicals to plaque, there is an indirect effect. Chemicals cause inflammation, promoting the release of calcium and cholesterol to buffer the inflammation. When the inflammation is in the arteries, the calcium-cholesterol plaque can build up, in some cases completely blocking the blood vessel.

Fluoride, routinely added to most municipal water supplies, has been shown to be a contributor to these conditions. A healthy body knows which collagen tissues need to be mineralized and which do not. Both aging and fluoride cause the body to pull calcium out of the bones and begin to mineralize soft tissue. Arteries then start to become calcified, a process known as arteriosclerosis, or hardening of the arteries.

Chlorine – Autopsies of American soldiers killed in Vietnam were compared with autopsies of men killed in the US in traffic accidents. Although the men in Vietnam were very physically fit, their arteries had a very high buildup of arteriosclerotic plaque compared with their stateside counterparts. The search for the reason narrowed down to one major factor: The men in Vietnam had to use water purification tablets before they could drink the water. Those tablets were chlorine. Chlorine irritates the blood vessel linings and causes the buildup of cholesterol to buffer the irritation, setting the stage for cardiovascular problems.[36] Even the lower levels of chlorine in US water could be contributing to the formation of plaque.

Stroke

The use of tobacco and alcohol, and an excess of cadmium (also found in tobacco), mercury and nickel are associated with an increased incidence of stroke.

Smoking – Women who smoke at least 15 cigarettes per day have three times the risk of stroke compared with nonsmokers.[37]

Aspirin – In a study that followed 79,000 women for 14 years, it was found that, although small doses of aspirin, a blood thinner, help prevent ischemic strokes caused by blood clots in the brain, women who took more than 15 aspirin per week were twice as likely to have a hemorrhagic stroke.[38]

Varicose veins

Varicose veins can be caused by nickel and other toxic metals, chemicals and allergy.

A swollen or fatty liver slows down the return of blood to the heart, contributing to varicose veins. A diet and supplementation program to support the liver along with liver cleansing can provide many health benefits, including the clearing up of varicose veins.[39] Both diet and liver cleansing are discussed in Part 4.

Constipation is a major cause of varicose veins, both because of the pressure of a loaded bowel against the veins in the lower abdomen, which damages the valves that keep the blood flowing in one direction, and because straining increases the pressure in the veins and breaks down the resistance in the blood vessel walls.[39] The dietary detoxification chapter discusses the importance of both fiber and water, as well as acidophilus bacteria and minerals, which are important in the prevention of constipation.

Blood problems

Mercury affects blood coagulation and can lead to easy bruising.[40] Mercury also has an adverse on red blood cells.[41]

Mercury binds to hemoglobin in the red blood cells, which is responsible for oxygen transport to the tissues, thus reducing oxygen carrying capacity.[42,43] This results in less oxygen reaching the tissues. The body attempts to compensate for this by increasing the amount of hemoglobin in the blood. A normal or increased hemoglobin (oxygen carrying) level combined with symptoms usually associated with low hemoglobin such as anemia are often indicative of mercury toxicity.[30] Such an increase in hemoglobin or reduction in oxygen carrying capacity can lead to fatigue and shortness of breath.

NSAIDS (non-steroidal anti-inflammatory medications) have a number of serious side effects including blood abnormalities.[44]

Many **pain-suppressing drugs** have harmful effects, including seriously interfering with the ability of the body to metabolize food properly, which leads to malnutrition. Some of the medications can interfere with bone marrow production and the replenishing of the blood supply.[45]

Iron – The blood disorder hemochromatosis, which is characterized by the uptake of too much iron by the blood, is the most common inherited disease, affecting one in every 300 Caucasians, and one in nine is a carrier.[46] People with hemochromatosis should not take iron supplements. Chelation, discussed in Part 4, is an effective way of reducing iron in the blood.

Anemia

Metals of various types can contribute to the development of anemia.

- Both nickel and mercury suppress iron, copper, and cobalt (found in vitamin B12), leading to anemia.[11]
- Lead can cause a type of anemia, raised serum iron with lowered total iron-binding capacity; i.e. more iron in the blood but lowered ability to use it.
- Doses of zinc over 150 mg/day can lead to an otherwise unusual condition called sideroblastic anemia, which has the symptoms of fatigue, anorexia, diz-

ziness, pale skin, and heart and liver failure[47], possibly by lowering the effective levels of copper and iron.

- Excess of aluminum, cadmium, copper, iron, fluoride, iodine, molybdenum, manganese, sodium, phosphorus, vanadium can all contribute to anemia.[48]

Bone and Joint Problems

Bone and joint problems in general

Fluoride is added to water to – in theory at least – boost the resistance of teeth to decay. However, fluoride has a deleterious effect on bone, and is considered here to be a chemical toxin. Bone and tooth disorders related to fluoride have been found in parts of India where levels are 0.7 to 2.5 ppm. For comparison, American cities and municipalities that add fluoride to their water do so at a level of 1 ppm.[1] Skeletal fluorosis occurs when fluoride disrupts the proper mineralization of bone, and is usually present along with dental fluorosis, white spots on the teeth. Osteoporosis and osteoarthritis result, as well as bone spurs and other anomalies. Calcification of the cartilage between the disks of the spine leads to fused vertebrae, with stiffness and loss of motion resulting. Fluoride is also associated with increased bone fractures.[2]

Lead can cross-fiber in bone, replacing calcium with resulting skeletal problems.[1]

Arthritis and joint pain

Solvents – Arthritis can be caused by solvents such as formaldehyde, which is found in many places, including carpets, cabinets, some furniture, and building materials.

Chlorine – It is not uncommon for swimmers to develop arthritis and other immune system problems, resulting at least in part from constant exposure to chlorine in chlorinated pools. Soaking arthritic joints in hot chlorinated water may ease the symptoms temporarily but make the arthritis worse in the long run, since chlorine will be absorbed through the skin, worsening the stiffness. Hot tubs are often a culprit, especially commercial ones (as in health clubs and apartment complexes), to which more chlorine is added than to home hot tubs.

Ankylosing spondylitis is a severe form of arthritis; although hereditary, its expression and severity can be correlated with external factors. Hot tubs which are often heavily chlorinated pose a particular risk as the heat opens up the pores, thus allowing even more chlorine to enter the body.

Patient profile

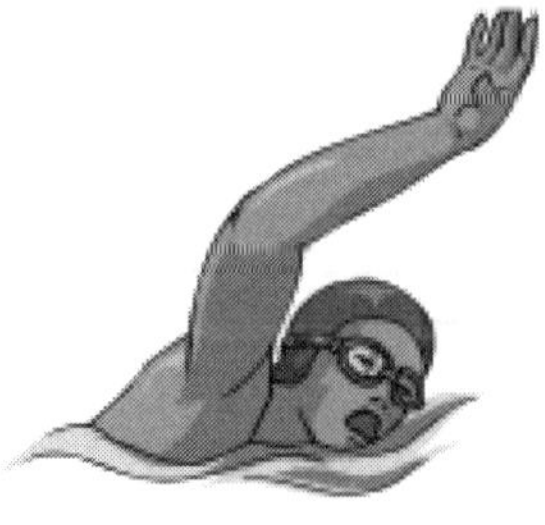

One patient, a man who was an Olympic gold medal swimmer, was exposed to a lot of chlorine from pools, and as a result may have developed ankylosing spondylitis, an autoimmune disease related to spinal arthritis. His illness improved when he later switched to using pools disinfected with filters, ozone, copper and enzymes rather than chlorine. He also changed his diet to one with fewer sweets and more healthful omega-3 oils, and made general lifestyle changes[1], in yet another example showing that multiple approaches usually give the greatest positive effect.

Fluoride, in addition to its harmful effects on bone in general, can play a part in arthritis. A healthy body knows which collagen tissues need to be mineralized and which do not. Both aging and fluoride cause the body to pull calcium out of the bones and begin to mineralize soft tissue such as ligaments and muscles, causing inflammation, arthritis and stiffness. Early stages of fluoride-induced damage to bones and cartilage are pain in the spinal bones, progressing to spine stiffness and limitation of movement. These symptoms are often labeled rheumatoid or arthritic.[3]

Metals and minerals – Iron can cause free radical damage, which can cause arthritis to flare up. In most cases, do not take iron supplements if you have arthritis, as iron can cause pain, swelling, and joint destruction.[4] Chelation can help to remove excess iron from the body, as can regular donation of blood.

Calcium can be taken from the long bones and muscles if there is inflammation elsewhere in the body, such as the arteries, since the body uses calcium to buffer inflammation. If you have joint pains, this may be the cause. It may be a good idea to have your arteries checked and take antioxidants for protection. Allergy, toxins, and waste byproducts of microorganisms can have the same effect on calcium as does inflammation, and in fact these things can cause or contribute to inflammation.

Many people with arthritis have high levels of copper and iron in their bodies.[4] Arthritic symptoms have been linked to mercury, the greatest source of which is dental amalgams.[5] Other metals and minerals whose high levels can contribute to arthritis include manganese, nickel, lead, silver, sulfur, and selenium.

NSAIDs (non-steroidal anti-inflammatory drugs), often taken for symptomatic relief of the pain of osteoarthritis, can actually make it worse. They can increase the rate of cartilage deterioration and joint damage.[6] NSAIDs inhibit the action of enzymes that are needed to make cartilage, which links them to more rapid joint destruction in arthritis.[7] Supplementation with enzymes could help to reverse this tendency.

Silicone breast implants can cause arthritis-like symptoms due to autoimmune reaction. In some cases, but not all, the symptoms disappeared when the implants were removed.[4] Rheumatic disorders have been linked to silicone breast implants.[8] In a follow up study of 50 consecutive silicone breast implant patients, a huge percentage, 78%, reported joint pain[9].

Vaccination, which, like fluoride, is considered by mainstream medicine to be beneficial, can also contribute to arthritis. Reactive arthritis has been reported following a flu shot.[10] Hepatitis B vaccine is linked to autoimmune rheumatoid diseases. These vaccinations are recommended for children even though the mode of transmission of hepatitis B is through blood and sexual contact, not an issue for children. The link with rheumatoid diseases is a powerful reason not to vaccinate children or adults who don't have the risk factors.[11]

Food sensitivities were found in nearly 78% of people with arthritis, with the most common being dairy, followed by caffeine, refined carbohydrates, wheat and oats.[12] If both wheat and oats, which contain plentiful gluten, cause problems, the issue might be gluten itself rather than sensitivity to the wheat or oat protein. Gluten intolerance is responsible for about 70% of autoimmune disease, which arthritis is considered to be, especially rheumatoid arthritis.

Nightshade vegetables, which include tomatoes, potatoes, eggplant, and peppers, can cause arthritis symptoms in susceptible individuals. Eliminating these from the diet, as in the detox diet in Part 4, can provide major relief to some arthritis sufferers; others may be affected little or not at all. 70% of over 5000 patients reported less pain when avoiding nightshade vegetables, including tobacco[7], which is in the nightshade family. Even if you don't smoke, avoiding secondhand smoke can make a difference if you have nightshade-sensitive arthritis.

Meat and dairy – Naturopath T. Michael Culp found that several of his rheumatoid arthritis patients were of blood type B and had high antibodies to chicken. Peter D'Adamo, ND, in his book ***Eat Right 4 Your Type***[13], stated that type B blood group people often had adverse reactions to chicken. Based on this Dr. Culp had his patients avoid chicken, with a rapid and remarkable improvement in their arthritis symptoms. The symptoms would then flare up again when chicken was eaten, further proving a connection.[14] Also, treatment for chicken by allergy desensitization, described in Part 4, may help. This is another example of individualizing treatment – if you are sensitive to chicken, eliminating it can make a huge difference, but elimination will make little or no difference if you are not. It's worth a try, though, especially if you are blood type B.

Food allergies and sensitivities may be a major player in rheumatoid arthritis.[15] Rheumatoid arthritis patients who were put on a vegan (no animal products at all, such as dairy or eggs)[16] or vegetarian diet[15] showed substantial clinical improvement. Such a diet can have nutrient limitations, but it is worth trying short term to see whether there is any improvement. Arachidonic acid, present in animal products, can promote inflammation, including joint pain. Those who eat the greatest number of cooked vegetables were about 75% less likely to develop RA than those who eat the least[17], possibly because eating more vegetables means eating less meat and dairy.

Patients with ankylosing spondylitis (AS) were shown to improve when they followed a dairy-free diet.[18] Certain fecal gram negative bacteria such as klebsiella are implicated as provoking factors in spondyloarthropathies (AS and related conditions), and these bacterial fragments may be present in milk and may trigger autoimmune responses in susceptible individuals.[19]

Gluten-containing grains can contribute to the joint pain of arthritis[20]; it is not uncommon for those with arthritis to report a flare-up of symptoms upon eating wheat. Gluten-containing foods should be avoided by those with rheumatoid arthritis; study results showed that eliminating these foods reduced pain and swelling and increased grip strength[15]; recall in the Assessments chapter that toxic and allergenic foods can cause muscle weakness.

Drugs can contribute to the development of arthritis, particularly rheumatoid arthritis:

- Smoking increases the risk of developing rheumatoid arthritis (RA). Current female smokers have twice the risk of developing RA compared with women who had never smoked; former smokers have a risk somewhere between the two.[21] Sore joints can be caused by the suppression of zinc and potassium by cadmium, which is found in cigarette smoke.
- A study in Finland showed that people who drink four or more cups of coffee per day double their risk of developing RA.[21]
- The regular use of aspirin by those with rheumatoid arthritis can actually hasten joint destruction. Aspirin produces very low plasma ascorbic acid (vitamin C) levels, and vitamin C is necessary for collagen formation. Taking vitamin C along with aspirin might counteract these harmful effects.[22,23]

Lyme disease, a bacterial illness spread by the deer tick, can cause a number of symptoms. One of the more common symptoms is arthritis-like joint pain. Specific testing is available for Lyme disease, although its accuracy is questionable, and antibiotic therapy can clear up the infection and reduce symptoms, especially if caught early.

Yeast and fungus can worsen arthritis, and a yeast-free diet can help – see the Detoxification diet and Maintenance diet chapters.

Osteoporosis

Fluoride – Several studies, including one which examined over 540,000 records of cases of osteoporosis, showed that the incidence of hip fracture increased by 27-41% in areas with water fluoridated at the 1 ppm level as compared with nonfluoridated areas. These studies were written up in the ***Journal of the American Medical Association*** and other respected journals.[24-26] Osteoporosis is increased and bone density is decreased with exposure to fluoride. Ironically, fluoride is being promoted as an osteoporosis *treatment*, which goes against common sense and study results.[27] Yes, bone is built, which is why these fluoride medications passed muster with the FDA, but it tends to be poor quality bone, brittle and porous and more prone to breakage.

Before fluoride and similar toxins were introduced into the environment, women went through menopause without being given synthetic estrogen for thousands of years. Estrogen is now routinely given to postmenopausal women to prevent osteoporosis and other disorders. It would be better to eliminate the causes of osteoporosis, including suppression of estrogen by fluoride, rather than dealing with the symptoms by introducing a pharmaceutical.

Both aging and fluoride cause the body to pull calcium out of the bones and begin to mineralize soft tissue, while bones and teeth, which should be mineralized, are mineralized insufficiently and begin to soften, a condition called osteomalacia, related to osteoporosis.

Excessive **alcohol** consumption is a known risk factor for osteoporosis, decreased bone formation, and defective bone mineralization[28], as well as bone marrow damage.[29]

Caffeine in coffee is linked to decreased bone mineral density.[30] Those who drink more than three cups of coffee per day increase their risk of osteoporosis by 82%.[31] Caffeine acts as a chelator to remove calcium, causing inflammation which pulls calcium from the long bones. Caffeine intake increases calcium excretion, and therefore the use of caffeine can promote or worsen osteoporosis.

Smoking – The Nurses' Health Study at Harvard, which followed 120,000 women for 25 years, found a 20% increased risk for hip fracture among smokers of all ages compared with nonsmokers. The risk persisted up to ten years after a woman quit smoking. Researchers postulate that smoking lowers estrogen levels, making the body less able to absorb calcium.[32] Smokers may also exercise less – especially the crucial weight-bearing exercise – than nonsmokers due to their lowered lung capacity, another risk factor for osteoporosis.[33] In addition, cadmium, found in tobacco, fights for the binding sites on cells with beneficial calcium.

Synthetic **steroids**, including prednisone, which is often used to reduce arthritis and other symptoms, steal calcium from the bones and body, possibly leading to osteoporosis after long-term use. Long-term steroid use is linked to the development of osteoporosis by causing premature death of osteoblasts, the cells that form bone.[34] One side effect of steroid use in teenage boys is stunting of growth, possibly by the same mechanism: the bones can no longer grow

Women who use inhaled steroids for asthma may have an increased risk of osteoporosis, according to a study in the ***New England Journal of Medicine***. Regular use of these inhalants is linked to bone loss in the hip.[35]

Estrogen Replacement Therapy (ERT or HRT) and contraceptives have a harmful effect on the growth of bone, which is ironic because these hormones are marketed as being beneficial in the prevention of osteoporosis. Bone is constantly being broken down and built up; it is a changing, not a static, system, even in adulthood. After menopause, the balance between these two systems is upset, resulting in more bone being broken down and resorbed than rebuilt. Estrogen replacement stimulates the activity of cells that rebuild bone, although it has many risks and side effects of its own. ERT helps conserve bone, but when it is discontinued there is a rebound effect, with a phase of accelerating bone loss.[36] Overall it is usually best not to start using it in the first place. Another reason to avoid starting hormone replacement is that, once exogenous (supplied from the outside) hormones are taken, whether estrogenic hormones, thyroid hormone, or others, the gland producing the hormone tends to stop functioning altogether and to atrophy because the body perceives that it is not needed for hormone production. A vicious cycle ensues, in which less hormone is made by the body, more hormone is needed as replacement, causing the gland to make less hormone, and so on.

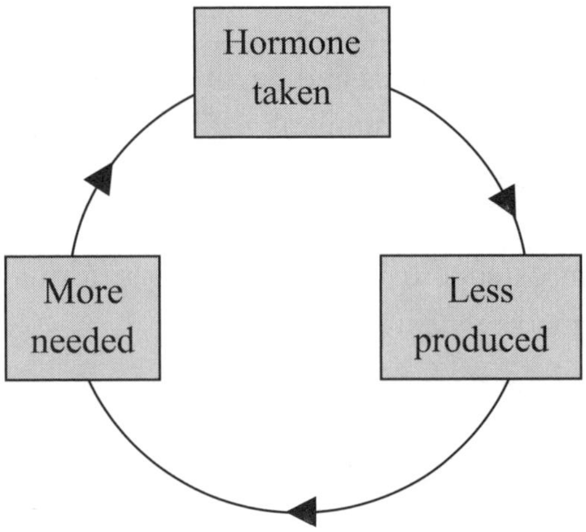

Contraceptives such as Depo-Provera that suppress ovulation reduce bone-protecting estrogen as well, setting the stage for osteoporosis at a relatively young age.[33]

Medications that can interfere with the body's use of calcium or adversely affect the bone building process include glucocorticoids (steroids), antiseizure medications, gonadotropin hormones used to treat endometriosis, heavy use of aluminum-containing antacids, some anticancer drugs, and excessive thyroid hormone.[37]

Metals – Bone loss may be due to interference with calcium and magnesium due to aluminum toxicity. An excess of the mineral calcium can contribute to osteoporosis, as well as can the better-known calcium deficiency; the mineral balance is what is important.

Ingestion of **gluten** grains is known to cause osteoporosis in those with celiac disease. The eating of foods to which one is allergic or sensitive can damage the intestinal lining, resulting in malabsorption of minerals needed for strong bones.[38] In such cases bone loss can be averted by adherence to a gluten-free diet, especially in those with celiac disease, i.e. gluten sensitivity. If those with celiac disease and osteoporosis follow a strict no-gluten diet, their osteoporosis may subside to a degree, but supplementation with magnesium will improve the results[39]; magnesium helps calcium go where it needs to go.

Phosphoric acid in sodas increases the risk of osteoporosis by interfering with the body's use of calcium.[40] If the phosphorus is too high relative to calcium, as when one consumes cheese, meat, processed foods, or phosphoric acid-containing soft drinks such as colas, the body, sensing a deficiency of calcium, may pull it out of the bones, which can lead to osteoporosis.[41] Calcium and phosphorus should be in an approximately 1:1 ratio, but the American diet provides about four parts phosphorus to one part calcium. Excess phosphorus can also bind magnesium, also critical in the making of bone.

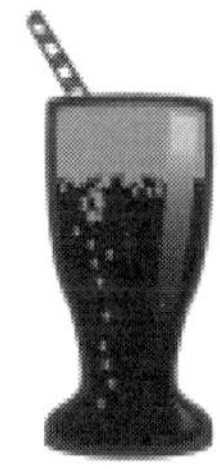

Diet can be a major player in the development or treatment of osteoporosis in ways besides avoiding gluten and soft drinks:

- Excessive salt consumption contributes to osteoporosis by encouraging calcium from the bones to pass through the kidneys into the urine.[42,43] Too high a magnesium level, rare unless high doses of magnesium supplement are taken without calcium to balance it, can cause this same effect.
- Since 1920, a high protein intake has been correlated with calcium loss, which can lead to bone loss.[44] High protein breaks down into amino acids which can chelate out minerals. In addition, high protein tends to make urine acidic, which pulls calcium out of the long bones to buffer it.
- Osteoporosis is a problem worldwide only among people who eat meat and dairy.[36] In the US, female meat-eaters had a bone mass loss of 35%, compared with 18% in female vegetarians.[45] Increasing vegetable protein and decreasing animal protein can decrease bone loss and lessen the risk of hip fracture.[46]
- Sugar is a major culprit in this and in many other conditions. Monkeys fed sweets and pastries develop bones that are porous, weak and brittle – this is osteoporosis.[47]
- Keep blood from becoming too acidic by avoiding stress, alcohol, tobacco, coffee, carbonated sodas and beef. If the blood is too acid, the body will remove calcium from bone to buffer the acidity.
- Isoflavone-containing foods such as tofu and other soy foods help guard against osteoporosis[48], in part because they stimulate estrogen production. However, soy is allergenic and has other down sides, such as suppression of thyroid function.
- Deficiencies of the minerals boron, manganese, and strontium, which are needed to utilize calcium in the building of bone, can contribute to osteoporosis.

- A 12-year study of over 77,000 women found that those who drank more than fourteen glasses of milk per week had 45% more hip fractures than women who consumed little or no milk.[49]
- Omega-3 oils, such as fish and flaxseed oils, are also needed for healthy bone; they transport calcium with albumin.

Gastrointestinal Problems

Gastrointestinal problems – metals

Metals are the cause of a number of gastrointestinal (GI) problems.

Digestive problems associated with **mercury** include constipation or diarrhea (by themselves or alternating), digestion problems, colitis, loss of appetite, ulcers, bloating and gas, loss of smell and taste due to the depletion of zinc, since mercury fights for the same cellular binding sites; poor eating and nutritional depletion can result. The effect of dental mercury on normal gut flora is well documented[1] and can cause a proliferation of yeast.

Many people with gastrointestinal problems are given **barium** to swallow or as an enema to visualize the upper or lower gastrointestinal tract respectively. Barium will enter the bloodstream and react, and even if the amount involved is very tiny due to the low solubility it is inadvisable to have something this toxic in the body. The benefit of the test may still outweigh the risk, but it is important to know the risk to help make this determination. Once in the bloodstream the barium cannot be easily excreted and must be chelated out like any other heavy metal, as described in the Metal Detoxification chapter.

Nickel such as that found in some dental work can cause digestive system difficulties such as nausea, diarrhea, colitis, ulcers, and poor digestion[2], as well as inflamed gums. Be careful with gold fillings – if there is nickel in the mixture, this can affect the colon.

Lead poisoning can cause gastrointestinal symptoms such as nausea and vomiting, diarrhea or constipation, colic, abdominal rigidity and pain, loss of appetite and weight loss.[3]

Gastrointestinal problems – microorganisms

Many microorganisms, discussed in the last chapter of Part 3, can cause gastrointestinal problems.

What are some specific gastrointestinal problems and their causes?

Anal itching

Anal itching is not so much an illness in itself; rather, its presence can help to identify what may be going on in the body.

Microorganisms – Some microorganisms, especially pinworms, can cause anal itching. The worms leave the body via the anus to lay their eggs just outside the anal opening, usually at night, and the accompanying sticky secretion can cause intense itching. This is a way for the worms to keep their life cycle going, as people scratch, pick up eggs under their nails, and then eventually put their fingers in their mouths or spread the eggs to the food they eat.

Chemicals that one is exposed to and to which one is allergic can cause anal itching and irritation as they are eliminated through the digestive tract.

Allergy to food or its breakdown products can also cause itchy anus, as the food may irritate sensitive anal tissues as it comes in contact with them on its way out of the body. Six common foods are most likely to cause anal itching: coffee (including decaffeinated), tea, cola, beer, chocolate, and tomatoes.[4]

Nickel – Itchy anus is often caused by nickel irritating the lining of the intestinal and anal mucosa as it is excreted. The itching and soreness is essentially the same reaction as sensitive individuals have on their earlobes from inexpensive earrings. Nickel can also come from stainless steel dental work, such as posts and the base of crowns. Traces of nickel can also be in margarine.

Appetite loss, anorexia

Anorexia, defined as loss of appetite and not necessarily related to the eating disorder anorexia nervosa, and resultant weight loss may be a result of cadmium replacing zinc, the mineral responsible for taste and appetite. Zinc, taken orally as a supplement, displaces cadmium and can stop and even reverse this and other symptoms of cadmium poisoning. Cadmium comes from cigarette smoke as well as other sources such as car brakes and tires, the dust from which can be a significant source of exposure to someone living near a busy road. The regaining of appetite after quitting smoking is often due to the lowering of cadmium levels and the return of smell, taste, and appetite.

Bloating

Although bloating can be caused by non-dietary factors, diet is a major player in the development of bloating. Bloating can be caused by eating too much fruit which can ferment; excessive cruciferous vegetables (broccoli, cabbage, Brussels sprouts) and asparagus, onions, and artichokes; lactose-containing milk and dairy products; any allergens such as gluten, soy, peanuts, or corn; and carbonated beverages.[5]

Bloating can also be caused by sugarless sweets sweetened with sorbitol and mannitol, which the body has trouble breaking down. Since these are then absorbed more slowly from the intestine, intestinal bacteria or fungus have more time to produce fermentation, which releases various gases.[5]

Other foods that cause bloating include insoluble fiber, found in oat bran, peas and fruit; and fatty foods. Shortage of digestive enzymes can cause bloating; ideally the enzymes will digest food, but if enzymes are insufficient the bacteria in the large intestine must do the job, releasing gas in the process. The gas in the lower intestine causes the bloating. Activated charcoal, available in capsules, can help break down and absorb the gas before it causes discomfort. If bloating is a persistent problem, keep a food diary to correlate foods eaten with the resulting discomfort.

A shortage of beneficial bacteria, which can occur during and after a course of antibiotics or exposure to dental mercury, can contribute to bloating. Supplements of these bacteria are available, but it is important to eliminate the cause of the loss of the body's bacteria.

Most of the bloat-causing foods are eliminated on the detoxification diet in Part 4.

Colitis, Crohn's disease, Irritable Bowel Syndrome (IBS)

Diarrhea that lasts for months or years can be a symptom of the potentially serious conditions of colitis and ileitis (Crohn's disease). These inflammatory conditions can be caused by **chemical** overload, as the colon is a major organ of detoxification. Anti-inflammatory **drugs** can cause ulcerative colitis; aspirin, for example, is a well-known stomach irritant.

Metals associated with colitis include aluminum, mercury and nickel.[6]

Dietary factors are a major cause of colitis. Certain foods are some of the most common triggers of colitis, and a food diary that notes both what is eaten and the onset or worsening of symptoms can be helpful in finding the individual food triggers. Common IBS triggers include lactose, caffeine, alcohol, aspartame, and foods high in insoluble fiber[7], as well as the common allergens corn, soy, and peanuts.

Food allergy or intolerance is a major contributing factor to Crohn's disease, especially lactose intolerance. About half of Crohn's disease patients treated achieved marked improvement with dietary modification alone. After a strict hypoallergenic diet is followed and improvement noted, foods can be introduced one at a time and symptoms of relapse related to the food are quite noticeable. The detoxification and maintenance diets in Part 4 are a good place to start.

See if eliminating gluten grains such as wheat helps. What manifests as irritable bowel syndrome may actually be the symptoms of celiac disease, or gluten intolerance.

Refined sugar may contribute to irritable bowel syndrome by shortening bowel transit time and increasing the fecal bile acid concentration, as well as by feeding yeast and klebsiella bacteria.

Constipation

Medications can contribute to constipation, including some antibiotics, anti-inflammatories, muscle relaxants, opiates / narcotics, analgesics, antacids, antidepressants, blood pressure medication, and diuretics.[8] A study of about 20,000 patients with constipation found that opiates and sedatives raise constipation risk by 60%, diuretics by 70%, antihistamines 80%, and antidepressants 90%.[9] Opiates and sedatives slow down the whole body's function, including the colon, while diuretics and antihistamines have a drying effect that can lead to hard stools. Antihistamines and decongestants, which dry out the tissues, can also make the stool drier, causing constipation.

Toxic **metals** such as mercury, iron, lead, arsenic and bismuth (found in Pepto-Bismol, which is named for it) can also contribute to constipation.[8] Ironically, supplements that are supposed to be helpful for overall health can contribute to constipation. Bone meal and dolomite, sources of calcium, are difficult to digest and may contain toxic lead. One patient, a 70-year-old woman, took bone meal, which not only did not help her osteoporosis but caused constipation.[6] Iron and calcium supplements can also cause constipation. Magnesium supplements, which work in part by countering excess calcium, can help ease constipation, although too much magnesium can lead to diarrhea, so these two minerals need to be in balance.

Diet – There are a number of possible dietary causes of constipation. Low fiber food and insufficient water are major ones.

Constipation, anal fissures, and pain with defecation in toddlers and young children have been shown to worsen with cows' milk and improve when cows' milk is eliminated. A study in the ***New England Journal of Medicine*** showed that cows' milk was the cause of constipation in two-thirds of the children involved in the study.[10] Wheat and dairy can cause constipation in adults as well.

Fermentation in the small intestine, which often occurs when sweet foods are eaten, draws water from the bowel, leading to hard stools and constipation. Sweet foods also tend to have little or no fiber, worsening the situation.

Food allergies can alter peristalsis, the normal downward-propelling motion of the GI tract, and contribute to constipation.[11]

Natural methods to increase bowel regularity are discussed in the chapter on Drugs.

Diarrhea

Diarrhea is one of the ways that the body rids itself of toxins, so it is best to deal with the root cause rather than suppressing this avenue of detoxification. However, diarrhea is often a sign of an infectious or toxic process within the gastrointestinal system. It can become dangerous if severe or prolonged due to dehydration, electrolyte (mineral) imbalance, and non-absorption of nutrients. Diarrhea that lasts for months or years can be symptoms of the potentially serious conditions of colitis and ileitis (Crohn's disease) or diverticulitis.

Antibiotics can cause diarrhea by killing the protective bacteria in the intestines.

Mercury, as from metal fillings, can also kill the protective bacteria and lead to diarrhea from an overgrowth of yeast and pathogenic bacteria in addition to other problems. Nickel, found in some dental work, can also cause diarrhea.

Diet – Other than toxicity or disease processes, dietary factors can cause or contribute to diarrhea. Foods that can worsen diarrhea include: alcohol, caffeine, beans, broccoli, apples, spicy foods, acidic foods such as citrus, fatty and fried foods, and dairy products for those who are lactose intolerant.[12] Some fruits, such as cherries, plums, grapes, and watermelon, can cause diarrhea in some people. Sweeteners of various types can cause diarrhea: aspartame artificial sweetener, sorbitol if consumed in large amounts, and sugar itself.

Very high doses of over 10 grams of vitamin C daily can cause diarrhea.

Magnesium supplements in forms other than glycinate can cause or worsen diarrhea.

Other than eliminating the causes, there are things that can be done for diarrhea. Ultra Flora IB is a probiotic (beneficial bacteria) supplement that can help ease diarrhea. Beneficial oils can also help, as can fiber, bentonite clay, and charcoal in capsules.

Gas, flatulence

Most of the causes of flatulence are dietary.

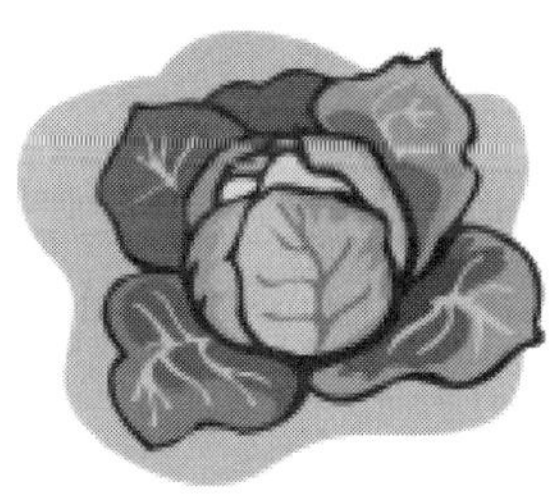

Flatulence (gas) can be caused by putrefaction in the large intestine. Putrefaction often occurs when undigested protein is broken down by bacteria or yeast, leading to fermentation. Certain foods such as beans and cabbage can be gas-producers. While it is a good idea to avoid these foods if they cause trouble for you, on a more basic level a properly functioning digestive system should be able to handle these foods without incident. Putrefaction often occurs when food stays in the intestines too long. Sufficient dietary fiber will speed up the digestive and elimination process. Ironically, too much fiber, or fiber introduced into the diet or increased too quickly, can also cause gas.

Dairy products are the most common cause of persistent flatulence. Gas after eating dairy products can be a sign of lactose intolerance.

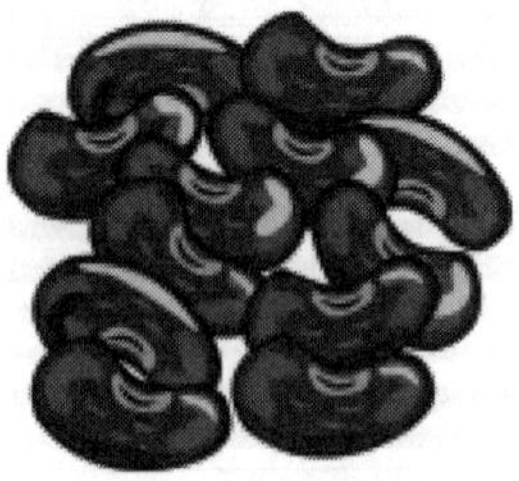

Beans have a reputation for producing gas, diarrhea, bloating, and other gastrointestinal symptoms. Many people do not digest beans well, resulting in fermentation and allergies. If beans cause discomfort, it is best not to eat them, or to eat them along with proteolytic or pancreatic enzymes or an enzyme product such as Beano, which can help digestion. Cooking beans with a seaweed such as Kombu has also been reported to help with the gas problem, as has rinsing and draining the beans frequently along with soaking overnight, before cooking.

For some people, gas caused by foods such as beans becomes less as the intestines get used to them. People who rarely eat beans because of the gas are ironically most likely to get gas from them.

Gas can be caused by eating too much fruit, which can ferment; high fiber foods, cruciferous vegetables (broccoli, cabbage, Brussels sprouts), asparagus, onions, and artichokes; milk; and carbonated beverages.[5] Cellulase enzymes, sold as a supplement, can help break down the fiber so it is less likely to be a problem.

Gas can also be caused by sugarless items sweetened with sorbitol and mannitol, which the body has trouble breaking down. Since these are then absorbed more slowly from the intestine, intestinal bacteria have more time to produce fermentation, which release gases.[5] Fructose can also cause flatulence[12]; high-fructose corn syrup is a major source of fructose.

It takes 2-4 hours for food to reach the lower colon to cause flatulence; keep a diary of food eaten and episodes of flatulence to make a dietary connection. If wheat is causing the problem, 6-8 hours can pass before the gassiness begins.[13]

Most of the gas-causing foods, with the exception of broccoli and cabbage, are eliminated in the detoxification diet in Part 4.

Heartburn and GERD

Most people experience heartburn at least once in a while. Despite its name it has nothing to do with the heart; it is so named because of the location of the discomfort. GERD, or gastroesophageal reflux disease, is frequent or even daily heartburn, which can cause ulcers and esophageal scarring. GERD can be quite severe and debilitating.

Diet – Most causes of heartburn are dietary. Avoid the most common trigger foods: alcohol, chocolate, tobacco, coffee, caffeine, tea, meat, milk, mints, tomatoes, orange juice, carbonated drinks, and sugar. Also avoid fatty, fried, salty, spicy, and sweet foods. After eliminating these from the diet for a month, add them back singly to determine your individual triggers.[12,14]

Mints, especially chocolate covered ones, relax the lower esophageal valve and increase the chances of heartburn. Ironically, mints are often served at the end of a restaurant meal, on the table or by the checkout counter.[12,15] In another mint-related irony, however, peppermint tea can ease heartburn.

Medications can contribute to heartburn. NSAIDs exert their activity by inhibiting the effects of prostaglandins. However, prostaglandins protect the stomach from digestive acids that can cause heartburn, so NSAIDs, by inhibiting prostaglandins, can cause or contribute to this condition.[16]

Antacids are often taken for heartburn, but can ironically worsen it in the long run. They are taken in the mistaken belief that excess hydrochloric acid (HCl) in the stomach is the culprit. However, fermentation from sweet foods and the waste products of microorganisms are more likely the problem. In addition, rebound heartburn can be caused by the chronic use of laxatives.

Other causes include dental nickel and root canals, helicobacter pylori (the bacteria that cause ulcers), and yeast.

Nausea and vomiting

Metals – Excess copper can cause nausea. Some people are so sensitive to copper that they can't even tolerate copper in nutritional supplements without becoming nauseated. Other metals that can cause nausea include mercury, nickel and lead. Continued excessive use of calcium can cause nausea.[16]

Diet – Gluten eaten by those with celiac disease can cause nausea. Caffeine and the artificial sweetener aspartame can also cause nausea in some individuals.

Gallbladder problems can cause nausea, especially when one eats oils and fats. The liver and gallbladder flush in Part 4 can help with this by cleaning out the gallbladder and improving its efficiency. Other symptoms of gallbladder problems are tight trapezius muscles, which manifest as tight shoulders, stiff neck, and pain between the shoulder blades.

Low salt intake can cause nausea; taking ½ tsp. mineral salt in water can relieve the nausea in about 20 minutes.

Pancreatitis

Alcohol is a major contributor to pancreatitis. Sugar becomes alcohol in the body of someone with a yeast overgrowth, sometimes called the auto-brewery syndrome, and is thus also a causative factor. In addition, because of the role of the pancreas in insulin production to metabolize sugar, the eating of sugar causes a load on the pancreas.

Pancreatitis has also been linked to pesticide exposure.[17]

Mental and Behavioral Problems

Mental and Behavioral, general

Chemicals – It is very possible that many psychiatric problems have chemical toxicity as their root cause. Carbon disulfide, used in rubber vulcanization, is an example of a chemical which can cause psychiatric disturbances.

Industrial solvents are intended to be solvents of fats, or degreasers. In the body, they are especially attracted to the fatty sheaths of nerve fibers and the lipid (fatty) membranes of cells. The partial dissolving of these nerve fiber sheaths leads to mental and behavioral nervous system effects such as memory loss, difficulty concentrating, and altered personality.

When you are exposed to certain chemicals, the sympathetic nervous system reacts to what it correctly perceives to be a dangerous invader, and signals the adrenal glands to secrete adrenaline to prepare for a confrontation. The rush of adrenaline (the fight-or-flight hormone) can cause a sudden feeling of anxiety, anger, depression, or tearfulness.

Drugs – Human brains are 60% fatty acids. Cholesterol lowering drugs, called statins, also lower the amount of fat available to the brain, and can thus have a negative effect on emotional stability. Studies show a rising death rate from suicide and violence in those taking these drugs.[1]

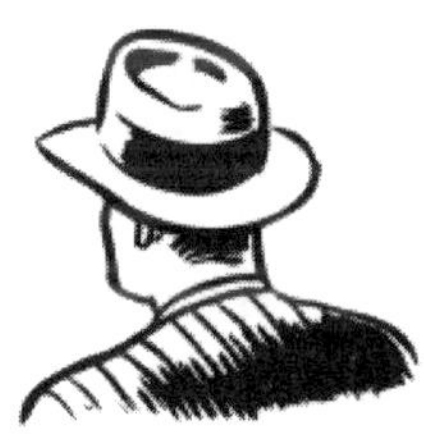

Mercury's effects on the mental and behavioral aspects of the nervous system have been well known for centuries. In the 18th and 19th centuries, mercury was used in the making of hats, which were then worn almost universally by men. Hat-making workers were so often affected by the mercury that the phrase "mad as a hatter" came into being. The character of the Mad Hatter in Lewis Carroll's well-known ***Alice in Wonderland*** book is taken from this phenomenon.

Mental symptoms of mercury toxicity affecting the posterior pituitary in the brain include[2]:

- Depression
- Timidity
- Rage
- Phobias
- Anxiety
- Lowered libido
- Indecisiveness
- Lack of self confidence
- Compulsions
- Mood swings

Mercury tends to accumulate in all tissues, but especially in the brain. It is one of the substances that can cross the blood-brain barrier. Brain levels of mercury are directly proportional to the number and size of amalgam filling surfaces in the mouth. Mercury accumulation in the brain leads to mental and nervous system effects such as brain fog, depression, vision difficulties, and others as listed above. Mental effects are among the most common due to mercury's special affinity for the brain. Mercury inhibits the effects of certain neurotransmitters:

- Dopamine — controls pain, well-being
- Serotonin — relaxation, sleep, well-being
- Adrenaline — energy and stamina
- Noradrenaline, melatonin — sleep cycles

Inhibition of these neurotransmitters by mercury can account in part for feelings of depression and loss of motivation.

Not surprisingly, dentists and dental assistants have been found to have neurological and behavioral impairments in direct proportion to their chelated and unchelated mercury excretion,[3,4] which in turn is related to the amount and duration of their exposure.

Other mental symptoms of mercury exposure include mental illness and psychological problems, including loss of function and memory, anger and emotionality, and timidity.[5,6]

Copper is a toxic nervous system stimulant, leading to low histamine levels (histapenia) in the brain, and in a vicious cycle the lowered histamine levels allow copper to accumulate. The results of high levels of copper include restlessness, insomnia, depression, violence, irritability, and paranoia.[1]

Hormones given to cattle to fatten them and increase milk production may be contributing to mental problems. Hormones in milk may well exacerbate the hormonal and emotional storms weathered by teenagers today – who tend to drink a lot of milk – as hormonal peaks and dips contribute to teenage depression, violence, and suicide. Dairy products are not recommended for a number of reasons, including this one. Anabolic steroid hormones, taken by some athletes, can cause "roid rage," uncontrollable and sometimes violent temper.

Yeast may be the causative agent behind some cases and types of mental illness. Researchers have found that certain cases of mental illness, unresponsive to psychotropic drugs, responded positively to a yeast-free diet and treatment for yeast.[7] Panic attacks, anxiety, depression, and irritability can be the result of candida yeast overgrowth.[8] Foods that contribute to the proliferation of yeast are eliminated from the diet in the detoxification and maintenance diets in Part 4.

Allergy – Mental illness is sometimes caused by allergies, especially to chemicals. Mental symptoms of allergy include anxiety, learning and memory problems, trouble concentrating, insomnia, depression, migraines, fatigue, irritability, crying, and anger.[9]

Diet – Those fats and oils that are harmful to the brain include[10]:

- Saturated animal fat
- Hydrogenated vegetable oils such as margarine and those in processed foods.
- Trans fatty acids such as those in margarine, processed foods, and fried foods.
- An overload or imbalance of omega-6 oils, such as corn, safflower, and sunflower oils.

What are some specific mental and behavioral disorders and their causes?

Anxiety disorders

Anxiety disorders include panic disorder, phobias, agoraphobia, hypochondria, social phobia, obsessive-compulsive disorder (OCD), post-traumatic stress disorder (PTSD), and generalized anxiety, as well as stress in general.

Stress and anxiety feed on each other – stress causes anxiety, and dealing with anxiety is stressful. Stress is not necessarily emotional stress – toxins are major stressors as well. Detoxifying and avoiding toxins are thus likely to have a positive effect on decreasing stress and anxiety.

Chemicals – Agoraphobia, fear of leaving the home (literally "fear of the marketplace"), is considered by many to be a psychological disorder, but it may actually be caused by exposure to toxins. Chemicals in the mall or store include formaldehyde in the carpets, sizing in new clothing, cologne, floor cleaner and floor wax. Fumes from cars and trucks on the highway include benzene, combustion products, and oils. Such exposure overloads the body of a person who is already stressed by the many toxins in their environment.

Panic attacks or agoraphobia may be brought on by allergy to substances in the environment. It is not coincidental that these panic attacks often occur while driving due to exposure to diesel fumes or road tar, or while in the store or at the mall due to the many chemicals found there.

In panic attacks, the body perceives a dangerous situation – the toxin – and the sympathetic nervous system signals the adrenal glands to secrete adrenaline to prepare for a fight-or-flight situation. This rush of adrenaline is perceived as a feeling of panic. After this happens a few times, the fear of having it happen again may be enough to trigger an attack on its own.

An unusual intolerance to stress can be related to chemical overload. A chemically toxic person can experience fear of any new assault or stress – an "I can't handle one more thing" feeling.

Panic attacks have been linked to organic solvents common in the workplace[11], and to sensitivity to other chemicals. Toluene, found in cologne as well as other places, can cause anxiety.[12]

Prozac®, the sleep aid and anti-anxiety drug, which initially calms people, has been linked to violent behavior, murders and suicides. The sleep aid Halcion® (triazolam), ironically named for a state of peace and serenity, can cause the side effects of agitation and rare thoughts of suicide.[13]

Metals – High levels of copper and low levels of histamine can contribute to paranoia.[1] Elevated serum copper levels are found in those who are paranoid and extremely fearful.[14] Mercury can contribute to shyness, manifesting in its extreme form as social anxiety.

Diet – Milk is a major culprit in food-related anxiety.[15]

Anxiety attacks and the consumption of sugar both cause similar symptoms such as racing pulse, rapid breathing, and high blood pressure; reducing or eliminating sugar can reduce feelings of anxiety in susceptible individuals.

Coffee and caffeinated beverages are a common cause of or contributor to anxiety attacks. Giving up these beverages could be beneficial if you are troubled by anxiety or panic, but withdrawal should be done gradually to minimize withdrawal headaches and fatigue. People with panic disorders are often extremely sensitive to caffeine, and should avoid it.

Food allergies can cause symptoms of anxiety and can trigger panic attacks. One fairly well known test for food allergies, described in the Assessment chapter in Part 1, is a quickening of the pulse after the suspect food is eaten; this pulse racing can be felt as anxiety.

Low levels of minerals, especially potassium, magnesium, or calcium, can cause feelings of anxiety.

Depression

Chemicals associated with depression include:

- Aspartame, the artificial sweetener
- Toluene, found in gasoline, and in cologne as well as other places[12]
- Formaldehyde, found in many places, including carpets and building materials

A Swedish study of 3521 women who had breast implants for cosmetic reasons (as opposed to reconstruction after mastectomy or accident), found that those with the implants were three times as likely to commit suicide.[16] The connection is unclear; perhaps the silicone triggers depression, or perhaps women who get implants are more unstable or insecure to begin with. But a three-fold increase in suicide risk is something for women to consider before getting implants.

Drugs – Some drugs are associated with depression:

- Some drug therapies, such as interferon, can cause major depression.[17]
- Alcohol is a depressant drug, in spite of the fact that in some people it can cause a temporary lift before the depression sets in.
- Smokers are more likely than nonsmokers to be depressed[18], although it is unclear whether smoking causes depression or whether depressed people are more likely to self-medicate with nicotine.
- Marijuana can contribute to depression and lack of motivation, especially with long-term use.
- Antidepressant medication itself can cause depression, both as a side effect and as a withdrawal symptom.

In a study done by the drug company that produces Paxil®, it was found that children and teens taking Paxil® experienced a higher incidence of suicidal thoughts than those taking a placebo.[19] Ironically, Paxil® is an antidepressant.

Metals – Depression is commonly found in people with mercury fillings. In a study of 181 patients with depression[20], all 181 (100%) reported improvement in this symptom after removal of the fillings. Studies have concluded that excessive mercury exposure, as from dental fillings, can cause depression.[1] Dentists lead the list in suicide frequency as ranked by occupation. Dentists have stresses similar to those of doctors, with mercury exposure as an added factor.

Nickel toxicity can contribute to depression. Bipolar disorder, also known as manic-depressive illness, can be caused by the nickel in dental braces.[21]

High copper levels were found in adults with depression.[14]

Manic depression can be caused by too much of the mineral vanadium. Four separate studies show that bipolar patients have higher than normal blood vanadium levels. High doses of vitamin C can help rid the body of some of this excess.[1]

Diet – Wheat gluten has been linked to depressive disorders; it may be best to eliminate wheat products.[18] Sugar consumption is also a cause of depression as the sugar high wears off.

Allergy – Brain allergies and sensitivities to foods and airborne chemicals can cause depression.[1]

Yeast – Candida and buildup of fungal molds can contribute to depression.[1]

Food dyes, especially tartrazine (FD&C yellow #5), have been shown to be responsible for sensitivity reactions, including clinical depression.[22]

Cognitive problems, Alzheimer's disease, brain fog, mental confusion

Chemicals – Exposure to pesticides and chemicals can cause brain symptoms which can mimic Alzheimer's disease. Farm workers exposed to pesticides show more mental decline than non-farmers[23] or organic farmers. Forgetfulness is one of the most common symptoms of pesticide exposure[24], especially organophosphate pesticides such as malathion; brain fog is also a symptom of such exposure. [25]

Solvents can cause cognitive decline by partially dissolving the fatty myelin sheaths of nerves, leading to memory loss, especially of short-term memory.

Toluene (found in gasoline and cologne as well as other sources), can cause brain fog[12], as can formaldehyde, found in many places including carpets and building materials, and other organic solvents. Methyl chloride, a solvent with multiple uses including decaffeinating coffee and the manufacture of rubber and plastics, can cause short-term memory loss as well as delusions and hallucinations.[26]

Medications and drugs – Medication, especially anti-anxiety medication and other mood-altering compounds, can cause Alzheimer's-like cognitive problems.[27] Chemotherapy patients typically have significant cognitive declines due to the high toxicity of the medication[23], a syndrome common enough to be called "chemo fog." Synthetic HRT doubles the risk of Alzheimer's disease in women who begin treatment at age 65 or older.[28]

According to the ***Physician's Desk Reference***, certain drugs are associated with the side effect of mental confusion. Some of the more common ones are[29]:

- Xanax (antianxiety)
- Dilantin (anticonvulsant)
- Wellbutrin tablets
- Xylocaine with epinephrine injections (local dental anesthesia)

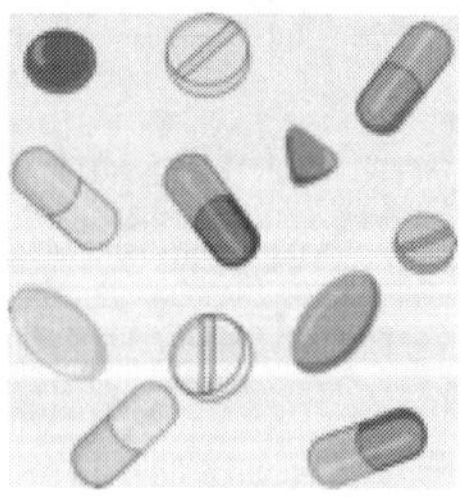

Other medications that can cause mental confusion include[30]:

- Sedatives and tranquilizers – Thorazine, Haldol, Valium, Librium
- Parkinson's medication – levodopa
- Antihistamines
- Antidepressants – Prozac, Elavil, Tofranil, Zoloft, Lexapro
- Antiseizure medication – Dilantin

- High blood pressure or heart medications – propranolol (Inderal), digoxin
- Painkillers – codeine, Darvon
- NSAIDs for arthritis – ibuprofen, naproxen, indomethacin
- Anticholinergic drugs – cold medications – atropine, Benadryl
- Anti-ulcer or acid reflux medications – Tagamet, Zantac, Pepcid

A study of 3000 elderly men found that those who smoked during their middle years were one-third more likely to have memory loss than those who had never smoked.[31]

Much cognitive function, such as the ability to focus attention, concentrate, remember and filter out irrelevant information, and the speed of information processing, were found to be adversely affected by marijuana smoking, with effects worsening with increased frequency and duration of use.[32] A marijuana smoker can take a long time to return to normal even after quitting. Sauna detoxification, discussed in Part 4, can help reduce brain fog and difficulty concentrating. Someone with a long history of marijuana smoking may temporarily feel stoned in the sauna as the drug, long stored in the body fat, reenters the bloodstream before being eliminated.

Metals – Mercury

Alzheimer's disease and/or senile dementia have been linked to mercury.[33] Mercury dental fillings in particular are linked to Alzheimer's disease, discussed in an article which itself had 62 scientific references.[34] Research at the University of Calgary in Alberta, Canada, has linked mercury toxicity with the formation of brain lesions found in Alzheimer's patients.[35] People with Alzheimer's disease have been found to have blood mercury levels three times higher than those without the disease.[23]

Mercury poisoning can cause memory lapses[36] and is a significant cause of memory loss. In a study of 109 patients with memory loss[20], 102, or 93.5%, reported improvement in this symptom after removal of the fillings. Memory and concentration problems related to diminished circulation improved after chelation for metals.[37]

Mercury blocks magnesium and manganese transport required for memory, resulting in lowered ability to concentrate.

Metals – Aluminum

Aluminum has been in the news for over a decade because high concentrations of aluminum have been found in the brains of Alzheimer's victims. Although the exact nature of the correlation is not known, the high aluminum concentrations are likely themselves a result of mercury toxicity, as the body is less able to clear out the aluminum when the body's filters (liver and kidneys) are clogged with mercury. Because mercury inhibits the body's ability to clear out metals, aluminum builds up. Aluminum, found in some antacids, adversely affects the cytochrome P450 (chemical) and metallothionein (metal) detoxification systems.

A study comparing aluminum levels in drinking water for 2344 patients with Alzheimer's disease or presenile dementia versus levels in the water used by controls without dementia found that the higher the aluminum in the water, the higher the correlation for Alzheimer's or dementia.[38]

In a placebo controlled trial of desferroxamine, a chelator which removes aluminum from the body, it was found that the use of the chelator (i.e. less aluminum in the body) was correlated with a reduction in the decline in function in patients.[39] Ten patients in Canada with Alzheimer's disease were chelated to remove mercury and aluminum; nine of them showed improvement. Chelation, discussed in the Metal detoxification chapter in Part 4, can often improve the condition by impeding further deterioration, but cannot reverse cellular damage.

High phosphorus can lead to loss of bone calcium, then to absorption of toxic aluminum.

Metals – other
Lead can cross the blood-brain barrier and contribute to senile dementia and Alzheimer's disease.[22] Iodine and lead can cause loss of alertness and slow mental reaction.[40] It was discovered in studies in Australia and at Harvard that too much zinc can cause the clumping of amyloid proteins characteristic of Alzheimer's disease.[41]

Fluoride – Aluminum-induced neural degeneration in rats, analogous to Alzheimer's disease, was greatly enhanced when the rats were given low doses of fluoride. The aluminum level in the brains of the fluoride-treated rats was double that of the non-fluoridated group. The fluoride enhanced the bioavailability of the toxic aluminum. Extrapolating these results to people, fluoridated water or other sources of fluoride are likely to initiate or worsen Alzheimer's disease or other dementias.[42]

Rats exposed to fluoride as adults showed cognitive deficits.[43] Rats drinking water at the recommended level of 1 ppm fluoride had dysfunctional blood-brain barriers that allowed more aluminum to enter the brain.[42]

Diet – Those who have a gene for developing Alzheimer's disease would be wise to watch their diet. A study of 263 elderly people with the Alzheimer's gene found that those who consumed a high-calorie, high-fat diet doubled their risk of developing the disease.[19]

Eating sugar contributes to brain fog; it causes insulin release, which lowers blood sugar, and less glucose is available to the brain. It also feeds yeast, which can cause foggy thinking.

Aspartame, an artificial sweetener, is linked to brain fog and memory loss.[44] Students at Texas Christian University who drank diet sodas sweetened with Aspartame experienced short-term memory loss.[31]

Allergy or sensitivity to a substance can cause mental or emotional impairment as well as physical symptoms. Brain fog is a fairly common symptom. For example, a person may be walking down the street, deep in conversation with a friend, and be exposed to diesel fumes, cologne, or insecticide. The person can become instantly confused and lose track of the conversation in mid-sentence. A day-to-day lack of mental clarity can likewise be due to food, inhalant, or other allergy.

Learning disabilities, ADHD

Chemicals – Learning disorders are more prevalent in children who live near heavily traveled roadways, implicating a chemical cause[22], such as cadmium from brake linings and tires.

A nationwide survey of children between the ages of one and twelve years who have taken over 20 cycles of antibiotics found that they are 50% more likely to have developmental delays, including speech and language problems and multisystem developmental disorders.[45] Yeast proliferation and digestive problems leading to malabsorption of nutrients are two possible connections.

Chronic exposure to chemicals in school contribute to learning disabilities, hyperactivity, and absenteeism. These chemicals include:

- Pencil lead, ink, chalk, dust, whiteboard markers, felt-tip markers
- Formaldehyde in particle board and plywood used to make desks and cabinets
- Cleaning materials such as rug cleaners and disinfectants
- Polyurethane insulating foam used in walls
- Chemicals in carpets such as formaldehyde, dirt repellents, fire retardants, and cleaning solutions

Pesticides can contribute to hyperactivity[46] due to their neurotoxicity.

The symptoms of fluoride toxicity are very similar to the symptoms of ADHD, indicating that fluoride in tap water, fluoridated toothpaste, or fluoride deliberately added to water marketed for babies and children may be a causative factor.[47] Rats exposed to fluoride prenatally showed hyperactivity,[43] and these study results might well be extrapolated to children.

Metals – Two of the best-known symptoms of lead poisoning are learning disabilities and mental retardation in children who usually ingest the metal by chewing on paint chips in older houses.

Lead based paint, although banned since 1978, is still a major problem. A child can attain a level of 35 mcg/dl of lead by ingesting an amount equivalent in size to one sugar granule per day during childhood. Children with 25-30 mcg/dl are six times as likely to have reading and learning disabilities.[48]

Mercury exposure has been linked to developmental problems.[49] High copper levels were found in hyperactive children.[14] Aluminum interferes with the electrical activity of the brain and contributes to slow learning.[26]

Diet effects are individual; for example, a wheat allergy can manifest as inability to focus. A food elimination diet, especially removing artificial food colors, preservatives, and sugar, is recommended; these have been shown to cause or contribute to ADHD in many cases. The detoxification and maintenance diets in Part 4 provide detailed guidelines. Follow the diet for 8-12 weeks and observe behavioral responses.[50] Hyperactivity and aggressiveness in children, which often accompany learning disabilities, can be brought on by diet and can therefore be controlled by dietary modification.

A diet which eliminated the most common allergens, including wheat, corn, dairy, yeast, soy, citrus, egg, chocolate, and peanuts as well as dyes and preservatives resulted in 73% of the children responding favorably[51]

Not surprisingly, researchers at Yale University School of Medicine found that sugar causes a noticeable physical and psychological reaction in normal healthy children. Children's adrenaline levels rose twice as high as adults' to counteract the effect of insulin which is released to offset the effect of sugar. The ability to pay attention is also affected by sugar.[52]

Removing sugar and other additives from the child's diet for a period of at least a week and monitoring the results is a risk-free, cost-free approach that can have benefits to the child's overall health as well as at least some potential for amelioration of ADHD symptoms. However, even if studies were to show that "most children" are not helped by this approach, it is worth trying due to the potential for great benefit for the individual child. 25 of 40 children, or 62%, of children with ADHD showed at least 50% improvement in behavior after two weeks of following a standard elimination diet.[53]

Patient profile

Mark, a preteen child with Attention Deficit Disorder (ADD), was taken off sugar, wheat and dairy and became calmer and was better able to study. He stopped disrupting the class, and the teacher was so amazed that she assumed that he was on the drug Ritalin.[40]

Artificial colors and preservatives were the most common provoking substances.[54] The removal of artificial food additives, salicylate-containing foods such as cucumbers and many fruits, and aspirin (a salicylate compound), can cause significant decrease in hyperactivity in some children.[55] According to a well-designed study published in ***Lancet***, 79% of hyperactive children improved when suspect substances were removed from their diet, then worsened when the substances were reintroduced. Artificial colors and flavors had the most significant effect on hyperactivity, and sugar also had a significant effect.[54]

Orange juice allergy is a common cause of behavior problems in children.[56]

Insomnia

Insomnia can be a sign of low serotonin; low melatonin from lack of light, aging, or deficiency of tryptophan, niacin (vitamin B3), or vitamin B6; high cortisol from high stress, or thyroid imbalance. Alcohol can help one get to sleep, but it is a poor quality sleep, and it can cause early waking. The most likely causes are low minerals and whiplash or other structural alignment issues.

Not all insomnia is the same. Distinguishing between patterns of insomnia can help point to a cause. For example, one person might have trouble getting to sleep but sleep well once asleep; another person might go to sleep with little or no problem but waken, perhaps to urinate, and be unable to go back to sleep. Yet another person might get to sleep fairly quickly, but the sleep is of poor quality with many small and brief awakenings.

Chemicals – Organophosphate pesticides such as malathion cause long-term alteration in brain waves and brain electrical activity, resulting in insomnia, irritability, and altered learning patterns and behavior.[25]

Insomnia can be caused by allergy to materials in the mattress and bedding, including dust, dust mites, and laundry detergent.

Insomnia has been linked to the use of silicone breast implants.[57] In a follow-up study of 50 consecutive silicone implant patients, 71% reported poor sleep.

Metals – A high level of the toxic metal aluminum, found in some antacids, aluminum cans, and other sources, can contribute to insomnia.[58]

Sleep medication – Ironically, sleep medications can cause insomnia. These medications disrupt the natural sleep patterns; taking such medication short-term can actually induce a long-term sleep problem. "…For every two-week period of sleep through medication, you just may be destroying your own natural sleep for months[59]."

Taking insomnia medication can perpetuate the insomnia. Once the body has become addicted to the medication, the body may be producing further insomnia in order to get its "fix."

Other medications can cause insomnia. These include[60]:

- Anti-inflammatories, especially steroids such as prednisone, have a stimulating effect
- Antihypertensive medication such as propranolol may cause insomnia through daytime lethargy
- Asthma medications such as theophylline are related to caffeine and have stimulant effects
- Antidepressants can have a stimulating effect.

Low minerals – Potassium deficiency is most likely to be the cause of insomnia if the insomnia is of the following pattern: Inability to fall asleep or get back to sleep with mind racing, fatigue, rapid or pounding heartbeat, muscle cramps, tightness or pain, kidney pain, twitching, muscle pain, anxiety, tossing and turning, difficulty breathing deeply. A potassium supplement can help you sleep within 20-30 minutes of ingestion if your insomnia is due to this cause.

A low level of magnesium, potassium, sodium, or calcium can cause frequent awakening at night and shallower sleep.[58]

Low amino acids – Low tryptophan, an amino acid, can cause insomnia. Tryptophan helps induce sleep and relaxation by producing the neurotransmitter serotonin. Tryptophan is no longer available as supplement in the U.S for political/legal reasons. When tryptophan was banned in 1989, many patients who couldn't sleep turned to Prozac instead, and many became addicted to it. Melatonin is a natural sleep aid that can be used instead. Tryptophan is now available by prescription. It should be taken at night. Tyrosine is another amino acid which is useful for sleep. While tryptophan is good for getting to sleep (PM sleep), tyrosine is good for staying asleep (AM sleep). However, tryptophan and tyrosine are antagonists and should not be taken together. Tyrosine should only be taken in the morning before breakfast, or it can actually interfere with sleep.

Theanine increases the neurotransmitter GABA, which can improve sleep.

Light – Exposure to full spectrum light during the day has eased insomnia.[61] Light on the skin, not only on the eyes, can affect the body's clock. Turning lights on during the night upsets the body clock. If necessary to get up, it is best not to turn on any lights. The use of a night light at night can have the same effect of confusing the body's internal clock.[62]

Other – Sufficient cholesterol is needed to make hormones that can help regulate melatonin production, which in turn can help alleviate insomnia.[63]

Skin Problems

General

Chemical toxins can contribute to skin problems such as rashes, acne and pimples, psoriasis, and eczema. This can be due to an allergic skin reaction from direct contact. A systemic link is that the skin is one of the major detoxification pathways of the body, and a chemical overload can clog this pathway, which can result in skin inflammation: acne, rashes, psoriasis, boils. Creams and oils of various types, often used to smooth dry or rough skin, or foundation used to conceal a skin problem, may actually be worsening the problem due to their clogging action.

Age spots

Age spots, or liver spots, are harmless in themselves, but they are an indicator of free radical accumulation in the body. They are called age spots because they tend to occur in the elderly, worsening with advancing age. This connection is less likely to be due to age itself, but rather to the additive and cumulative exposure to toxins over decades. Causes of age spots include chemicals in general, excess sun exposure, lack of exercise (due to the lymph detoxification connection), poor liver function (hence the name liver spots), and ingestion of rancid oils.[1] A liver cleanse is recommended. Both the liver cleanse and the connection of the lymph system with detoxification are described in Part 4.

Athlete's foot

Athlete's foot is caused by the tinea fungus. Avoid yeast products, described in the chapter on the Detoxification Diet in Part 4, since athlete's foot is a fungus.[2] Any fungal infection that appears to affect the outside of the body, such as athlete's foot, toenail fungus, skin fungus of whatever type, or vaginal yeast infections, is actually an indicator of internal yeast overgrowth. The underlying problem needs to be addressed in the form of diet and other healing modalities to keep the external symptoms from recurring.

Rash, dermatitis

Dermatitis is usually caused by toxins that are being eliminated through the skin.[2] Contact dermatitis is a skin reaction to contact with certain chemicals and natural substances, including those in the air. Toxic byproducts of microorganisms and fungus can also cause dermatitis.[3]

Nail polish and acrylic nails can cause an allergic rash on the face and neck from touching the skin with the nails.[4]

Formaldehyde and the artificial sweetener aspartame can also cause rashes.[5]

Nickel, found in some dental work and stainless steel, is the most potent allergen of all the trace elements, accounting for more contact dermatitis and other allergic reactions than all other metals combined, especially eczema or dermatitis on the eyelids, groin, elbows, and elsewhere.[6]

Eczema

Eczema in children is usually caused by allergy to wheat, corn and B vitamins; allergy desensitization (NAET) for these foods often brings about healing of the condition[7], although avoidance of allergens may be preferable. NAET can also help to prevent the later development of asthma.[7] Allergy desensitization is described in Part 4.

Eczema is almost always associated with candida yeast overgrowth[8], as well as giardia or bacteria. The yeast-free diet described in the Detoxification Diet chapter in Part 4 can help to control yeast and thus may have a beneficial effect on eczema and other conditions caused by yeast.

Eczema often results from an oil metabolism problem. The gallbladder aids in the processing of oils, so anything that adversely affects the gallbladder, such as fungus, giardia, or helicobacter, can lead to eczema.

Grayish skin color

Liver problems can cause a grayish-blue skin coloring, as the liver filters out toxins and a poorly functioning liver causes toxins to accumulate in the blood.

Taking a large amount of colloidal silver internally can cause a permanent grayish skin discoloration known as argyria, the accumulation of silver under the skin. Colloidal silver works well as an immune system booster and antiviral agent, but should only be taken for a short time as needed, not as a daily supplement.

Itchy earlobes

Up to 33% of women and 17% of men are allergic to nickel.[6] A sign of nickel allergy is the development of hot, red, itchy earlobes soon after putting on inexpensive earrings. Inexpensive earring wires or posts are usually made of stainless steel, which contains nickel; this is also the case with cheap gold-colored earwires. Expensive earrings are likely to be made of gold or silver, which rarely cause a reaction. Lack of a noticeable reaction, however, does not mean that one is not allergic to nickel.

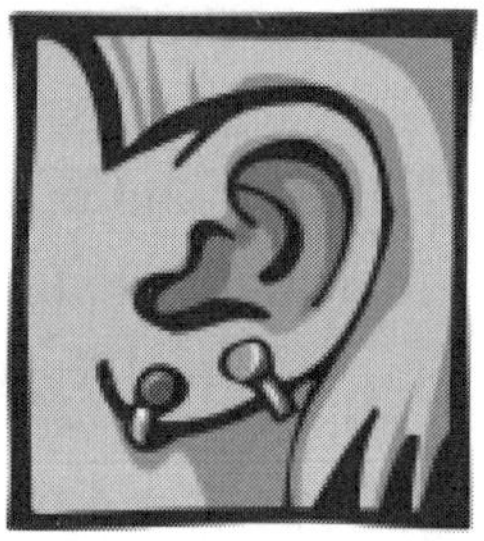

The wearing of cheap earrings does more than just provide a visible means of identifying nickel allergy. They can actually cause nickel allergy by sensitizing earring wearers to a metal they might not otherwise contact. Men with pierced ears have thirty-three times the nickel sensitivity as men without pierced ears.[9] Women are even more likely to have nickel allergy because of earrings, jewelry, and nickel oxides in cosmetics which sometimes contact sensitive mucous membranes.

Jock itch, tinea cruris

Jock itch, a common name for red, scaling, itchy areas in the groin, is caused by a tinea fungus, related to ringworm. The anti-yeast diet aspect of the Detoxification Diet can help with this, as yeast or sugar in the diet can cause or contribute to yeast problems elsewhere in the body.

Jock itch is sometimes spread from a case of athlete's foot. One mode of transmission occurs when men put on their shorts before their socks, and fungus from their feet is transferred to the groin. For this reason, one should put on socks first if athlete's foot is present or suspected.[10]

Pimples, acne

Pimples and acne are the result of blocking and inflammation of the sebaceous glands caused by internal and/or external toxins. The toxins accumulate faster than the sebaceous oil can clear them out, resulting in visible inflammation. Acne, a severe condition of pimples that can be painful and lead to permanent scarring, may be caused by an allergic systemic or skin reaction, in which case identifying and eliminating the offending substance will do more good than putting something on your skin or taking an antibiotic.

Treatments for acne can cause other problems. Tetracycline, taken orally for acne, can kill and deplete the good bacteria in the intestinal system, leading to fungus and yeast infections. Fungi can double in number every 24 hours when not controlled by the protective bacteria, so runaway yeast overgrowth doesn't take long to develop. As your face gets clear from the tetracycline, your mind gets fuzzy from the fungus – not a good tradeoff.

When an area around the mouth repeatedly breaks out, this is often due to dental metals, especially nickel and mercury, in nearby teeth. Acne-like eruptions around the mouth have also been linked to the use of fluoridated toothpaste.[11]

Diet is a frequent contributor to acne and pimples. Acne may be caused in some people by an allergic reaction to dairy products or to sensitivity to sugar. Try eliminating these products from the diet for a month and watch for improvement. Iodine, found in fish, iodized salt (also used in many processed foods), kelp, and onions, is known to worsen acne. It is also found in some supplements and nearly all sea vegetables (seaweeds). The foods that most commonly cause or aggravate acne are wheat, dairy, tomatoes, and the seasonings mustard, pepper, and paprika.[12]

Other common causes of pimples are microorganisms, allergy, sugar, and the metals cadmium, mercury or excess selenium.[5] Some drugs can contribute to acne, especially steroids (oral or topical), lithium, oral contraceptives, and some anti-epileptic drugs.[1]

Psoriasis

Psoriasis is an itchy, unsightly skin disease. It often shows up as reddish to gray thickened scaly patches, usually starting on the elbows. The patches can itch severely. An overgrowth of yeast in the digestive tract can be involved in some cases of psoriasis[13], and can be helped by eliminating yeast and yeast-feeders from the diet.

The parasites giardia and helicobacter pylori can cause psoriasis. A lack of oils or poor functioning of the gallbladder, which processes oils, can also be a cause; in this case, the liver/gallbladder flush in Part 4 can be of benefit.

Sunburning easily, sunlight sensitivity (photosensitivity)

Some drugs, cologne, and some chemicals can cause sensitivity to sunlight (photosensitivity). Increased sunlight sensitivity can occur on the part of the skin of an allergic user where the scented product or cream was applied.

Wrinkling

Wrinkling, although an expected part of aging, is not necessarily inevitable. There are things that one can do to minimize wrinkling:

- Fluoride is a major cause of wrinkling and of collagen breakdown in general. Avoid fluoridated drinking water where possible; most city water is now fluoridated.
- Low beneficial oils such as olive and fish oils can lead to wrinkling.
- Insufficient water (hydration) is linked to wrinkling.
- Sugar stiffens collagen and causes skin wrinkling and loss of flexibility.[14]

- Smoking is a major cause of premature wrinkling, which is due to the lowered level of oxygen to the skin.[12] Acetaldehyde, found in both cigarette smoke and smog, is a strong cross-linking agent. Cross-linking of skin causes premature wrinkling.
- Be careful what you drink; alcohol and caffeine have a diuretic, or dehydrating, effect, drying the skin and leading to wrinkling. Salt and other minerals to help retain water to moisturize skin from within, as well as healthful oils, can help with some age-related skin changes, including wrinkling.

Endocrine System Problems

What is the endocrine system and what does it do?

The endocrine system consists of ductless glands which produce hormones and release them directly into the bloodstream. The blood then carries the hormones to their target organs to perform their function. There are six different endocrine glands, although some of them are in multiples:

- The **pituitary** is sometimes called the master gland. Located deep in the brain and only the size of a pea, it secretes hormones that control the other glands.
- The **thyroid gland**, located in the neck, is responsible for the metabolic rate. A malfunction of the thyroid can affect the entire body.
- The four tiny **parathyroid glands** are located next to and around the thyroid. Their primary function is to regulate calcium and phosphorus metabolism, and their primary action is on bone.
- The **pancreatic islet cells** produce insulin, which regulates glucose metabolism and its storage as glycogen. Underfunctioning of the pancreas and insufficient insulin production (type 1 diabetes), along with insulin resistance (type 2), is known as diabetes, discussed in this chapter.
- The two **adrenal glands** lie just above the kidneys. They secrete adrenaline (also called epinephrine). Adrenaline is produced in reaction to stress, and is responsible for the "fight, flight, or freeze" response involving the sympathetic nervous system.
- The **gonads**, ovaries in women and testes in men, secrete the hormones responsible for sex drive and reproduction.

The endocrine glands are extremely important in the functioning of the body. They are also interdependent; if one is working suboptimally another can take its place up to a point, although the endocrine system can go down like a row of dominoes if there is enough stress on the system.

What chemicals can affect the endocrine system in general?

The Endocrine Society has stated that "Results from animal models, human clinical observations, and epidemiological studies converge to implicate EDCs [endocrine disrupting chemicals] as a significant concern to public health.[1]" Pesticides and herbicides are associated with disruption in endocrine, reproductive and sexual function.[2]

Mercury from amalgam binds to -SH (sulfhydryl) groups, which are used in almost every enzymatic process in the body. Mercury therefore has the potential to disturb all metabolic processes.[3] Electrically generated nerve impulses, such as those produced by the battery effect (metals in the mouth) can travel to the hypothalamus and pituitary of the brain and affect these structures that control the autonomic nervous system and hormone-generating endocrine glands.[4]

Gland problems (thyroid, gonads, adrenals) can have chronic **parasitic infection** as their source.

If certain hormones are supplied or oversupplied by food, especially **meat and dairy** products, the glands which normally make these hormones become dysfunctional and even atrophied with disuse. Testosterone and progesterone are lowered, resulting in women and men with low motivation and sex drive. Milk may well exacerbate the hormonal and emotional storms weathered by teenagers today, since hormonal peaks and dips contribute to teenage depression, violence, and suicide.

What are some of the endocrine system problems and their possible causes?

Thyroid problems, hypothyroidism

About 30 million people in the US, almost all of them women, have malfunctioning thyroid glands; half of these people may not know it.[5] Low body temperature may be even more effective than blood tests in determining hypothyroidism.

Environmental toxins can disrupt thyroid functioning.[6] Chemicals such as dioxin and PCBs (found in plastic pipes and elsewhere) interfere with normal hormone function, including that of the thyroid.[7]

Iodine is needed for proper thyroid function. **Chlorine** and fluorine (as **fluoride**) are in the same column of the chemical Periodic Table as iodine, and thus have similar binding characteristics in the body, i.e. can replace iodine in the cell's function. Chlorine is typically found in city tap water, which should be avoided; this includes showers, since chlorine in water can be absorbed through the skin. A shower filter can help, as can avoiding the drinking of tap water. If you start taking supplemental iodine and start feeling worse, this can be due to the dumping of toxic bromine from the iodine receptors in the cells. This is temporary and is a sign of detoxification and resulting ultimate benefit. However, if you feel worse with iodine, have your doctor test you to rule out sensitivity to iodine.

Fluoride, found in most tap water and in most commercial toothpaste, can block iodine receptors in the thyroid, resulting in symptoms of low thyroid function. According to the ***Merck Index***, fluoride was at one time used medically to depress thyroid activity. As little as 5 mg (1/6000 ounce), the amount consumed daily by the average person drinking fluoridated water, has a thyroid lowering effect, with associated symptoms that include fatigue.[8] A study done in Switzerland with mice has also found that fluoridated water depressed thyroid function 30-40%.[7] Fluoride competes with T3, the active form of thyroid hormone converted from the T4 produced by the thyroid gland; a study of 123 people with varying degrees of thyroid function revealed this link, leading researchers to believe that fluoride in drinking water speeds the development of thyroid disease. More than 60% of Americans use fluoridated water,[9] which may well be related to the increase in hypothyroidism in the US population.

Perchlorate, a chemical contaminant found in some water supplies from a fertilizer that leaches into ground water, blocks iodine from entering the thyroid and prevents synthesis of thyroid hormone. Long term exposure to perchlorate, even small amounts, can interfere with thyroid function.[9,10]

The drug **lithium**, used for bipolar disorder, can have an adverse effect on thyroid function.[10]

Smoking – Past or present smokers have an increased risk of hypothyroidism. Tobacco contains thiocyanate, a chemical that suppresses thyroid function. The association may work the other way around: hypothyroidism may contribute to smoking in certain people because the nicotine artificially and temporarily raises metabolism and masks the fatigue and weight gain from the hypothyroidism. After quitting smoking, these effects of hypothyroidism are felt.[10]

Mercury slows thyroid function.[9] Endocrine problems such as low body temperature often improve rapidly when amalgam is removed, a sure sign that the amalgam was causing the problem in the first place. Normal body temperature is about 98.6 F orally. People reacting to amalgam components often have a temperature range of 96.2 to 97.6 degrees, which can rise to 98.2 in as little as one day after amalgam removal and to 98.6 soon afterward.[11] A low body temperature is a sign of low thyroid function, and many people have mistakenly been given thyroid hormone to remedy a symptom caused by amalgam fillings.

Decreased thyroid function can result when **cadmium** blocks the copper and zinc that, along with iodine, promote proper thyroid function.

A **yeast** overgrowth can contribute to a low-functioning thyroid.[12]

Soy, sometimes in the form of soy protein powder, is often recommended for menopausal women because of its estrogenic effect; however, it can reduce thyroid function. Hypothyroidism is common in menopausal women, and soy, ironically recommended for this population, can help one problem but worsen another. Soy can interfere with intestinal absorption of ingested prescription thyroid hormone. People on thyroid hormone supplements should therefore avoid soy products.[13]

Diabetes

Diabetes has been linked to **pesticide** exposure.[14]

Aspartame – One of the complications of diabetes is diabetic retinopathy, or degenerative loss of sight. One contributor to this may be the artificial sweetener Aspartame, used often by diabetics because their condition causes both an intolerance of sugar and a craving for sweetness, has been linked with nerve damage, and its breakdown products methanol and formaldehyde are associated with irreversible eye damage.

Smoking – A Yale University study shows that smoking may increase type 2 diabetes risk. Smokers' muscle cells did not absorb glucose as well as those of nonsmokers by a large (74%) margin.[15] Cellular resistance to glucose is the hallmark of type 2 diabetes. Smoking also has a negative influence on carbohydrate and lipid metabolism. In a group of insulin-treated diabetics, 114 smokers had a 15-20% higher insulin requirement (30% higher in heavy smokers) and serum triglyceride concentration, as compared with that of nonsmokers.[16]

Medications – Calcium channel blockers, ironically taken to reduce heart attack risk, can increase them nearly ten-fold in diabetics who take the drugs.[17] This is especially significant since diabetes itself raises the risk of heart disease. Diabetes drugs themselves can cause serious problems; the diabetes drug Rezulin (troglitazone) was pulled from the market in March 2000 after 89 cases of severe irreversible liver failure and 61 associated deaths.[18] This is yet another reason to focus on natural methods such as diet in the control of diabetes and other ailments rather than depending on drugs.

Aluminum buildup is implicated in diabetes. Elevated aluminum has been found in many diabetics, and it adversely influences glycolysis, a major part of glucose metabolism. The drinking of large amounts of soda from aluminum cans is a major source of dietary aluminum.[19]

Mercury, particularly from metal fillings, hinders the body's detoxification of aluminum by taking up the activity of the metal detox pathways, and both the mercury itself and the secondary buildup of aluminum can contribute to the development of diabetes.

Women with high levels of **iron** are at greater risk of developing type 2 diabetes.[20]

Microorganisms – Cytomegalovirus can destroy the cells of the pancreas and limit their ability to produce insulin, and so has been implicated in playing a triggering role in diabetes.[21]

Because of the high levels of blood sugar found in diabetes, fungus and **yeast** can be a problem, as sugar feeds these parasitic organisms. Sugar and other yeast feeders, as well as yeast itself, are eliminated in the Detoxification Diet in Part 4.

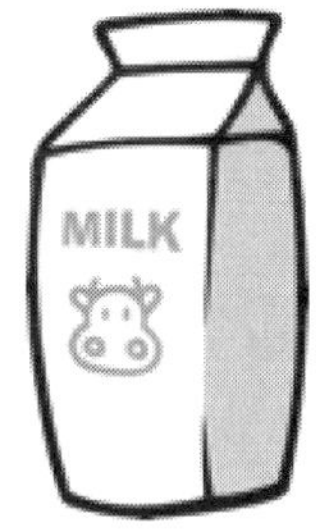

Consumption of **cows' milk** by infants has been linked to juvenile onset (insulin-dependent) diabetes. Cows' milk is a possible trigger of the immune response that starts the cascade of events culminating in Type 1 diabetes (IDDM); cows' milk protein (casein) appears to cause an autoimmune reaction with the pancreas.[22]

Overweight

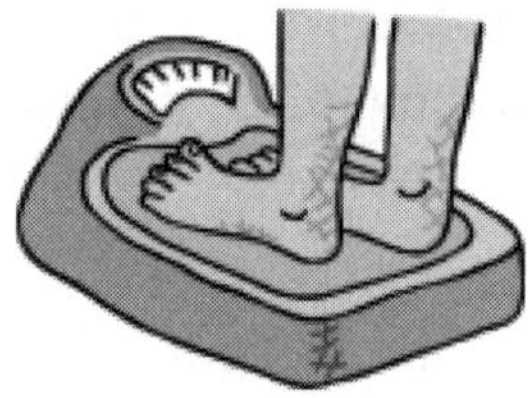

Problems with overweight are widely thought to be a simple calories in / calories out equation, an imbalance between food and exercise. However, chemical toxicity can have a major influence on the gaining and retaining of weight. Diet has a major effect on weight, no surprise, but there are dietary factors other than calories or carbohydrate grams to consider.

When weight-loss dieting isn't a good thing

If the overweight is due primarily to toxicity, dieting can make things worse. The problem lies in the way the body deals with fat-soluble toxins such as solvents and pesticides. The body stores these in fat cells, like storing waste oil in barrels. As the fat cells shrink, the toxins are released into the bloodstream, producing feelings of fatigue and illness. In this case, the body may have held onto the fat to try to dilute the toxins, and dieting is defeating that purpose. After you have dieted and reduced the mass of fat cells, the body may do all it can, by decreasing metabolic rate and/or increasing appetite, to increase and enlarge the fat cells back to where they were in order to cope with the toxins. This is likely a major reason why there is a 95% chance of rebound weight gain after dieting.

So should a person with toxic overweight not try to lose weight? Yes, but first the problem of toxicity must be identified and dealt with, which is the purpose of this book.

Another problem with dieting is that some diets do not meet the dieter's needs nutritionally because it may be too depleted in calories or limited in food types.

<u>Chemicals</u>

Chemicals can contribute to unwanted weight gain in a number of ways.

Much overweight (about 70%), but not all, is due to retention of excess fluid, rather than fat caused by overeating, although both can be, and usually are, combined in one person. Toxins in the body can lead to fluid retention as the body attempts to dilute the toxin. Allergies can cause the same effect, since the body perceives the allergen as a toxin and tries to dilute it.

If toxins are present, such as pesticides, mercury, or the waste byproducts of microorganisms, the body's natural response is to try to dilute the poison with water or fat, depending on whether the toxin is water- or fat-soluble. Both responses will be seen as a gain in weight, and/or difficulty losing it.

If a person who loses water weight on a detoxification diet, such as the one in Part 4, stays away from food allergens and toxins, much of the weight should stay off.

Chemicals can contribute to hypothyroidism, a lowering of metabolism and consequent difficulty in burning off calories as described in the Endocrine chapter. Puffiness and swelling of parts of the body, such as eyelids, face, and sometimes feet and hands can be symptoms of hypothyroidism[1], along with overall weight retention.

Medications

Quite a few medications – including, ironically, weight loss aids – can cause weight gain by a variety of mechanisms.

As is the case with any toxin, drugs can cause water and fat weight gain as the body tries to dilute the toxin.

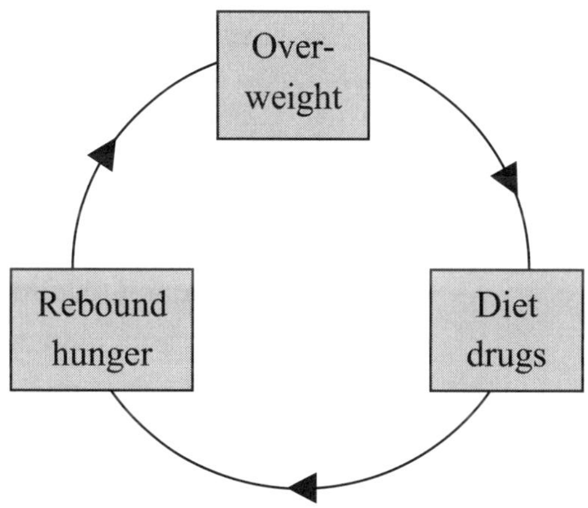

A number of both prescription and over-the-counter (OTC) weight loss aids are available, many of which contain phenylpropanolamine (OTC) or amphetamines (prescription). These drugs artificially suppress appetite, regardless of the body's food needs. Weight loss resulting from the use of these drugs is rarely maintained, since healthy eating habits and lifestyle changes have not been learned, and a rebound effect of increased appetite may occur when the drugs are discontinued. Those who take diet drugs will usually experience reduction in hunger, then no effect, then rebound hunger as the cellular starvation causes a ravenous hunger that is stronger than the drug. Eating less by any means can reduce levels of nutrients in the body, and increased hunger is the body's way of attempting to get sufficient nutrients.

Prescription hormone drugs can cause weight gain, especially birth control pills, estrogen replacement therapy, prednisone (often used for arthritis), and others. These drugs can cause weight gain through water retention and increased appetite.

In addition to those mentioned, other medications can cause weight gain by slowing metabolism and increasing fat storage; these include diabetes drugs and antidepressants[2] and drugs for bipolar disorder.[3]

Certain medications can cause metabolic resistance to losing weight even with calorie restriction. These medications include psychotropic drugs such as Prozac®, steroid hormones such as estrogen and prednisone, and NSAIDs for arthritis and other pain.[4]

Some medications – either the medications or their sweetened base – tend to raise insulin levels, including anti-inflammatories, antacid tablets and liquids, breath fresheners, cough drops and syrups, and stool softeners. It is best to combine these with meals to reduce the insulin impact.[5]

Metals

An excess of the metals and elements silver, cadmium, mercury, iodine, potassium, nitrogen, sodium, nickel, or selenium[6] can contribute to water retention. The biggest source of mercury is metal dental fillings.

Food additives

Many food additives contribute to weight gain since they are typically toxic – i.e. don't belong in the body – and the body will retain water and/or fat to try to dilute them, as would be the case with any toxin.

Artificial sweeteners can actually cause weight gain for the following reasons:

- Artificial sweeteners obviously taste sweet, and the sweet taste signals the pancreas to produce insulin. Blood sugar drops without any or enough actual sugar to buffer the insulin, and the hunger level rises. More food is then eaten.
- Psychological factors can also cause one to eat more, as the person using artificial sweeteners may give her/himself permission to eat more of other things to compensate, such as apple pie with their artificially sweetened coffee.
- Artificial sweeteners are not simply inert substances with an absence of calories. They are toxic substances that the body is not designed to use. As mentioned, the body will often retain water and fat to attempt to dilute toxins, resulting in weight gain.

Animals given **MSG** became obese, even though they were not eating more food. Those animals on MSG showed high insulin levels, which stimulates the body to make and store fat[7], as well as increasing hunger to take in sugar to counteract the insulin. A steady diet of processed foods with MSG can damage areas of the brain that regulate food intake and fat production.[7]

Microorganisms

In addition to toxins, time and metabolism, microbiology is an important player in the weight gain and loss game. Fungus often grows out of control due to diets that are too high in sugars and refined or intermediate carbohydrates, combined with a shortage of protective bacteria. As the fungi ferment, they give off toxic waste products that the body tries to dilute by holding water. A vicious cycle is created as the body craves more sugar to feed the hungry fungi. Women are more likely to have a fungus problem than men due to their higher estrogen levels. Estrogen promotes the storage of sugar, leading to lower blood sugar levels, sweets cravings (especially premenstrually), and more fungal growth.

Mercury, whose primary source is metal tooth fillings, can contribute to fungus growth by killing the protective bacteria that help keep the fungus under control.

Nutritional deficiencies

Cravings in general can result from a lack of a related nutrient, as described below. Cravings often come from the body's need for a substance related to that craved such as a nutrient; counterfeit substances may temporarily relieve symptoms of deficiency, but create greater deficiency in the process. Food cravings are often linked to chemical allergies[8], as well as to food allergies. Allergic addiction is possible, especially for the common allergens wheat, milk, eggs, soy, corn, tomatoes, peanuts, yeast or sugar. Most or all of these are present in most carbohydrate foods, which helps to make such foods among the most commonly craved.

Salt and minerals – Interestingly, in some cases water retention can be caused by too *little* salt, although people commonly believe that only too much salt can result in water retention. If there is a deficiency of salt and other minerals, the body may hoard water, knowing that releasing water also means releasing some of this less-than-optimal amount of minerals dissolved in that water. Increasing both salt and mineral intake and water intake can, in these cases, actually cause the body to eliminate excess water and contribute to weight loss. Also, salt and other minerals allow water to penetrate and be used by the cells. Low minerals can cause the cells to perceive insufficient water even if plenty is present, leading to the body's retention of water.

Patient profile

One patient, a doctor, was overweight (260 pounds) and had very high blood pressure (240/130). His doctor had put him on a low salt diet, which didn't help. Another doctor, who was more knowledgeable about the way the body really works, took note of the low sodium level on the patient's blood test. He *increased* the patient's salt intake, going against conventional wisdom in doing so. The water weight was quickly dropped and his blood pressure returned to near normal. The kidneys may not let water out of the body until the electrolytes such as so-

> dium and potassium are rebalanced, a process complicated by the fact that sodium is lost in sweat. It is desirable to let water out of the body so new water can come in, much like an oil change allows your car to run better and protects the engine.[6]

A craving for chips, salted nuts, or processed foods might actually be the body's way of trying to get the salt it needs.

Water can be considered to be a nutrient, and a deficiency of water can lead to the retention of water weight. Paradoxically, one way to encourage the elimination of too much water is to drink even more of it. The body will sense that there is plenty of water available, so it is not necessary to hoard it. Additional water also flushes out excess salt and some water soluble toxins, which is beneficial both weight-wise and health-wise and is an important part of detoxification.

Oil, typically vilified in the weight-loss wars since it is high in calories and limited for this reason, has another surprising role in loss and gain of weight. A deficiency of oil can result in the absorption, as with a thirsty sponge, of oil-based chemicals such as solvents and pesticides from the environment, which in turn can cause more chemical-related weight gain. Beneficial oils such as fish and olive oil can in fact help to carry oil-soluble chemicals out of the body, and are an important part of both losing weight and gaining health.

Another way in which oil deficiency contributes to weight gain is that, if you are deficient in the healthful oils, you may crave anything with fat in it, including unhealthy choices such as fried foods and ice cream. However, if the wrong kind of fat is eaten, the body's needs are still not satisfied and the craving continues and worsens. The use of healthful oils reduces the oil deficiency and thus can ease the craving. In this way the *addition* of oil to the diet can result in the ingestion of *less* oil and fat.

Chocolate – No, chocolate is not a nutrient, although it might feel like it to some people who crave it, and is thus the subject of many a PMS joke. Chocolate is a source of magnesium and of oils. Eating almonds may be helpful if you are having a chocolate craving – they contain both magnesium and good oils. Magnesium, 300mg twice a day, can help counteract chocolate cravings.[9]

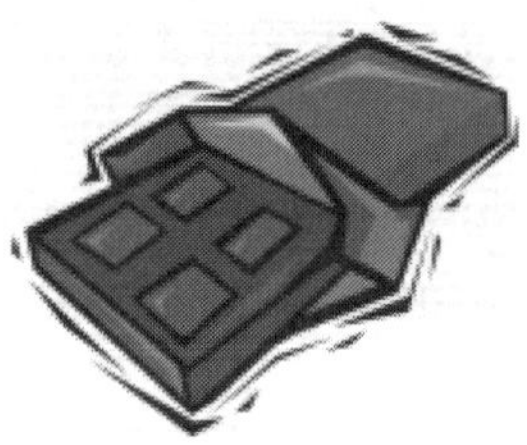

Food allergies

Food allergies can cause weight gain and retention in a number of ways:

- An allergen, interpreted by the body as being a toxin, will have the same effect as a toxin because the body will tend to retain water and fat to dilute it.

- Food allergies can cause unstable blood sugar, which interferes with weight loss, in part by causing insulin levels to yo-yo up and down; high insulin levels cause increased appetite.
- Food allergy causes nervousness, which causes overeating in an attempt to escape the nervousness. Thus "nervous eating" may have a physical more than a psychological base.
- Food allergies often cause an allergic addiction, in which the body craves that which is causing problems. Adrenaline released due to the stress of the food allergy causes the blood sugar to rise and then fall, increasing both appetite and the desire for another adrenaline "fix" in the form of the problematic food.

Because of these several mechanisms, weight loss after eliminating allergens, as with the detox diet, can be dramatic. This may explain the success of limited, low-allergenic diets like the rice diet, grapefruit diet, or cabbage soup diet. But the weight is often regained, and then some, because an allergy can develop to the single food eaten daily. Also, since a diet composed of a limited number of foods is difficult to stick to for very long, as well as being nutritionally unwise, the person is likely to resume "normal" eating, including allergens, and the weight comes back on as rapidly as it was lost. The Detoxification diet, maintenance diet, and rotation diet in Part 4 give guidelines to healthy low-allergenic eating.

Other causes

If the body is holding onto excess matter, resulting in constipation, this can contribute to weight gain. A colonic can cause a several-pound drop in weight as well as a flattening of the abdomen by removing this accumulated fecal matter, but the root cause of the constipation still hasn't been addressed.

Large breasts can come from holding toxins. Breasts are a mixture of lymph tissue (milk glands) and fat, and both of which can hold toxins. Soreness of breasts is another indication of toxicity. Bras constrict the lymph channels and keep toxins from draining, predisposing the woman to breast problems, including breast cancer and swollen, lumpy breasts. Underwire bras in particular constrict the lymph channels and should be avoided.

Parasites can contribute to overweight in a couple of ways. Parasites put out toxins as part of their life and death cycle, which the body attempts to dilute by retaining water. Also, parasites consume much of the nutrition intended for your cells, and your starved cells will send the message to your brain that you need to eat more, usually carbs and sugar.

Sugar cravings can be caused by – in addition to allergic addiction and yeast – the consumption of corn syrup, which is found in a huge and sometimes surprising array of products, especially when it is cheaper to use in a product than sugar. Its consumption causes the release of insulin, which in turn increases appetite for sweets, but unlike sugar itself, it doesn't satisfy.

What is cellulite, and what causes it?

The skin over the areas of overweight in some people, especially women, is lumpy, puckered, and dimpled rather than smooth. This is often referred to by the nonmedical term "cellulite." These dimples and lumps are actually swollen lymph nodes and toxic damaged fatty tissue between dermis and epidermis. Heavy rope-like fibers surround the fat cells; the buildup of these causes the characteristic appearance of cellulite.[10] You can starve yourself and exercise faithfully but the cellulite will remain until the toxins are cleared.

Cellulite is caused by poor lymphatic drainage. Lymph should flow freely, but when it doesn't, it congeals like jelly and the proteins separate out and form thick fibers. These slow the flow even further in a vicious cycle. The normal flow of lymphatic fluid can be disrupted by tight clothing such as bras, especially underwire; lymphatic blockage can lead to cellulite.[10] The lymphatic exercises and massage discussed in Part 4 can help facilitate proper lymph flow, and can thus potentially eradicate some of the cellulite.

In diagnosing the cause of cellulite, it is helpful to pinpoint when the problem started. If it started at puberty, the cause is likely to be hormonal, estrogen in particular[10], although there can be other causes and contributors.

A sedentary lifestyle can lead to cellulite in a couple of ways. First, sitting around without exercising and working the lymph nodes can cause them to swell. Secondly, sitting for long periods of time compresses blood vessels and lymphatic vessels.[10]

A three-step plan to fight cellulite is

- Identify and eliminate toxins
- Detoxification diet
- Lymphatic exercises and massage

What about liposuction?

Liposuction, the surgical removal of fat via a hole made in the skin, can actually worsen cellulite by damaging the fine network of capillaries and lymph vessels on the outside or back of the thighs. Results may initially be cosmetically pleasing, but then cellulite in those areas may end up worse than before the surgery[10] since future toxins won't be carried away effectively.

Patient profile

One patient, a woman who was overweight and had heavy cellulite on her thighs, tried many diets and up to two hours a day of exercise with no success. An eight-day detoxification diet helped her get rid of both the excess weight and the cellulite. Treatment for allergies and microorganisms allowed her to keep the weight off.[6]

How can I tell whether my weight problem is due to chemicals?

There are a number of ways you can tell whether your weight problem is due to chemicals, microorganisms, nutrient deficiencies, or other non-caloric causes.

If you feel worse instead of better when you force your body to lose weight by strenuous dieting, the reason may be that, by shrinking the fat cells, the toxins stored within them have been released into the bloodstream, causing a feeling of ill health.

Blood tests and other tests can help to determine the root cause(s) of overweight, and whether they are chemically or nutritionally based[6]:

Blood tests

- Thyroid function can show whether food is metabolized at the proper rate. See Endocrine chapter for discussion on hypothyroidism.
- Triglyceride level can show whether weight is due to fat (if elevated over 100 or the triglyceride to thyroid ratio is over 10:1) or water (triglycerides are low – below 80 – or normal). When one is insulin resistant, sugar is stored as medium chain triglycerides, which then convert back to sugar, a precursor to diabetes.
- Glucose – if it is high, this could indicate diabetes, which is sometimes associated with obesity. Diabetes is discussed in the Endocrine chapter.
- Liver function levels, such as low or high LDH, SGOT, SGPT, or GGTP, show how well chemical and metal toxins are eliminated, and toxins can cause water retention. The liver cleanse is covered in Part 4 of this book; this cleanse can improve the way in which the liver handles toxins.
- High LDL (so-called bad cholesterol), total cholesterol, or triglycerides can indicate fatty liver or fat-based overweight.
- Nutrient deficiencies can be determined by low albumen (protein), glucose (sugar), triglycerides (fat) and assay of individual minerals.

- Allergies – a five day rotation diet and other allergy tests. A low A/G ratio, high chloride, or high eosinophils (white blood cells) on a blood panel are other indications.

Other tests

- Urine pH, taken towards the end of the first urination of the morning after dawn, can indicate chemical or metal toxicity or low minerals if less than 5.5. Again, toxicity can cause water retention.
- Bowel tests for parasites. Their toxins can cause the retention of water to dilute them, as well as a number of other problems.

What should I do to correct for chemical and dietary causes of overweight?
Detoxify the body via detox diet, chelation to remove toxic metals from the body after they are removed from the teeth, sauna to eliminate chemicals, and colonics to clean sludge out of the digestive tract.

In the cases of food cravings and overeating, following the Detoxification diet in Part 4 can help to dramatically lessen cravings, and thus overeating and weight gain, in a number of ways:

- By eliminating most allergens, allergic addiction can be curbed.
- Nutrient deficiencies, such as low oils, are addressed, so cravings for unhealthy sources of these nutrients will ease.
- Yeast overgrowth is brought under control, lessening cravings for sweets and other carbohydrates. Aloe 7000 and other supplements can also help with the control of yeast.
- The psychological habits of eating certain (non)foods, such as the morning donut and coffee or the midnight snack, will be broken to a certain extent after eight days of eating in a different manner.

Once biological sources of your cravings are taken care of, the amount of willpower needed to resist such tempting foods may lessen to the point that, after as little as a few days, you simply don't have as much desire for them. A program of healthful eating becomes much easier to follow. Your appetite will change – really! Once you eliminate sugar, you will start to taste the natural sweetness of fruits and even vegetables. Get yeast under control and nutrients built up, and cravings will start to go. Once you are healthier, you may well find that you actually prefer the more healthful foods.

Chronic Fatigue, Fibromyalgia, and Chemical Sensitivity

Chronic fatigue syndrome (CFS), fibromyalgia syndrome (FMS), and multiple chemical sensitivity (MCS) are three ailments that are discussed together because they often occur together in various combinations. Brain fog, a feeling that you can't think clearly, concentrate, or remember, often occurs in tandem with these. These ailments are discussed in much more detail in a book on these subjects, written by the authors of this book.

Chronic fatigue

What are some of the most common causes of CFS?
Chemical overload is a common cause of CFS, along with metals, allergens, and microbes, although whiplash / bite problems and dental work are more likely causes.

Chemicals can be defined here and throughout this book as any substances that can be ingested, inhaled, or absorbed through skin contact, and that aren't something that the body needs or is designed to handle. This excludes clean air, clean water, and beneficial food, but can include pretty much anything else – pesticides, solvents, metals such as dental work, drugs, and more.

Dr. Dworkin, one of the authors of this and other books, developed a severe case of chronic fatigue in the early 1990s, accompanied by chemical sensitivity and brain fog. Her story is recounted in the Sauna Detoxification chapter. With Bachelor's and Master's degrees in Chemistry, she had spent years in laboratories in both school and work settings being exposed to solvents and other chemicals, as well as pesticides and paint at home, and dental mercury. She needed extensive detoxification before she got her life back.

Pesticides – Fatigue, brain fog, and forgetfulness are some of the most common symptoms of pesticide exposure.[1]

Breast implants – Chronic fatigue syndrome has been linked to silicone breast implants.[2] In a follow-up study of 50 consecutive silicone implant patients, 87% reported fatigue. The silicone can easily migrate into the body following a rupture or leak, both of which are common. Mold, present in all implants, can be another complicating factor if there is a leak and the mold enters the bloodstream.

Nearly any chemical overload can cause or contribute to chronic fatigue; the above are just a few specific examples.

What can be done about chemical overload?

The best way to deal with an overload of chemicals is to:

- First, identify and remove from one's immediate environment those chemicals, including mercury from metal dental fillings, that can be continually entering and overloading the body.
- A complete sauna detoxification program can help remove chemical triggers from the body. Other detoxification procedures such as colonics and lymphatic massage and exercises can also help. These are all discussed in Part 4.
- Support the body with nutrients as needed, including glutathione complex, sulfur aminos, cystine, NAC (n-acetylcysteine), molybdenum, and lymph support. Red root tea, which promotes lymphatic cleansing, along with omega-3 oils and Adva-Clear, are also useful.

To take the poetic approach:

Take out the bad stuff and put in the good,
The body can then work as it should.

This is simple…but not easy.

Drugs and medications

Drugs are often thought of as being the illegal mind-altering substances on the news, but for the purposes of their effect on the body the category is much broader. Drugs include:

- Illegal (street) drugs
- Alcohol
- Tobacco
- Caffeine
- Over-the-counter drugs
- Prescription drugs

Drugs are chemicals that, regardless of their beneficial or desired effects, the body has to clear out in addition to any other toxins. As with other chemicals, fatigue can result from drug use. Many drugs cause side effects similar to the symptoms of chronic fatigue.[3]

Excess sugar, for some, has drug-like effects, including addiction and increasing tolerance. Artificial sweeteners, although used as and in food, are more like drugs in their toxic effects.

A large percentage of adults with Chronic Fatigue Syndrome (about 80%) have a history of frequent and recurrent antibiotic treatment in childhood or teen years.[4] The antibiotics themselves, the yeast overgrowth that often results from their use, and the disruption of digestion from the destruction of beneficial bacteria can be the culprits.

Vaccination is also linked to Chronic Fatigue Syndrome in young adults.[5]

Metals

One can be exposed to metals in a number of ways, but one of the most common is through dental work, especially mercury fillings.

Fatigue associated with mercury toxicity can result from several of mercury's effects, including reducing adrenaline and neurotransmitter effects, reducing oxygen to tissues, and interfering with coenzyme A, which converts sugar to energy. In a study of 325 patients with fatigue[6], 310, or 95%, reported improvement in this symptom after removal of the fillings from the mouth and mercury from the body through chelation.

In addition to the direct toxicity, mercury can suppress necessary minerals such as potassium, calcium, magnesium, zinc, copper, and iron.

Nickel[7], found in stainless steel root canal posts as well as other sources such as PFM (porcelain fused to metal) crowns and bridges, is a potential cause of CFS. Nickel is toxic and allergenic, as well as carcinogenic (cancer causing), and the body's dealing with detoxification or immune response to a constant allergen can cause fatigue. We estimate that 33% of women and 17% of men have a nickel allergy. One way to determine a nickel allergy is soreness, itchiness, and swelling around the site of inexpensive (non-gold) earrings. Urinary tract infections, endometriosis, red receding gums, stomach and digestive problems, and stiff joints are also signs of nickel toxicity.

Heavy metal poisoning can cause daytime sleepiness.[8]

Testing can be done to determine whether metals are a significant problem. Provocative chelation, in which an IV chelating solution such as DMPS or DMSA binds to metals so they can be excreted in the urine, can be done to evaluate the presence of mercury, lead, aluminum, cadmium and other metals. Hair analysis can also be done, although it is not as effective in detecting mercury.

Urine pH testing, described in the Assessments chapter, can help detect metals indirectly. Optimal urine pH is around 6; a pH of less than 5.5 (acid) can be an indicator of metals or chemicals in the body, or low minerals.

If either testing or personal history of exposure indicates that metals are a major contributor to health problems, detoxification geared to metal removal from the body can be done, such as chelation, described in Part 4.

Microorganisms – Are you bugged?

There are six major types of microorganisms, any of which can cause fatigue. The six types are:

- Worms
- Fungi, mold, yeast
- Viruses
- Amoebas and protozoa
- Bacteria
- Mycoplasma

These are discussed in greater detail in the Microorganisms chapter in Part 3.

An overgrowth of any of these can cause or contribute to fatigue because they take nutrients and other resources that the body needs. In addition, they put off toxins as part of their life cycle that, like any other toxins, can overwhelm the body and cause fatigue.

In some cases of chronic fatigue, the fatigue comes on after a viral illness; you get sick and then don't get better. Other times the symptoms sometimes occur following apparent recovery from an acute viral infection or flu, and especially mononucleosis, caused by the Epstein-Barr virus.

Given that there are geographical clusters of CFS, some believe that CFS is infectious, although widespread exposure to a local toxin is also a possibility. Because CFS has so many causes, which can vary by person, it follows that only some, but not all, cases of CFS might be due to an infectious agent.

Yeast overgrowth is a common cause of, or at least contributor to, CFS.[4,9] Candida yeast and other fungi are most often secondary to mercury from dental fillings and other sources; the mercury kills the beneficial bacteria that help to keep the yeast under control, in an example of the upstream thinking discussed in the introduction. Yeast overgrowth can be secondary to overconsumption of large amounts of carbohydrates, especially sugar, which is yeast's food, or to low levels of beneficial bacteria which can be replaced through supplementation. Parasites and mercury need to be dealt with first, however, or the beneficial bacteria consumed will meet the same fate as the original bacteria. Antibiotic use, especially long-term, can upset the delicate balance of intestinal flora and cause yeast to overgrow.

Urine pH testing, described in the Assessments chapter, can help detect fungal overgrowth indirectly. Optimal urine pH is around 6; a pH of 6.5 or greater (alkaline) can be an indicator of fungal overgrowth in the body, although a high pH can also indicate bacteria, allergy, or fermentation. You can take a visual saliva test for fungus: spit into a clear glass of water and if it hangs down with root-appearing rhizoids, fungus can be indicated. Another visual test is to observe the tongue – if it has white or yellow patches, this can also indicate fungus.

A number of bacteria have been linked to CFS in some people, including klebsiella and helicobacter pylori. Lyme disease[10], caused by a spirochete bacteria carried by the tiny deer tick, can cause fatigue, especially if it is untreated. Lyme disease mimics a number of other ailments such as arthritis, and is notoriously difficult to diagnose.

Root canals

Although those who do root canals claim that harmful bacteria from the tooth are eliminated, research dating back to the 1930s[11] has found otherwise. Root canalled teeth are often a continuing source of bacterial infection in the body, which can be a major cause of or contributor to fatigue and related disorders. It is often best to extract an infected or root canalled tooth, sacrificing the tooth to save the body.

Food sensitivity and allergy

Allergy or sensitivity to foods and other substances can contribute significantly to fatigue. The drop in energy that can affect even those without CFS a couple of hours after lunch is often due to an allergic reaction. If a person is continually taking in something to which she is allergic, that drop in energy can be pretty much continuous.

In the case of allergy or sensitivity, the body is reacting to something that may be relatively harmless to most people. The body sees that substance as a toxin, and reacts accordingly, attacking the allergen as if it were a foreign invader, keeping the body in fight-or-flight stress mode.

The detoxification diet in this book, free of the most commonly allergenic foods such as dairy, wheat, corn products, soy, yeast, peanuts, tomatoes, sugar, citrus, vinegar, and additives, is a common recommendation for those with CFS. Improvement in symptoms can be noted to the degree that food reactions are that individual's cause of symptoms. It is important to break the allergy cycle with a four-day schedule of food rotation.

Food itself can be the problem, but so can what you eat it with (dental work) and what's eating it along with you (microbes).

How are other diseases tied to fatigue?

Many illnesses, both those caused by microorganisms and those caused by autoimmune dysfunction, have severe fatigue as a component. These diseases include iron-deficiency anemia and lupus[10], which is often associated with chemical toxicity. Multiple sclerosis (MS), which can itself have multiple causes, is also commonly accompanied by fatigue. Hypothyroidism, discussed in the Endocrine chapter, has fatigue as one of its major components

Fibromyalgia

What is fibromyalgia?

Fibromyalgia is a condition characterized by pain in the muscles, joints and tissues. The word fibromyalgia is not a disease diagnosis; rather, it is a restatement in Latin/Greek of the symptoms. "Fibro" refers to connective tissue, "my" refers to the muscles, and "algia" means pain.

Fibromyalgia differs from most types of pain in that the pain doesn't have an obvious organic cause, such as an injury or organic illness. This complicates the task of finding an obvious starting point for treatment. The diagnosis of fibromyalgia is only a starting point, however. It is still necessary to know what, in a particular individual's case, is the cause(s).

What are the causes of fibromyalgia?

The triggers, as with nearly any chronic illness, are typically additive and cumulative. Reducing the total body burden can help eliminate the underlying cause. Keeping track of your activities, toxic exposure and diet and how they correlate with worsening or improvement in the pain can help to pinpoint possible individual causes. You can then take measures to avoid the offending substances or activities.

Toxic triggers can include

- Chemicals and heavy metals
- Allergies
- Dental problems and dental work (mercury, nickel, root canals)
- Microbes

Other triggers can include:

- Structural problems such as whiplash, bite (e.g. high crowns), or concussion
- Deficiencies of minerals, oils, exercise, oxygen, sleep, or water
- Regulators such as hormones, metabolic enzymes, and neurotransmitters
- Stress

Although structural problems like whiplash and bite balance are often at the base of fibromyalgia, discussion of these is beyond the scope of this book.

How do chemicals and other stressors do their damage?

Toxins can cause poor blood or lymph circulation, or clumping of blood, which is visible under the microscope. This clumping reduces the oxygen to the muscles and tissues, causing aching similar to that experienced by runners who push themselves too far due to accumulation of lactic acid in the muscles.

Toxins include, but are not limited to:

- Formaldehyde from glues in home furnishings, carpet, and cabinets
- Solvents and other chemicals
- Perfume
- Pesticides
- Diesel fumes
- Heavy metals
- Mold and microbial waste
- Radiation and EMF

What are some of the most common allergies, and how do they cause pain?
Allergies such as nickel, foods, molds and airborne allergens can cause tightening of the meningeal mediated system, which can affect the head, neck and back. Meningeal contraction is felt as head pressure or tightness in neck and trapezius (between shoulder and neck) muscles. Such contraction is felt as pain in many people.

What about the role of microorganisms?
An overgrowth of any of the six types of microorganisms can cause or contribute to pain, as they take nutrients and other resources that the body needs, plus they put off toxins as part of their life cycle that, like any other toxins, can overwhelm the body and cause pain. Pain can either be caused directly or in the form of rheumatoid arthritis or other diseases.

Because fibromyalgia patients often have flu-like feelings, and because fibromyalgia symptoms often follow a bad cold or flu, an immune-suppressing infection, possibly viral such as the various herpes infections, may be involved in some cases. A dental abscess or infection, including that from root-canalled teeth, can also cause flu-like feelings that then lead to fibromyalgia. The immune response to infection can cause symptoms similar to those of the flu – backaches, overall achiness, skin hypersensitivity.

Fibromyalgia patients may suffer from an intestinal overgrowth of Candida yeast due to overuse of antibiotics and other drugs. Dr. Teitelbaum, who is known for his work with fibromyalgia, has a protocol for fibromyalgia that includes antifungal treatment, which has proven effective in clinical trials with fibromyalgia patients.[12]

Silicone breast implants

Fibromyalgia has been linked to the use of silicone breast implants.[13] In a follow-up study of 50 consecutive silicone implant patients, 75% reported overall joint and muscle stiffness. In a study reported in the ***FDA Consumer***, women with silicone gel that had migrated outside the fibrous scar around the breast implant were nearly three times more likely to report that they had been diagnosed with fibromyalgia or other connective tissue disease than women without extracapsular silicone gel.[14] Fungus, one of the causes of fibromyalgia, can grow in implants, and enter the body if the implants rupture, or even if they don't.

> **Patient profile**
> Jenny, a patient, had breast cancer and she had implants put in during reconstructive surgery. She was having severe pain, mostly in her back, arms, and neck, and fatigue. The breast implants had suppressed her immune system, leading to autoimmune problems and dental infections. The breast implants were removed, along with her root canalled teeth, and the dental infections cleared up. She then underwent sauna detoxification and structural realignment to allow her lymph glands to drain properly, and had physical therapy on her frozen shoulder that resulted from the shoulder pain. She had been on strong painkillers, which further suppressed her immune system and hindered detoxification and made her sicker; her health improved as she was able to stop taking the medication.

What are some other correlations?
Aching and stiffness in joints and muscles, especially of the hands and feet, is a symptom of hypothyroidism. This aching and stiffness can be severe enough to be mistaken for arthritis or fibromyalgia.[15]

Multiple chemical sensitivity

What is Multiple Chemical Sensitivity?
Multiple Chemical Sensitivity (MCS), also called Environmental Illness (EI), is an immune system disorder characterized by heightened reactivity to many different chemicals, usually by inhalation. The term Universal Reactor is also used for a more severe case in which the person appears to react to almost everything. A National Academy of Sciences workshop estimated that 15% of the U.S. population are chemically sensitive to some degree.[16] Many of the chemicals that the person is sensitive to would be toxic to anyone, but someone with EI would have a more immediate and severe reaction and/or would react to a much smaller amount than would affect the average person. EI can dramatically limit the lifestyle of the person who has it.

What does the experience of MCS feel like?
Symptoms can be roughly broken down into acute or chronic. Acute symptoms are easily recognizable and come on almost immediately after exposure to the chemical. Because of the rapidity and distinctness of the symptoms, the chemical(s) responsible are usually fairly easy to determine. Symptoms can include[17]:

- Seizures
- Asthmatic attacks
- Headache
- Nausea

- Flu-like symptoms
- Difficulty sleeping
- Loss of balance
- Gastrointestinal problems
- Irritated eyes, nose, or throat
- Panic attacks
- Rapid or irregular heartbeat, shortness of breath, chest pain
- Abrupt drop in blood pressure, which can cause fainting
- Fatigue, which may come on suddenly
- Hypersensitivity to odors
- Confusion, memory loss, and brain fog that come on suddenly
- Fear of any new assault or stress – an "I can't handle one more thing" feeling
- Emotional reactions, including sudden tears, anxiety, anger, or a feeling of being trapped

Some people just know they're reacting but are hard-pressed to describe specific symptoms.

The causes of chronic symptoms are usually more difficult to pin down. Such symptoms are usually more vague, and may not come on immediately after exposure, so the sufferer may not even realize that s/he is chemically sensitive, much less the particular chemical(s) involved.

Who is most likely to develop MCS?
People who are most likely to develop MCS are those who have the greatest occupational or other chemical exposure, including:

- Chemists
- Industrial workers
- Those living near toxic waste sites
- People who work in sealed buildings, especially new buildings
- People who have moved into an all-new house
- Artists working with toxic media such as paints and metals

How does Multiple Chemical Sensitivity start?
MCS/EI usually starts when the body's detoxification pathways are overwhelmed by more chemicals and other burdens (emotional, structural, parasites such as helicobacter or other bacteria, or mold, for example) than it can handle. For some people the precipitating event is a single massive exposure, such as an industrial accident (rare), having one's house sprayed for termites or other bugs (quite common), living near a golf course (heavily sprayed with pesticides), or in an area with aerial spraying. With other people, the exposure is so prolonged and so subtle that they find it difficult to pinpoint a *year* of disease onset. Gallbladder problems brought on by helicobacter, giardia or fungus, which themselves can be set up by mercury dental fillings among other causes, can set the stage for intolerance to oil-soluble chemicals by leaving you so oil-deficient

that your cells start soaking up oil-based chemicals like a sponge. Mercury from metal fillings can overload the metal detox pathways, allowing metals to build up in the body.

60 percent of all MCS patients are able to identify the specific exposure that set off their initial reaction.[18] This can be, for example, spraying for insects, or a chemical spill at work.

So where is the problem, and what can I do about it?

Chemicals – Formaldehyde and general chemical overload are common triggers. Chemicals from plastic food containers or plastic wrap can set off symptoms in those with chemical sensitivities.[19] Patients exposed to pesticides have been reported to have more severe symptoms than those exposed to chemicals during a building remodeling.[20]

Fungus – Those who are chemically sensitive may have yeast overgrowth as a root cause; the chemicals triggering the symptoms may just be the trigger, not the cause itself. Mold and mildew in the home often worsen symptoms in a person with MCS.

Other root causes include gluten intolerance, microbes, and dental work.

What can be done?

The first step is to identify the chemicals involved. Keep a diary of exposures and reactions. Then reduce or eliminate exposure to the greatest extent possible. Elimination of other toxic suppressors can also help reduce chemical sensitivity by reducing the total body load.

Those with MCS have usually reduced their chemical exposure as much as they can, since there is a strong correlation between exposure and symptoms. However, chemical sources are often overlooked due to lack of information. Part 3 of this book discusses the many sources of toxic chemicals, including chemicals and sources with which many people may be unfamiliar, such as cologne and building materials.

Some of these detoxification modalities – most of which are discussed in Part 4 – include:

- Sauna for chemicals and metals
- Lymphatic massage and tissue cleansing exercises, in combination with colonics
- Colonics to help carry out the toxins
- Removal of mercury, nickel, and root canals
- Chelation to remove metals
- Gallbladder flush to remove gallstones and sludge and to break down oils
- Detoxification diet
- Acupuncture to help rebalance the body
- Homeopathics

- NAET allergy testing and treatment to identify and eliminate chemical allergies
- Adjusting bite and whiplash injuries

Sauna is one of the most helpful techniques for removing an overload of chemicals from the body.

A powerful argument for the efficacy of avoidance and detoxification is the large number of people who have eliminated or lessened their MCS symptoms following extensive detoxification.

The most difficult patients

Clearing the chemicals from the body is simple in concept but not easy. Detoxification is a two-step process: first the chemicals must be removed from their storage depots in fat, muscle, lymph, liver, kidneys, and elsewhere. During this stage the chemicals are dumped into the bloodstream. In the second stage, the chemicals in the bloodstream are removed via sauna, colonics, chelation, and other modalities. The chemicals in the bloodstream from detoxification can cause reactions just as if increased levels of chemicals were in the bloodstream from outside exposure. For this reason, detoxification typically causes symptoms to worsen before improving. Bear with the discomfort, however; relief usually follows. Keeping electrolytes (minerals) up while detoxing is crucial, as unbalanced minerals can cause one to feel worse. Because many MCS patients are already at their limits as far as what they can handle, and detoxification temporarily, and ultimately beneficially, raises the level of chemicals in the bloodstream, detoxing for MCS should best be done with professional supervision.

What are some important food and nutritional considerations?

It is crucial that food be as pure and additive-free as possible to reduce exposure to food-related chemicals. Organic foods should be used when possible. Water should be filtered by a reliable method such as reverse osmosis.

The detoxification diet, followed by a rotational diet – both discussed in Part 4 – can help lessen food allergens. A detoxification diet eliminates the most common allergens, including dairy, corn, wheat, soy, nuts (especially peanuts), sugar, and others. In a rotational diet, no food is eaten more than once every four days in order to give the body an opportunity to clear it out before re-exposure; this reduces allergic reactions.

Patients with MCS are known to have a higher likelihood of nutritional imbalances[21] despite oral supplementation. Intravenous (IV) infusions of certain vitamins and minerals (especially vitamin C and the B vitamins, magnesium, and trace minerals) can be beneficial.[22]

Nutrients, discussed in Part 5, that are most likely to be helpful for MCS include those that do the following:

- Help the body to eliminate toxins
- Help the liver detoxify chemicals to the greatest extent possible
- Support the kidneys in eliminating the toxins
- Support the immune system
- Increase sweating, and the elimination of toxins via sweating, with ginger and niacin
- Support the body's health in general

It is important to obtain nutritional supplements from a reputable company, and to avoid any artificial colors, flavors, fillers, and preservatives, to which a person with MCS might be sensitive. Such sources are listed at the end of Part 5.

Healthy oils – omega-3, omega-6, and lecithin – help carry out and eliminate oil-soluble toxins such as solvents and pesticides.

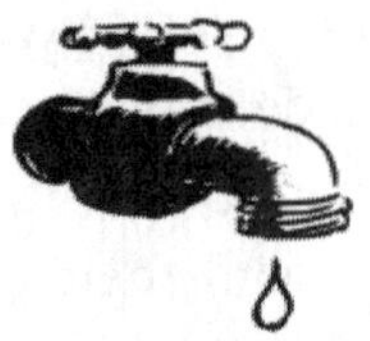

Water hydrates the body systems for optimal function. In addition, water helps to carry out water-soluble toxins for elimination in the urine.

Sulfur-containing amino acids such as glutathione, N-acetylcysteine, and methionine help in detoxification. When taurine is low, extreme sensitivities to chemicals can develop, especially to chlorine, aldehydes, alcohols, solvents and ammonia.[23]

How can exercise help?

Exercise can, among other benefits, help to remove toxins from the fat, muscles, and the lymphatic system. Exercise works the lymphatic system to remove toxins from that system; lymph nodes are concentrated in areas that are most affected by movement such as the armpits and behind the knees. Lymphatic exercises are covered in Part 4.

Part 3
Suppressors

General Information about Toxins

Why is the avoidance of new toxins so important?
The previous book section discusses many examples of the ailments that can be caused by chemicals, and the next section discusses detoxification. This section discusses the importance of recognizing and eliminating specific chemical toxins.

As discussed in the Introduction, it is vital to eliminate the influx of new toxins as well as detoxifying from the ones that exist in your body. If this is not done, it would be like draining the tub while the faucet is running – after all the work of detoxification you may well end up no less toxic, and no healthier, than before.

However, so many of us are not fully aware of the toxicity of the products that we use; some of them, such as cologne, medications, fluoridated water, and some furniture, may come as a surprise. The chapters in this section cover the three aspects of eliminating new toxins:

- Recognizing how important it is to do so
- Recognizing and identifying the sources of toxins
- Learning how to avoid these toxins, and what substitutions can be made

Clean and green
There has been much in the news lately about global warming and environmental issues, and a consequent trend in "green" living. Large numbers of books, magazine articles, TV shows, and Internet websites are available on the subject. Awareness has been and is being raised, and alternatives are given. Happily for our purposes, the measures that are best for the planet are, for the most part, the measures that are best for our bodies and our health as well. Air and water pollution, for example, are harmful to both the planet and to us, and anything that raises awareness and promotes cleaner water and air is good for all of us, collectively and as individuals.

Such books, programs, and articles contain much useful information that could be used to help to reduce the influx of new toxins into our bodies; such sources should be utilized where possible in addition to using the information in this book.

How do chemicals cause problems in the body? What makes toxins toxic?
Chemicals can affect the body in different ways. Some chemicals are necessary in order to maintain the many bodily functions, and are needed in specific amounts. However, poisonous chemicals are toxic because they disrupt the proper functioning of the body. They do this by:

- **Damaging** the cells directly, like asbestos, which is formed of microscopic spikes – think of a dog's nose full of porcupine quills.
- **Interfering** in one or more of the complex biochemical processes that keep the body going.
- **Substituting** for a necessary substance, such as cadmium in tobacco smoke replacing necessary zinc.
- Adversely **affecting** the body's **filters** which help to cleanse the body: the liver, kidneys, lungs, and lymph.

What determines how chemicals affect us?
Many things influence the way chemicals affect a particular person.

- Some chemicals target a particular organ, system, or type of cell, such as kidneys or nervous system.
- Other effects are determined by individual genetic "weak links" in each person; for example, a tendency towards cystic fibrosis or cerebral palsy.
- One way in which chemicals do their damage is by exerting a specific effect, such as central nervous system depression or anoxia (lack of oxygen to tissues).
- Other toxic effects are caused by the interruption of one of the many thousands of biochemical processes in the body.

What are the two primary types of chemical exposure?
It is important to understand the difference between the two types of chemical exposure:

- **Acute** exposure is a one-time event in which the body is exposed all at once to more of a chemical than it can handle. With acute exposure, both the symptoms – including death – and the cause are usually readily apparent. Some examples of acute exposure are chemical burns, drug overdose, and food poisoning
- **Chronic** exposure occurs when a person is exposed to a toxin in small quantities over a long period of time, in a total amount greater than the amount the body can eliminate over time. Effects are cumulative and additive, and tend to worsen if the cause is not eliminated. The previous book section gives many

examples of the diseases and symptoms that can be caused by chronic exposure to various chemicals.

Why is it sometimes hard to track down the cause of chemical toxicity?

With chronic exposure, it usually takes some detective work to find the cause. Even the symptoms may not be initially obvious; you may just feel "off." Your symptoms may be due to exposure to more than one chemical, or to causes other than chemical exposure.

To further confuse matters, symptoms fluctuate in type and severity because the total body burden is in a state of constant flux. You will probably be more severely affected when the total body burden of stressors is highest. It may take careful observation over a period of time to figure out what is really going on. The Assessment chapter in Part 1 gives ways in which chemical overload and type of toxins can be determined.

What makes some chemicals more toxic than others?

A number of factors influence toxicity, in addition to whether the exposure is acute or chronic. The type of chemical dictates what parts of the body will be affected and how severely. Other factors are:

- The dose – how much and over how long a period of time
- The body's ability to process and excrete the toxin
- Individual susceptibility, genetics
- Potency – how toxic the chemical is
- Route of entry into body – inhalation, ingestion (swallowing), or topical (skin)

How does the body prepare poisons for excretion?

Once a chemical is in the body it is metabolized, or broken down, into byproducts. Detoxification systems within the body such as cytochrome P450 and the sulfur-containing compounds glutathione and metallothionein aid in this process, which is necessary for eventual elimination of the toxic substances. The organs and pathways of elimination are discussed in the beginning of Part 4.

How is nutrition involved?

Nutrition plays an important role in the effectiveness of these systems. Like any other systems in the body, the detoxification systems work best with the right kind of food, just as your car runs best with the right kind of fuel. General nutrition guidelines can be found in many sources, including ***Thriving in a Toxic World***, written by this book's authors. Nutritional and other supporters specific to detoxification are covered in Part 5 of this book.

The subjects of the following chapters

A great many types of chemicals can cause harm when one is exposed to them. Many of these listed can be found in the home, and thus you have considerable control over their use.

A lot of the information in the chapters in this section is taken from, and is covered in much greater detail in ***Surviving the Toxic Crisis***, written by the authors of this book.

Pesticides

What are pesticides?

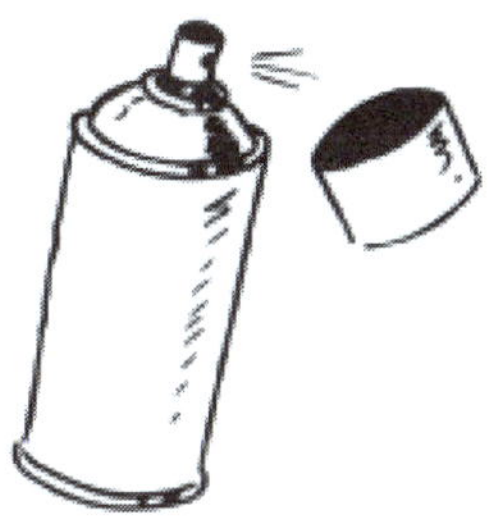

The category of pesticides includes insecticides, rodenticides, fungicides, herbicides, and repellents. The suffix "-cide" means "to kill," as in "homicide." These pesticides work by damaging the cells of the target animal, insect, or plant. However, they can also damage our cells and penetrate our nervous systems. There is not much difference between our cells and tissues and those of members of the animal kingdom, and to some extent even the plant kingdom.

What is the difference between humans and bugs?

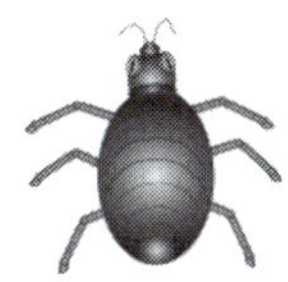

Pesticides are toxic to both bugs and people. People, who are warm blooded, have fat in their bodies for insulation, and, since pesticides are oil soluble, they are stored in our fat. Bugs are cold blooded and have no fat in their bodies, and so the pesticide attacks their nervous systems directly. The effect on bugs is acute, or short term. The effect on people is chronic, or long term, unless there is a large single exposure, because the pesticide is stored in our fat and elsewhere in our bodies and released slowly rather than affecting us all at once. However, when our fat is loaded with toxins, we lose this advantage.

Some people are oil deficient, so this causes them to react more like a bug, i.e. suffer from more severe (acute) symptoms. Even an overweight person can be oil deficient. Oil deficiency can result from an insufficient intake of beneficial oils, and also from gallbladder problems, since the gallbladder digests and processes oils. Parasites such as giardia, which themselves may be secondary to mercury amalgam fillings due to the antibiotic (killing) action of mercury on the beneficial bacteria which protect us from parasites, can also cause gallbladder problems.

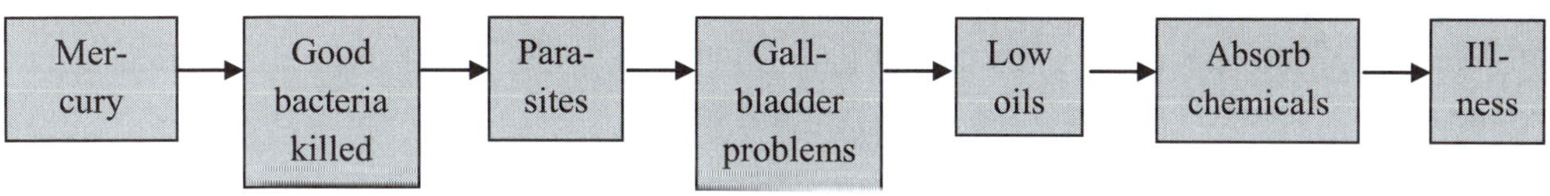

How can people be exposed to pesticides?

People can be exposed to pesticides in a number of ways.

- Inhaling sprayed pesticides
- Eating produce and grains that have been sprayed
- Drinking water contaminated by runoff from sprayed fields.
- Eating meat and poultry which have been fed pesticide-sprayed grain

A large number of patients at the Center for Advanced Medicine have pesticide exposure, whether recent or decades past, at the root of their health problems:

Patient profiles

Ron, a lawyer in his early 40s, who lived in an agricultural, produce growing area that used pesticide sprays, developed kidney and liver problems.

Another patient, an interior decorator in her 50s, lived in the agricultural San Joaquin Valley. She developed a number of symptoms which kept her from working, including brain fog, fibromyalgia (whole body pain) and fatigue. Diesel fumes, pesticides and perfumes brought on headaches. After sauna and other detoxification procedures, she recovered.

A number of people came into the clinic with health problems following Malathion spraying in California. One of these, a female top athlete with low body fat, came in with brain fog and low energy related to pesticide exposure. Her low body fat may have worsened her symptoms, since body fat acts as a buffer.

How long are pesticides toxic?

Pesticides are long-lived and fat-soluble, so they can remain in the soil and in our bodies for decades, leaching out slowly and causing chronic damage. Release of these fat stored chemicals could explain why some people get sick when they lose weight. The fat acts as storage barrels for toxic waste, and when the fat/ storage barrel is removed, the toxins enter the body systems via the bloodstream, causing symptoms.

It is not uncommon for a person undergoing sauna therapy to release pesticides and other organic chemicals in their sweat to such an extent that a person nearby can smell the chemicals. This can happen even if the initial exposure was years or decades ago.

What are some of the effects of chronic pesticide exposure?

Pesticide exposure can cause a number of harmful effects, which are discussed in greater detail in the relevant chapters in Part 2.

- **Fatigue and forgetfulness** are common symptoms of pesticide exposure.
- **Carcinogenicity** – The cancer-causing potential of pesticides is further discussed in the chapter on Cancer.
- **Central nervous system** (CNS) effects include headaches, dizziness, loss of motor control, learning disabilities, and behavioral disorders.
- **Skin problems** of various types, which makes sense since the body tries to eliminate these toxins through the skin.
- **Gastrointestinal** symptoms such as nausea, appetite loss, abdominal pains, and excessive salivation.

- **Pancreas** effects – Pancreatitis (pancreas inflammation) and diabetes have been linked to pesticide exposure.[1]
- **Liver** effects – jaundice, fatty liver, necrosis (cell death), and increased susceptibility to viral hepatitis.
- **Kidney** effects – albumin or protein in urine, which can be detected during a routine urinalysis; tubular necrosis, which is tissue death of the toxin-filtering tubules in the kidneys.
- **Endocrine/Reproductive** – Pesticides and herbicides, being pseudo-estrogenic, are associated with disruption in endocrine, reproductive and sexual function.[2]
- **Respiratory** effects – pulmonary edema, chest tightness, bronchial constriction or spasm, wheezing, or cough.
- **Muscle weakness**

Some of these effects, especially nerve damage, are irreversible, as stated in a medical journal article as early as 1958[3], yet pesticide use continues.

Are ingredients labeled "inert" on the pesticide label safe?
A warning when label reading – ingredients are listed as active or inert. Active ingredients are those which have the effect suggested by the label; in the case of pesticides, they kill pests. Inert ingredients are those that do not kill pests, but the name is misleading in that they are not necessarily inert in the body. Some of them may in fact be more toxic than the "active" ingredients.

Don't herbicides only harm plants?
Herbicides are formulated to kill plants. However, there is reason to believe that they are not harmless to humans, despite what their manufacturers want you to believe.

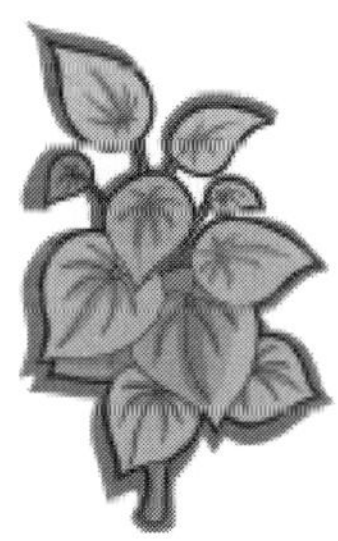

Most plants have chlorophyll, which give them their green color. Humans and other mammals have hemoglobin in their blood, which gives it a red color and is involved in oxygen transport. The chemical structures of chlorophyll and hemoglobin are startlingly similar, consisting in both cases of a structure called a porphyrin ring with a single metal atom in the middle which gives the substance its characteristic color – iron in the case of hemoglobin and magnesium in the case of chlorophyll.

When a plant is sprayed with an herbicide, it goes from a healthy green color to a sickly brown color. Since hemoglobin is so chemically similar to plant chlorophyll, it seems reasonable that herbicides can also damage our hemoglobin, and thus adversely affect oxygen transport to our tissues. Lowered oxygen to the tissues and brain can lead to fatigue and impairment of mental function, depression and anxiety .

What are some alternatives to chemical pesticides?

Now you have plenty of good reasons to avoid chemical pesticides. However, pests happen, so what do you do now? Alternatives to petrochemical and toxic pesticides include[4-6]:

- Plants such as marigolds repel certain harmful insect species. Chrysanthemums are another plant that can repel and even kill insects. Pesticides made from chrysanthemums are called pyrethrins, and are less toxic than commercial pesticides.
- Helpful insects such as ladybugs which eat aphids, and praying mantises, can be obtained from stores that supply organic gardeners.
- An invasion of ants in the house can be controlled by keeping food where they can't get at it. If they find it, they touch feelers to communicate with the rest of the nest that there is a party going on at your house.

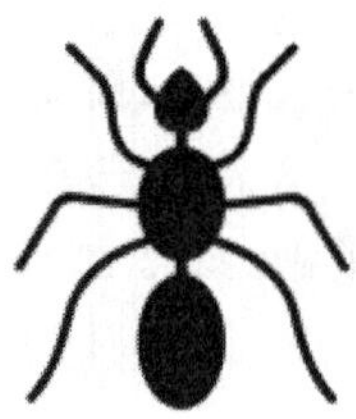

- If ants still get out of hand, they can be vacuumed up using the crevice tool on a vacuum cleaner.
- Boric acid, a granular white solid often sold as a laundry cleaner, repels many bugs. It is not entirely nontoxic, but is safer than most insecticides.
- Daily thorough vacuuming helps to keep the flea population down.
- Brewer's yeast and B vitamins fed to your pets will make them less attractive to fleas.
- Another method which is sometimes successful against certain pests is heat. Close all windows, remove pets and plants, plan to stay elsewhere for a few days, and crank up every safe source of heat you have.
- Some companies now use liquid nitrogen, which is much colder than your household freezer, to freeze a wide variety of pests, as well as starving them of oxygen.
- Some companies now use microwaves to kill or repel household pests. As long as you and your pets are not present for the treatment, there is no residual adverse effect.
- Tobacco water, made by soaking cigarette or pipe tobacco in water, can be used to water plants to kill some insects that infest plants. It makes sense that

tobacco is harmful to both ourselves and insects, since cellularly we have a lot in common.

- Rubbing alcohol can be wiped, or detergent solution can be sprayed, on plant leaves to kill plant pests.

Attitude adjustment

Another solution is to look at pests in a different way. If all else fails when you, for example, have ants in the kitchen, and it looks like a spray can of commercial pesticide is the only way to go, there's another possibility: just live with the ants. That would be the lesser of two evils, and requires only an attitude adjustment.

How can the right type of fertilizer discourage plant pests?

It is helpful to fertilize plants using natural materials. Just as our bodies are stronger on natural and healthful foods, so do plants respond better with natural fertilizers such as manure and compost. Considering experiments with natural vs. artificial fertilizers, it seems that plants produce their own natural bug and disease repellent when fed as intended, and then toxic pesticides are not needed.

Solvents

What are solvents?

Solvents are used to dissolve chemicals that do not dissolve in water, although water is technically a solvent. The solvents discussed here are typically used to keep chemicals such as paints, glues, and laminates in liquid form until they are applied where desired and the solvent is allowed to evaporate. Alternatively, they are used directly as a solvent as in paint thinner or remover, or a degreaser. While evaporating – which can take minutes, months, or anywhere in between – the solvent is in the air and can be inhaled and cause health problems.

These solvents can also be taken into the body by absorption through the skin, and sometimes by drinking contaminated water.

Solvents are oil-soluble and thus can be stored in fatty tissue, to be released into the bloodstream over time or when the fat is unable to hold any more. They are particularly attracted to individuals who do not take in sufficient dietary oils, or who have gallbladder problems since the gallbladder helps to process oils, in the way that a dry sponge is more likely to attract water.

Industrial solvents are intended to be solvents of fats, or degreasers. In the body, they are especially attracted to the fatty sheaths of nerve fibers and the lipid (fatty) membranes of cells. Nerve fibers conduct impulses from the brain to the muscles like electric cord wires. The myelin sheath acts like the outer insulation of an electrical cord. The erosion of the myelin sheath is like the fraying of an electrical cord, and nerve impulses can dissipate by shorting into nearby tissue rather than speeding up and reaching their destination. The partial dissolving of these nerve fiber sheaths leads to nervous system effects such as:

- Memory loss, difficulty concentrating, altered personality
- Impaired dexterity, reduced motor function
- Multiple sclerosis (MS)

What other problems do solvents cause?

Other solvent effects, discussed in greater detail in the applicable chapters in Part 2, include:

- **Carcinogenicity** – Many solvents are linked to the development of cancer, since they can penetrate the lipid (fat) membrane around the cells and damage the DNA (blueprint for reproduction).

- **Skin irritations** due to skin contact with liquid or vapor are caused by removal of oil from the skin.

- **Liver** – The liver is damaged by chloroform, ethanol (beverage alcohol, also a solvent), and other alcohols. Cirrhosis (drying, scarring, and hardening) of the liver is a well-known effect of chronic alcoholism for this reason. Alcohol also increases liver damage from other solvents.

- **Immune system** – Solvents suppress lymphocyte (white blood cell) function, adversely affecting the body's ability to fight off disease organisms.
- **Cardiac effects** – Certain solvents and related compounds can cause cardiac arrhythmias (irregular heartbeat).

What is one of the worst and most prevalent solvents?

Formaldehyde is one of the most common solvents, and is one of the most likely to cause health problems, in part because it is found in so many places. It is used primarily as a bonding material, but it has many diverse uses. Products that it can be found in include[1]:

- Paints
- Nail polish
- Glues
- Fuels
- Plastics
- Particle board, paneling, plywood
- Pesticides
- Air fresheners
- Textiles
- Cosmetics
- Mattresses, couches, cushions
- Cleaning supplies
- Foam insulation
- Tobacco smoke
- Carpeting, carpet pads

Although formaldehyde can be found in high levels even in an unfurnished home, especially if new, one study showed that the addition of furniture to an otherwise empty house tripled formaldehyde levels.[2] Formaldehyde and other chemicals found in carpeting have been found in tests to kill mice that are kept in newly carpeted cages. Babies that crawl around on carpet, especially new carpet, can absorb considerable amounts of these chemicals due to the closeness of their nose and mouth to the carpet, and also due to the comparatively large amount of skin contact with the carpet.

Formaldehyde, also used as embalming fluid, suffocates the cells, or prevents oxygen from reaching them, so they don't decay. This is good for preserving a corpse, but bad for preserving your health.

Health effects from chronic exposure to formaldehyde include[3,4]:

- Headaches
- Fatigue
- Arthritis
- Depression
- Nausea
- Cancer, especially lung, pharynx, nose sinus, kidney, and brain[5]
- Immune system suppression
- Chronic cough, asthma
- Brain fog, inability to concentrate
- Chemical and food sensitivities
- Eye, nose, and throat irritation, burning

Much of this discussion of formaldehyde applies to other solvents and chemicals as well.

What are some other solvents to watch out for?

- **Methyl chloride**, used in rubber and plastics, can cause nerve damage in the hands and feet, blurred vision, and short-term memory loss.
- **Acetone**, a common solvent used in nail polish remover, can cause vertigo (dizziness) and weakness.
- **Methylene chloride**, a solvent with multiple uses including decaffeinating coffee, can cause delusions and hallucinations.
- **Alcohols and glycols** such as antifreeze can kill pets that are attracted to the sweet tasting antifreeze and lick it from the driveway or road; children may also be attracted by the sweet taste and such poisonings are not uncommon.
- **Benzene**, a toxic chemical, can be formed by the reaction of the preservative sodium benzoate and ascorbic acid (vitamin C), a combination that is found in some sodas and other products.

BPA, short for bisphenol A, is a chemical used to harden plastics. An article in ***JAMA*** published in Sept. 2008 discussed a study involving 1455 American adults which linked high urinary BPA levels to heart disease, type 2 diabetes, and liver problems. Heat causes the chemical to leach into food, so to be safe, do not heat plastic containers in the microwave or put hot food or drinks into them.[6]

What can be done to avoid or minimize solvent exposure?

Solvents have a characteristic smell, although there are many variations on the exact smell. Most people, once they have been made aware, are able to notice that there is a smell in the air that should be avoided. Keep in mind that if you can smell something, that is because you are breathing in molecules of it, to the detriment of your health in the case of solvents. Knowing the likely sources of the solvent should help increase awareness of risk.

Since the goal is to avoid, to the greatest extent possible, the inhalation of solvents, it is best to avoid exposure whenever possible by avoiding the sources. To this end, find less harmful sources of building and remodeling materials – the publicity and awareness surrounding green building can provide considerable useful information. Paints are available that are low-VOC (volatile organic compounds), which should be used when painting, along with plentiful ventilation. Bamboo rather than particle board can be used for cabinets and floors, and tile or natural wood are healthier alternatives than carpet for flooring. An air filter or cleaner can help to detoxify solvents and other chemicals in the air.

Sauna detoxification, discussed in Part 4, is one of the best treatment modalities for removing solvents from the body.

Air Pollution

Air pollution is defined as anything in the air other than oxygen, nitrogen, and naturally occurring gases. These pollutants can be

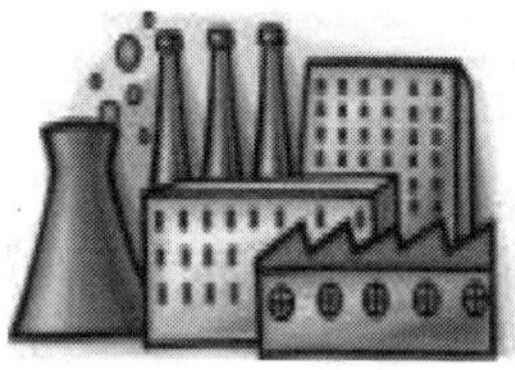

- Fine solids (particulates) like soot
- Organics such as pesticides or solvents
- Corrosives such as in acid rain
- Radioactive matter
- Excess carbon dioxide, in the news as a cause of global warming

Air pollution sources can be either

- Primary, directly from sources, such as carbon monoxide or sulfur dioxide
- Secondary, from reactions of primary pollutants with other atmospheric components and pollutants; examples are sulfates and ozone

Is all air pollution outdoors?
One most often thinks of the smog or ozone layer when air pollution is mentioned; however, not all air pollution is outside. The air indoors is often more toxic than the air outdoors. This is especially true in newer, tightly sealed buildings which seal in the pollutants generated indoors. However, old buildings have their dangers, especially mold and mildew spores, and chemicals and materials such as asbestos insulation and lead paint which are banned from use in newer construction. Most of the focus of this chapter is on indoor air pollution, since more can be done to correct and avoid sources of such pollution.

Most people in industrialized countries spend nearly all of their time indoors. The term "indoors" refers to any enclosed space, including homes, vehicles, workplaces, offices, and stores.

Patient profile
In one case a whole family got sick from formaldehyde exposure in a new house. The child had rashes and inability to concentrate. The mother and child underwent sauna detoxification, eliminating the child's rashes and problems studying.

What are some types of indoor air pollutants?
Types of indoor air pollutants include:

- **Formaldehyde** from urea-formaldehyde foam insulation, plywood, hardwood paneling, carpet, and fabric, discussed in the previous chapter on Solvents. Emission of formaldehyde is at its worst when the building is tightly sealed, when the product is new, and when the air is humid.

- **Aerosol spray products** – cleaners, hairspray, deodorants, paints, and insecticides
- **Air "fresheners,"** an ironic name, work by covering up one odor with another chemically created one, by coating the nasal passages with an undetectable film of oil, or by chemically deadening the nerves in your nose which are odor receptors.[1] They don't actually eliminate or neutralize the chemicals causing the odors.
- **Microbes and mold spores** in the air come from breathing, air ducts, humidifiers and dehumidifiers, vacuum cleaner exhaust, and human and animal skin scales.
- **Asbestos**, consisting of tiny sharp particles which pierce lung cells and can cause irreversible lung disease, is found in insulation of old buildings and appliances, building tiles, roofing shingles, and brake linings in cars.
- **Carbon dioxide** (CO_2) is a metabolic waste product that can accumulate in the air of a crowded, poorly ventilated building. It is not very toxic in itself, but a person who is breathing more CO_2 is getting proportionately less oxygen, and is likely to be sleepy and think less clearly.
- **House dust** varies greatly in composition according to location (urban, rural, near road) and indoor activities. It can contain animal hair and scales, aerosol spray components, dust mites, mold spores, and other pollutants.
- **Cooking gas** and carbon monoxide (CO) from furnaces and water heaters can rob the body of oxygen. Some patients are so sensitive to cooking gas that they need to switch to electric appliances in order to get their health back.
- **Colognes** and other scented products, discussed in a later chapter, contain many harmful chemicals which enter the body of anyone who wears or smells them.
- Many **cleaning products** are toxic. A 15-year study in Oregon showed that women who stayed at home during the day had a 54% higher cancer death rate than women who worked outside the home. The study suggests that chemicals in household products might be a causative factor.[1]

Patient profile

One patient who did domestic work, a woman in her late 50s, got sick from her cleaning products. She started getting better after she switched to less toxic products in addition to doing sauna detoxification, taking glutathione (an oral chelator), and being on a good supplementation program for support, as well as other treatments.

What are some symptoms of air pollution exposure?

Symptoms of chronic pollution exposure depend on the pollutant and individual sensitivity, but some general symptoms include:

- Pulmonary (lung) irritation and cough, asthma and chronic bronchitis
- Burning eyes, throat and nose
- Increased susceptibility to cancer

How can I reduce indoor air pollution?

Many things can be done to reduce exposure to indoor air pollutants, particularly in your home where you have some control over ventilation and creation of new pollution.

- Open windows to increase ventilation, which reduces humidity, which in turn reduces mold and mildew growth and the release of formaldehyde.
- Clean and maintain heating ducts, air filters, air conditioners, humidifiers, and dehumidifiers.
- Filters for vacuum cleaners are available, as are central vacuum systems which exhaust vacuumed air to the outside, but they can be expensive.
- Green plants absorb carbon dioxide and some pollutants.
- Keep use of aerosol sprays, commercial cleaners, and other chemicals to a minimum.
- Photocopy machines, which contain harmful toners and chemicals, can be vented to the outdoors or kept in a room in which nobody works regularly.
- Furnaces, water heaters, and gas stoves should be cleaned and maintained regularly to reduce gas leaks and carbon monoxide emissions.
- Air cleaners of various types can be used.
- Choose building and remodeling materials carefully and avoid exposure when possible; try to arrange to stay elsewhere during the remodeling, including during the dusty demolition phase.

What are some other pollutants, and their sources and effects?

Corrosives in the air cause a constant, cumulative irritation to the lungs. Eroded lung tissue puts up less of a barrier to harmful chemicals and infectious agents than healthy lung tissue, much as abraded skin is more likely to let in bacteria and chemicals than intact skin. Abraded skin and lung tissue are roughed up, causing more surface area to be exposed to irritants. Damaged lung tissue is also slower to heal.

Tobacco smoking causes damage from the smoke and chemicals contained in it. In addition, due to the lung irritation, a smoker is more susceptible to the effects of other airborne toxins. The damaged lungs are then less able to filter out these toxins.

Nitrogen oxide, also called nitric oxide (NO), is produced by all high temperature combustion (burning) processes involving air. It is quickly oxidized (chemically changed) to nitrogen dioxide (NO_2), a corrosive gas, in sunlight. The lungs are especially affected, and nitrogen oxides can cause respiratory disease, bronchitis, and pulmonary edema (water in the lungs). The edema is the body's retention of water in an attempt to dilute toxins.

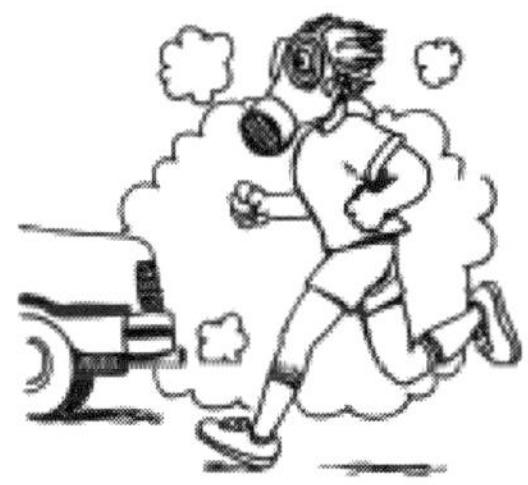

Carbon monoxide (CO) is a product of incomplete combustion (burning). It interferes with oxygen transport by binding hemoglobin, the oxygen-carrying component of blood, 250 times more efficiently than oxygen, so oxygen hardly has a chance. Too much CO can be fatal; a car engine running in a closed garage is a classic example. Carbon dioxide (CO_2) is far less toxic, but can be an asphyxiant (prevents breathing of oxygen) and blood acidifier in large quantities. It is also thought to contribute to global warming; if it's bad for the planet, it can't be good for us.

Sulfur dioxide (SO_2) and sulfur trioxide (SO_3) are the major air polluting forms of sulfur, along with small amounts of sulfides and mercaptans, which are other sulfur compounds. They are released by the burning of coal for heat and electric power and by other burning processes. Sulfur dioxide and the water in the lungs combine to form sulfuric acid (H_2SO_4), a strong acid that can eat away stone and so can do a lot of damage within the body.

Smog is air pollution made visible. The word smog was originally coined to combine the words <u>sm</u>oke and f<u>og</u>. Today, smog is a mixture of smoke, water vapor, particulates, and primary and secondary pollutants. Motor vehicle exhaust is the largest source, followed by industrial emissions. Many people who get sick in smoggy places like Southern California regain their health when they move to a place with comparatively clear air such as Montana.

Patient profile

One patient, a nurse in her 30s from Ohio, became environmentally ill (EI) after she moved to San Diego, California. She also developed brain fog, fatigue and seizures. Moving away from San Diego was what she needed to do to get better, which took about three months in her new environment. She still had allergies but they were not nearly as severe.

What can be done to minimize outdoor air pollution?

Unlike indoor air pollution, outdoor air pollution is largely out of our control. However, some measures that can help include not compounding the problem with indoor pollution, using an air filter or cleaner, and moving to an area with cleaner air if possible. Detoxification methods such as those in this book keep your internal environment as clean as possible and help to maximize your body's ability to deal with the air pollution that remains.

Water Pollution

Like air, the water we encounter in everyday life is usually full of contaminants.

What contaminants might be in water?
Many contaminants can be found in water. These include:

- **Chlorine** added as a disinfectant
- **Chlorocarbons** and **chloramines**, formed from the reaction of chlorine and organics, can be more harmful than either of the original constituents, and can be liver and kidney toxins.
- **Fluoride** added for the dubious purpose of preventing dental cavities
- **Organic molecules**, most of which are harmful, like gasoline and solvents
- **PVCs**, which are plastics from water piping
- **Copper** from piping and **lead** from pipe solder in older homes
- **Other harmful metals and rust**
- A variety of **microorganisms**, including bacteria, parasites, fungi, and algae
- **Pesticides** (discussed in an earlier chapter) and fertilizers that seep into underground water supplies.
- **Minerals**, which can be beneficial but can adversely affect the taste
- **Radon** from natural radioactivity
- **Nitrates** from fertilizers and decomposing plants
- **Dirt**

How can I tell if my water is acceptable?
If you have a private well or an older house, it may be wise to have your water tested at your tap rather than at the source to pick up contamination from household pipes. Private companies do this for a fee. You can possibly have your water tested free by a company that would like to sell you an expensive water treatment system; however, their results may be biased towards finding problems – correctable, of course, by their product. The best testing laboratory is one that is independent and state certified. State or local health departments sometimes test for bacteria free of charge.

Chlorine

What about chlorine?
Chlorine is often added to public water supplies for disinfectant purposes, since it is toxic to potentially infectious microorganisms. Because all cells, whether bacterial or our own, have much in common, it is not surprising that chlorine is toxic to us as well. Chlorine therefore has both benefit and a down side. The best way to deal with chlorine is to let it do its job on bacteria, and then don't drink the water without filtering, as in bottled water or reverse osmosis.

Is showering safe?

If you are unwilling to drink your tap water, you probably should not be showering in it.

It is possible to absorb more chlorine into the body from showering in chlorinated water than from drinking it. The largest organ in the body is the skin, which contains many pores that are opened wider when exposed to warm or hot water. The pores that have been opened from the shower or bath will then let in more chlorine. There are shower filters that attach between the piping and the showerhead that will remove most of the chlorine.

Patient profile
A 40 year old woman switched from tap water to bottled water and used a shower filter, and lost 20 pounds. Chlorine toxicity and sensitivity was causing her weight gain, as her body retained water to try to dilute the toxin. There was also improvement in her energy level and joint pains.

How can chlorine be removed from the body?
Chlorine can be cleared from the body through a supervised sauna program, as chlorine exits through the pores when sweating. Care must then be taken not to then absorb more chlorine; a filter should be used on your after-sauna shower. Exercise also helps to clear chlorine by working the lymphatic detoxification system and by inducing sweating.

Fluoride

What's the story on fluoride?
Fluorine is routinely added to drinking water, usually in the form of sodium fluoride, for the highly dubious purpose of preventing dental cavities in children. Fluorine is very toxic, causing deaths from acute exposure and many types of chronic health problems in a large number of people. Some researchers believe that fluoride, like Prozac®, makes the population more compliant and less aggressive. This is actually a more accurate analogy than one might suppose: Prozac's generic name is fluoxetine, a fluoride compound. Another interesting and scary factoid

about fluoride: they started putting it into the drinking water in Germany in 1933. It is unknown how much this may have contributed to the complacency of much of the populace during the Holocaust.

The amount – more accurately, concentration – of fluoride used in water is usually 1 part per million (1ppm), said to be an effective amount; however, it has been found that as little as 1ppm of fluoride can be toxic, so there is little or no margin for dosage error. However, this is only a concentration, not an absolute amount; the tipoff is the word "per." As an example, if you put a drop of ink in a glass of water, the concentration of ink is one drop per glass. However, a person who drinks two glasses of water will be getting two drops of ink, twice as much as someone who drinks one glass of water, and someone who drinks more tap water will get more fluoride than someone who drinks less. Therefore no two people end up getting the same amount of fluoride even if the concentration is consistent, and the bottom line is that saying that a particular concentration of something is optimal is meaningless. But back to the "optimal" 1ppm concentration – this amount has been shown to be toxic and carcinogenic.

What are some of the symptoms of fluoride exposure?

Symptoms of fluoride exposure are varied, depending in part on the genetic weak link of the person affected. Since certain parts of the body are more affected, most notably the skeletal system and collagen, certain symptoms show up predictably with chronic or acute exposure:

- Gastrointestinal – nausea, stomach cramps, increased salivation, constipation, appetite loss
- Collagen – bone and joint aching, stiffness
- Skin – wrinkling, rashes, mouth and lip sores
- Skeletal – dental fluorosis (mottling of teeth)
- Tiredness, weakness
- Neurological
- Emotional – lethargy, compliance

This list sounds a lot like premature aging. For this reason, fluoride has been called the Aging Factor.[1] The ***U.S. Pharmacopoeia*** and the ***Physician's Desk Reference*** (PDR) are also quite familiar with the symptoms of fluoride toxicity. Fluoride's toxic effects are so well known that its use has been banned in most European countries.[2]

Fluoride mineralizes the collagen by pulling calcium out of the bones. Collagen, found in skin and in many body tissues, is supposed to be supple, but when mineralized, it becomes stiff and less useful. Fluoride also interferes with proper collagen formation, which can lead to wrinkling. Early stages of fluoride-induced damage to bones and cartilage are pain in the spinal bones, progressing to spine stiffness and limitation of movement, followed by the development of a characteristic hunchback (kyphosis).

Fluoride affects the immune system by weakening the cells which attack foreign invaders, opening the door to increased infections. Fluoride confuses the immune system's ability to distinguish between self and non-self by combining with the body's tissues, leading to autoimmune diseases such as rheumatoid arthritis, lupus, and skin conditions. Fluoride can also contribute to the development of cancer by inhibiting DNA repair.

How can fluoride be avoided?

Water and shower filters that get rid of chlorine do not necessarily remove fluoride, which is a smaller molecule that is not as easily filtered out, although reverse osmosis and distillation do remove it. Bottled water, and water from the water dispensing machines found in some parts of the country, may or may not contain fluoride. It is a good idea to call the companies involved to find out. Such a call, in addition to getting the needed information, can have the effect of letting manufacturers know that fluoride in the water is not acceptable. Filtercon, a company that sells water filters, can be contacted at 800-550-1995.

You should be able to find a non-fluoridated toothpaste at your local natural foods store, or you can use either plain baking soda alone, or a baking soda/salt combination. Do not allow your child's teeth to be fluoridated. Avoid nonstick cookware coatings, since these are typically made from a fluoride compound; glass pots are best overall.

Personal Care Products

What personal care products can cause problems?

Colognes and personal care products are in such common use and contain so many toxic chemicals that they deserve a discussion of their own. Personal care products include:

- Colognes, perfumes
- Cosmetics, makeup
- Acne medications
- Powders
- Nail products
- Creams and lotions
- Deodorants
- Sanitary pads and tampons
- Hair dyes, sprays, shampoos
- Toothpaste, mouthwash

Colognes are particularly harmful. Unlike the other products listed which expose only the user, colognes and other scented products expose other people, by design, to their odor and therefore to the toxic penetrating chemicals causing the odor. These are particularly toxic for the user, however, since s/he is both inhaling it and absorbing it through the skin almost continuously.

Why are colognes and scented products so toxic?

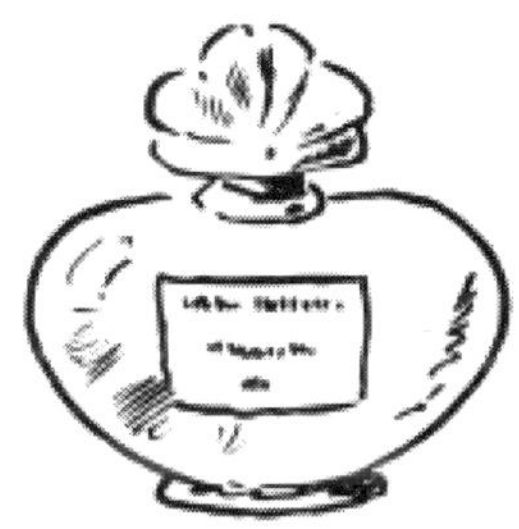

Up to 5000 different chemicals are used in various combinations in scented products, and 84% of these have had little or no human toxicology testing.[1] A single brand of cologne contains dozens of chemicals, none of which belong in the human body. 95% of chemicals used in fragrances are synthetic compounds derived from petroleum, including many toxins and sensitizers that are capable of causing cancer, birth defects, central nervous system disorders and allergic reactions.[2] The FDA is unable to police the fragrance industry since it is exempt from listing product ingredients.[3]

Sensitivity to cologne components is quite common, and can affect both the wearers and those around them. The allergy sufferer may or may not be aware of the allergy or the cause, or that the allergy may be self-induced. Some common symptoms are:

- **Brain fog** – This may be slight and chronic, or can be sudden and severe.
- **Emotional** – The sympathetic nervous system reacts to what it correctly perceives to be a dangerous invader, and signals the adrenal glands to secrete adrenaline to prepare for a confrontation. The rush of adrenaline (the fight-or-flight hormone) can cause a sudden feeling of anxiety, anger, or depression.
- **Rashes** and increased skin sunlight sensitivity where the product was applied
- **Fatigue** and muscle weakness

- **Increased sensitivity** to other toxins or allergens as the body is overloaded with more than it can handle.
- **Meningeal system contraction** similar to that caused by other toxic chemicals. Structural misalignments can then occur from the pressure, with a multitude of accompanying symptoms such as headaches and light sensitivity.

What other scented products may be toxic?
Cologne is one of the strongest scented products, but many other scented products contain lesser amounts of these chemicals. Penetrants in the products are especially hazardous. These scented products include other personal care products such as:

- Deodorants, makeup, lotion, and bath salts
- Soaps, shampoos, and detergents
- Household cleaning products
- So-called air fresheners
- Baby powders and oils
- Clothes-dryer sheets

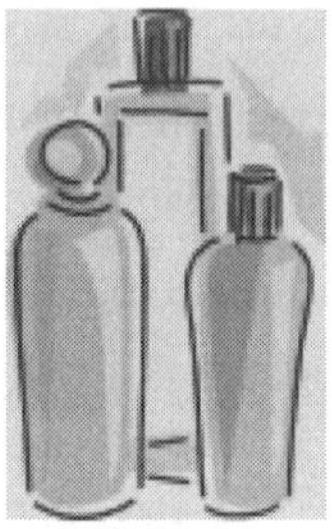

Can cosmetics be harmful?
Cosmetics are made up of petrochemicals, metal salts, fragrance, penetrants, and other chemicals which do not belong in or on the body. These chemicals are both absorbed through the skin and inhaled.

Metal salts, which are compounds made from metals, are commonly used to color cosmetics; most heavy metals and their salts are toxic.

Nearly all cosmetics contain oil-based petrochemicals, which accounts for their greasy feel and staying power. Fragrance is usually added to cover up the oil-refinery smell that would otherwise be noticeable.

Lipstick, as wearers know, must be frequently reapplied throughout the day. Where does it go? It is ingested as the wearer licks her lips, eats, or drinks. The oils and metals in the lipstick vary by product, but it is safe to say that they do not belong in the human digestive tract.

Mascara and eyeliner sometimes have lead or coal-tar dyes for intense color. They are necessarily applied very close to the eye, a very sensitive part of the body that can absorb chemicals from its immediate surroundings and send them elsewhere in the body via the tiny eye capillaries. Mascara wands and eyeliner brushes, and the product itself, can harbor infection and for this reason should never be used by another person or kept for very long (2-3 months).

Hair dye, like mascara, contains coal-tar dyes and metals. They can also contain aniline dyes, known to cause cancer in animals. Studies showed that women who used synthetic hair dyes had a 50% greater chance of developing non-Hodgkin's lymphoma, a type of cancer of the lymph system, than women who never dyed their hair. Hair dyes have also been implicated in leukemia and multiple myeloma.[4]

Shampoos contain dozens of chemicals with unfamiliar and unpronounceable names, most of which are listed on the bottle. Shampoo components may not be as dangerous as those in other hair care products, but they are deliberately scrubbed into the scalp and can be absorbed into the bloodstream from there. Sodium lauryl (or laureth) sulfate is commonly used in shampoos as a wetting and foaming agent. There is some suspicion that this compound, also used as a driveway degreaser, a pesticide and herbicide, and a food additive in products such as marshmallows[5], has irritating or even carcinogenic potential. For these reasons it might be wise to avoid it.

Nail polish is lacquer, similar to that used to lacquer furniture. Used habitually, it can keep the nail bed (where the nail meets the finger, and where new nail growth is generated) from breathing properly. If the nail and nail bed get too little oxygen, this may set up conditions conducive to fungus growth. Both nail polish and polish remover contain acetone, a strong solvent which is strong enough to dissolve lacquer so it certainly dissolves lipids (fats and oils) in the body's cells and nerves. The chemicals from nail salons where acrylic nails are applied and polish is in regular use make such places very toxic environments.

What about non-cosmetic personal care products?

Underarm **deodorants** usually contain aluminum, a toxic metal used for its drying properties. An excess of aluminum has been linked to Alzheimer's disease. Antiperspirants, usually combined with deodorants in a commercial product, deliberately clog up the sweat glands under the arms. Sweat is one of the body's ways to eliminate toxins, and antiperspirants interfere with this.

Tampons are made of a combination of cotton and synthetic fibers designed to be absorbent. Cotton is usually heavily sprayed with insecticides which can be absorbed into the body. Deodorant tampons contain a scent which serves no useful purpose and may cause irritation.

Face, body, talcum, and baby **powder** are made of tiny particles of talc or other substance. This fine powder is inhaled when used, and the particles can lodge in the lungs, causing scarring of delicate lung tissues.

What else can I do to avoid these toxins?

You can look at the pros and cons of any particular product and make an informed decision, based on the risks described in this chapter versus the perceived benefit to yourself, to continue using a particular product.

Treat the root causes that may be contributing to unhealthy-looking skin, body odor, bad breath or other cosmetic or aesthetic problem.

In general, safer versions of all of the mentioned products can be found in stores geared towards natural foods. However, be an informed label reader; tiny amounts of vitamins and herbs are sometimes added more for advertising appeal than to convey any real benefits, and harmful ingredients may still be present.

Deodorant alternatives – A person who is well past puberty may not even have underarm odor, but habitually uses deodorants every day for years just in case. Try going without deodorant on a weekend or day when you will be alone – you may find that you can do without it. Another consideration is that body odor often comes from unclean living. Eliminating tobacco, alcohol, meat, and unhealthful food will lower the amount of odorous material that needs to be detoxified through the skin. If you still feel you need deodorizing, there are alternatives to commercial deodorants:

- In many cases simple hygiene such as a daily shower is all that is needed.
- Rubbing alcohol will kill the bacteria that cause odor, and a once a day wipe with alcohol may do the trick. Alcohol is not harmless, but once it dries it is gone, unlike deodorants and antiperspirants.
- Magnesium is less harmful than aluminum, and magnesium-based deodorants such as deodorant crystals or rocks are available in health stores.
- Tea tree oil (melaleuca) and oils of pine, lavender, geranium and peppermint fight bacteria and can be used as deodorants.
- Dry baking soda, which is often used to deodorize refrigerators and sink drains, can also be applied to the underarm area.

Safer natural **hair dyes** include henna (red/brown), chamomile or lemon juice to brighten blonde hair, and walnut husks (dark brown).

Let's think about some of these messages

One advantage of personal care products compared with other toxins is that most of them are optional. Now that you are more aware of the down side of perfuming and coloring your body, you may well decide that you will cut down on or eliminate such products.

One way to approach this is to evaluate advertisers' messages, which are, after all, designed to sell products by creating an artificial need or desire. Primarily aimed at women, these messages convey the idea that the Real You is foul-smelling and unattractive, and that you are offensive to others if you appear in public without covering your hair, face, skin, armpits, and teeth with purchased products. Internalizing these messages can cause real damage in addition to that from physical toxicity. Think about it, and challenge these messages. As a result, you will keep more of your money in your wallet, improve your self-esteem, and – getting back to the theme of this book – eliminate a significant source of toxicity in your life.

Drugs

What is a drug?

Although people would tend to disagree on the definition of a drug, for the purposes of this chapter, a drug is defined as a chemical substance that is not naturally found in the body or needed by the body – so this excludes foods and nutrients – and that is deliberately taken into the body to produce some functional or perceived change in the body or mind. A drug overrides and does not support or enhance the body's natural healing mechanisms, and may interfere with them.

Drugs include substances that do at least one of the following:

- Attack a disease causing agent, such as an antibiotic which kills bacteria
- Artificially change one's mood or energy level
- Relieve symptoms
- Affect the function of an organ or system, such as the heart (rhythm regulators) or kidneys (diuretics).

The word root *pharmaco*, referring to drugs, is taken from the Greek word *pharmakos*, meaning *poison.*[1] It seems that the ancient Greeks knew something about medications that we are just rediscovering.

Doctors recognize many different classes and subclasses of drugs. Drugs can be classified by organ system affected (cardiovascular or psychoactive drugs, for example), by major action (antibiotics, cancer chemotherapy), or by method of ingestion or application (dermatologicals). Most self-prescribed drugs, and the large majority of drugs of abuse, legal and illegal, are the psychoactives, which help to calm, energize, or improve mood.

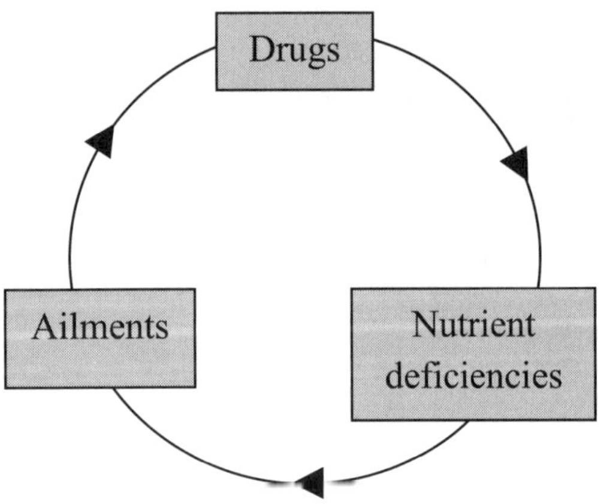

What are side effects and what is their significance?

Side effects have been defined as unwanted effects of a drug, such as the tendency of aspirin to promote stomach ulcers. In actuality, drugs have only effects, which we designate as actions (good) and side effects (bad). Aspirin's ulcer-promoting effect is as much a part of its character as its headache relieving effect. Another type of side effect is the loss of nutrients caused by most drugs[2]; nutrient deficiencies can then cause many symptoms of their own.

All drugs have at least the strong potential for side effects. It is therefore important to understand what drugs can and cannot accomplish, and what their side effects are, in order to make an informed decision about taking them, the risk vs. the benefit.

Another type of side effect is that many drugs cause a loss of nutrients, and those who take any drugs for any reason need to be particularly vigilant about nutrient deficiencies. One of the problems with drugs is that they are often used to suppress the symptoms of ailments that are caused at least in part by nutrient deficiency and could be helped by nutrient supplementation.

> **Important: Despite the down side of medications and your hopefully increased awareness of these stemming from the following discussion, it is crucial that any intentions to discontinue or modify your prescription medication routine should be discussed with your physician rather than undertaken on your own.**

What can be wrong with taking symptom suppressing drugs?

Many, if not most, medications are taken for the suppression of symptoms. In many of these cases, the underlying disease process is not corrected or even addressed. The reasoning appears to be that if the symptom is gone, the disease is gone, which is often not the case. In general, the problems involved in taking symptom-suppressing medications are:

- Masking a serious underlying problem – Pain and some other symptoms are signals that something is wrong, and masking the symptoms may cause a dangerous or even fatal delay in finding out what is really causing the problem.
- Many symptom-suppressing drugs suppress the body's mechanisms for dealing with the underlying problem. Coughing, running nose, and mild diarrhea are the body's way of expelling undesirable matter, and fever helps the body to fight infection, so drugs that work against these work against healing.
- The rebound effect – With regular use, many symptom-suppressing drugs cause the very symptoms that they are used to treat, such as aspirin causing rebound headaches.
- Side effects and/or allergic reactions are possible with any drug.
- Interaction with other drugs and even foods can occur, with serious effects or inactivation of the drug. The antibiotic tetracycline, for example, is rendered less effective by taking it with milk.
- They can pose a danger to a developing fetus, in spite of pre-release drug testing, which, for obvious ethical reasons, can't be done on pregnant women.
- So-called "inert" ingredients in these medications, such as alcohol and sugar in syrups, artificial colors and flavors, and tablet binders that hold the tablet together can cause problems of allergy and toxicity.

- Children seeing their parents take, or give them, medication for every little thing are more likely to self-medicate. This can take the form of a young child getting into the baby aspirin and eating them like candy, or the teenager who turns to alcohol or other drugs as a quick fix for emotional pain.

The common side effects and down sides of any prescribed or OTC drug are easy to find in product literature, advertising, online, or the PDR. Knowing these effects can help you to make an informed decision regarding using these drugs. In the case of prescription medications, this decision should be between you and your doctor.

What are some of the alternatives to symptom-suppressing drugs?

The choice is not necessarily between toughing it out and taking risks. There are safe, non-drug alternatives for most of the symptoms mentioned. Since toxin buildup can cause pain and other symptoms, removing toxins and detoxifying the body, followed by replacing minerals, should be the first step in relieving almost any chronic problem. Identifying and eliminating the problem at its source, toxic or otherwise, would be the next step. There are also techniques and supplements that can help in symptom management; for example:

- **Pain relief** – Massage of the sore area, acupuncture and acupressure, use of homeopathic remedies, "superfoods" such as Life Solubles and Sun Chlorella, and the omega-3 oils, and bioflavonoids such as quercetin and pycnogenol that help to balance the eicosanoids (inflammatory chemicals).

- **Colds** – Your mother was right – chicken soup helps reduce nasal congestion. So does breathing steam, by itself or with peppermint oil or Vicks Vapo-Rub, but be careful of scalding. Liquid germanium may also be useful, especially in a nebulizer which converts the germanium to a mist to be breathed, releasing oxygen.

- **Laxatives** – If your bowels move only once every two or three days or longer, this can be a sign that your body is not working optimally or your diet is deficient in fiber, oils, enzymes, or protective bacteria, all of which help the food move down the digestive tract. As with all symptoms, it is better to look for and treat the root cause of constipation rather than subjecting your colon to violent contractions induced by harsh, habit-forming laxatives.

- **Diet aids** – Overweight is a symptom, rather than a primary problem, and it is important to recognize and treat the causes, some of which are discussed in the chapter on Overweight. If your adrenals and DHEA are depleted due to the use of diet drugs or other causes, adrenal function can be supported using wild yam cream, tyrosine, pancreatic acid, vitamin B6, PABA, and GLA oils.

What about drugs that truly make a difference?

A few classes of drugs can truly be life-saving rather than just symptom-suppressing. Drugs that actually attack a disease-causing agent include antibiotics and cancer-fighting drugs. However, their benefits should be weighed against their down sides to provide a balanced picture. The purpose of these drugs is to kill cells (bacterial or cancer). In doing so, they inevitably also kill necessary, useful cells and protective microorganisms in our bodies.

Antibiotics

What are the down sides of antibiotics?

The word antibiotic comes from the roots "anti," meaning against, and "bios," meaning life (as in biology, the study of life). Antibiotics, therefore, are drugs against life.

Although antibiotics can be useful and even lifesaving in managing an acute bacterial infection, they have a number of other drawbacks, including immune system suppression in the long term, the killing of beneficial bacteria that help control yeast, and the potential for serious, even fatal, reactions.

Ideally the doctor will do a culture before prescribing an antibiotic to identify the specific bacterium and best antibiotic for it, but this is not often done because doing a culture can take days.

It is usually a good idea to take protective bacteria (sometimes called probiotics) such as acidophilus (preferably) or bifidus, as capsules, liquids, or in quality yogurt. Ideally they should be taken as far away as possible from the antibiotic, for example in mid-day if the drug is taken morning and evening, but in any case at least two hours away from the antibiotic. If they are taken too closely together, the antibiotic will simply kill the beneficial bacteria that have just been taken instead of going after the bad guys. These bacterial supplements help to replenish the body's protective bacteria which are killed by the antibiotic. Most acidophilus is derived from milk, so use caution if you are allergic to dairy products. Dairy free brands of acidophilus, such as Ultra Flora and BifidoViden, are available.

Cancer chemotherapy

What are some of the side effects of cancer drugs?

Anti-cancer drugs can be lifesaving, but they can be very potent and toxic. They can suppress the immune system so that it can no longer fight the cancer on its own, and the drug must therefore be strong enough to kill all of the cancer cells and not just most of them. Cancer cells are mutated fermenting body cells rather than foreign invaders, so drugs that kill fermenting cancer cells will also damage normal respiratory cells, especially fast-growing cells such as those in hair follicles and the mucous lining of the mouth, which explains the typical hair loss and mouth sores. When the body detects a strong poison, the liver reacts by trying to expel it; violent nausea, vomiting, and diarrhea usually accompany chemotherapy for this reason.

Does cancer chemotherapy always do more harm than good?
Certainly not. Building up the immune system naturally so that it can fight the cancer would be ideal, but this process takes time, and time is something that one may not have if one is dealing with a fast-growing cancer. Some cancers, such as Hodgkin's lymphoma, respond well to chemotherapy, and in such cases the benefits outweigh the risks.

Is there another approach to supporting the body in fighting cancer?
The body usually successfully dispatches mutated cells, technically cancer cells, all the time before a tumor can form when the immune system is strong and working optimally.

An important part of cancer treatment is the identification and elimination of the cause of the cancer. Eliminating toxins, both environmental and dietary, are key in treating and preventing cancer. This will enable the body and its immune system to function optimally. Optimal nutrition is another important aspect. A number of natural cancer remedies exist as well.

Recreational drugs

What are recreational drugs?
The term refers to self-medication used to artificially change one's mood, raise one's energy level, lift one's spirits, cope with problems by dulling the associated feelings, or let down inhibitions. The use of substances for this purpose goes back to the beginnings of recorded history, and includes illegal "street drugs" like marijuana, heroin, barbiturates, cocaine, and LSD, as well as legal substances such as alcohol, tobacco, and caffeine. It is important to understand that a drug has whatever effects it has regardless of its legal status, which usually has more to do with politics and powerful lobbies than with public health considerations or common sense. Therefore, the categorization of illegal drugs as evil and alcohol, tobacco, and caffeine as harmless has no basis in fact, and consumption of even legal drugs should be taken seriously.

Are you addicted?
Many of the recreational drugs discussed here are or can be addictive. Are you addicted? Your judgment on the matter may be impaired by the drug(s) you are taking. Try going without the substance for 90 days. If you can't seem to do so, there's your answer. If you can and do give up the substance, look back and ask yourself whether you would like your life to be the way it was before, when you were using the drug. The answer will rarely be yes.

Depressant drugs

Depressant drugs include strong painkillers, barbiturates, sleep aids, and alcohol. Overdose of depressant drugs can be fatal; these drugs can slow and stop the heart and respiratory functions. Use of these drugs can suppress the immune system and can slow down the body's detoxification pathways, allowing toxins to build up in the body; for example, the constipation that results from the use of depressant drugs. Withdrawal from these drugs can be dangerous and should be done only with medical supervision.

Stimulant drugs

Stimulant drugs, which are used for a feeling of increased energy and alertness, include cocaine and amphetamines...and caffeine. Stimulant drugs are usually addictive. Overdose can be fatal due to cardiac (heart) overstimulation. Withdrawal can be unpleasant, and brings to mind the saying: "What goes up must come down." Coming down can bring fatigue and depression as the drug brought energy and elation.

> With drugs, what goes up must come down.

Marijuana

What are some of the effects of marijuana?
Although illegal, marijuana is almost as much a mainstream drug as it is a street drug. Reported subjective effects vary, with users reporting euphoria, relaxation, and other positive effects. Marijuana has been shown to be useful medically, as are many herbs, and the relief of nausea from chemotherapy is one of the best known benefits, although certainly not the only one; it has also been shown to be useful for decreasing glaucoma, killing pain, and lowering blood pressure.[3]

Negative long term physical effects include lung damage and even cancer caused by the inhalation of any kind of smoke, made worse by the fact that marijuana smokers usually inhale deeply and hold the smoke in their lungs as long as possible. Negative psychological effects of marijuana include memory and concentration loss, brain fog, mood changes, and decline in motivation. One can take a long time to return to normal even after quitting.

Appetite, especially for sweets, is usually triggered, as marijuana's use can lower the level of hydrochloric acid in the stomach, which allows fungus and helicobacter pylori to proliferate, and this then depletes blood sugar. Yeast overgrowth can occur fast enough to cause sugar cravings – the "marijuana munchies" – within hours of smoking, followed by drowsiness, brain fog, and sleepiness. Fungal overgrowth, or ongoing yeast infection, can continue long after the drug has been given up. Marijuana's appetite stimulating effect is one reason for what some consider to be its benefit to cancer patients, who often drop weight at an alarming rate.

Problems are introduced by the illegality of growing and selling marijuana, primarily the use of adulterants of various types, including herbicides used by law enforcement, other drugs added to increase the effect, and leafy matter of whatever type to increase the weight and thus profit before sale. These adulterants are, or can be, toxic, and may account for many of the side effects attributed to marijuana. They certainly don't belong in your body.

What if I would like to quit?

Although marijuana has not been proven to be physically addictive or deadly, it is far from harmless. If not used medicinally, the down side might outweigh the upside. If you are a user, you might like to quit.

The active ingredient, tetrahydrocannabinol (THC) is fat soluble and is stored in body fat. This means that its effects are present for a while, although not to a debilitating degree. A regular user has an ever-increasing amount being stored in the body. It can take months to get back to normal after quitting since the drug is released from the fat cells and excreted very slowly. For this reason, the desire to smoke it can linger. Often the removal of the substance, whether a drug or a food that is linked to allergic addiction, from the body will cause the cravings to cease.

Sauna detoxification, described in Part 4, has been shown to be quite useful for detoxification from marijuana. Feelings of being "stoned" have been reported by ex-marijuana users who undergo sauna detoxification, even years after the drug use, as the fat-stored chemical is released into the bloodstream during sauna. Once the drug has been removed from the body, the fungus can clear up – although diet and perhaps medication might be needed to accomplish this – and cravings for marijuana should diminish or cease.

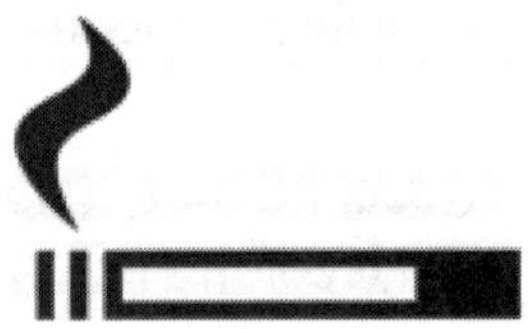

Tobacco

How addictive is tobacco?

Nicotine, the active ingredient in tobacco, is nearly as addictive as crack cocaine. If this sounds hard to believe, consider that nearly everyone who smokes has an addictive relationship with it: tobacco is smoked multiple times every day, it is very difficult to stop smoking, and there are strong cravings and anxiety if tobacco is not available. Very few smokers can truly take it or leave it, although self-delusion about this is common.

Smokers say they like the relaxing effect of tobacco, but this relaxing effect is due to the alleviation of the withdrawal symptoms, which can start within 30 minutes to three hours after the last cigarette. Smoking is relaxing only in comparison to withdrawal, and a heavy smoker is either smoking or withdrawing almost constantly.

Why is smoking harmful?

Some of the negative effects of smoking have been discussed in Part 2 in connection with particular ailments. Immediate physical symptoms experienced by smokers include coughing, burning in the chest, dizziness, nausea and loss of appetite. Withdrawal symptoms include obsessive craving for cigarettes, extreme irritability, sleeplessness, depression, and inability to concentrate.

Smokers have a higher death rate at all ages compared with nonsmokers. Men who smoke less than half a pack a day have a death rate 60% higher than nonsmokers at a given age; one to two packs a day, about 90% higher; two or more packs a day, 120% higher.[4] About one thousand Americans die of smoking-caused illnesses per day. Smoking will kill more Americans than AIDS, heroin, crack cocaine, alcohol, car accidents, fire, and murder combined.[5]

Other long-term effects include:

- Heart attacks and strokes, vascular diseases, high blood pressure
- Cancer, especially lung, mouth, larynx, and bladder
- Emphysema and chronic bronchitis; a smoker's risk of death from these is 6.5 to 15 times that of the nonsmoker[4]
- Decreased resistance to other toxins and microorganisms due to liver overload and overall immune system suppression

What are some of the harmful components in tobacco?

- **Nicotine** is the active ingredient in tobacco. It is responsible for both the relaxing or stimulating effects of tobacco and the high addictiveness.
- **Carbon monoxide** allows less oxygen to get to the brain and cells.
- **Tar**, the brownish-yellow stuff that can be seen on the cigarette filter, clogs the alveoli in the lungs and is carcinogenic (cancer causing). Sticky blackish deposits on the lungs, like road tar, can be seen at autopsy on a smoker.
- **Metals** – A number of toxic metals are found in tobacco smoke. Nickel is a carcinogen and allergen. Cadmium lowers levels of zinc, a mineral necessary for the senses of smell and taste, explaining in part the increase in appetite after quitting smoking.
- **Nitrogen oxides** can damage throat and lung tissues and oxidize the body's fats, making them carcinogenic.
- **Acetaldehyde** is a strong cross-linking agent, which causes premature wrinkling, and cross-linked arterial tissue toughens and leads to cardiovascular disease.

What about exposure to tobacco other than cigarettes?

Passive smoking is a danger. The term refers to the smoke inhaled by a nonsmoker who is in the vicinity of a smoker. The EPA has officially linked passive smoking and increased risk of lung cancer[6], which is otherwise rare in nonsmokers.

Smokeless, or chewing, tobacco contains nicotine which makes these products nearly as addictive as smoked tobacco. Although smokeless tobacco is less likely to cause lung cancer than cigarettes, it is associated with a high incidence of mouth and throat cancers.

Cigar smokers often claim that they don't inhale, but many of them are deluding themselves. The smoke, even if just held in the mouth, can cause or contribute to oral and other cancers.

How can I quit smoking?

If you don't smoke, don't start! There are many drawbacks, including a major daily hit in the vicinity of the wallet, and no advantages. If you smoke but would like to quit, you can take a number of approaches. Almost all smokers have tried to quit at least once but didn't succeed for long, as this is a powerful addiction. Don't give up. You may need to try a different approach; some of these include:

- Cutting cigarettes out altogether, also called "going cold turkey." This is usually more effective than gradual withdrawal.
- Aversion therapy, hypnosis
- Different types of formal stop-smoking programs
- Nicotine patches or gum, available by prescription, to relieve the worst of the physical withdrawal symptoms while you deal with the psychological withdrawal.
- Support groups
- Nutritional support, including vitamin and herbal support for the adrenals, minerals such as zinc and chromium, and amino acids such as glutamine to stabilize blood sugar. Zinc, by replacing the toxic cadmium from cigarettes, can reduce cravings and withdrawal symptoms.

Is there anything to do to reduce risks before, during, and after quitting smoking?

It is not uncommon for a long-term smoker to develop smoking-related health complications, especially cancer, several years after quitting. Several things can be done while or after quitting smoking to reduce these health risks:

- Chelate out the metals cadmium and nickel, both of which are in tobacco smoke. Chelation is discussed in the chapter on Metal Detoxification.

- Sauna detoxification can help remove cigarette toxins from the body.
- Take beneficial minerals, especially zinc.

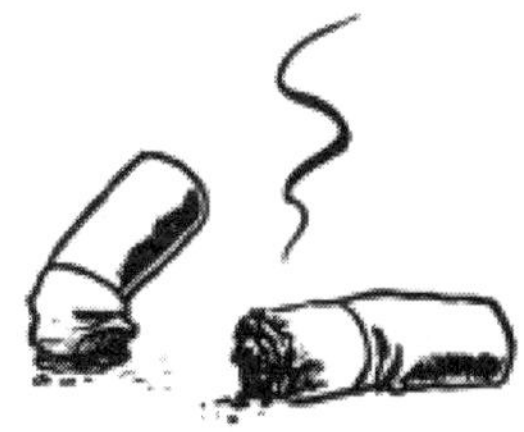

- Have the Adrenal Stress Index (ASI) test done to determine whether additional adrenal support is needed, such as the hormone DHEA or pregnenolone, or vitamin B5 (pantothenic acid).
- Take omega-3 oils such as flax oil to increase levels of hormones such as adrenaline, which are usually diminished from smoking.
- Take antioxidants such as vitamins A, C, E, bioflavonoids, and selenium to counteract smoking damage.
- Life Solubles and Kona Gold minerals contain many of the above nutrients.

This is where a knowledgeable practitioner can help you by putting together a support program that encompasses these measures, individually tailored to your needs.

<u>Alcohol</u>

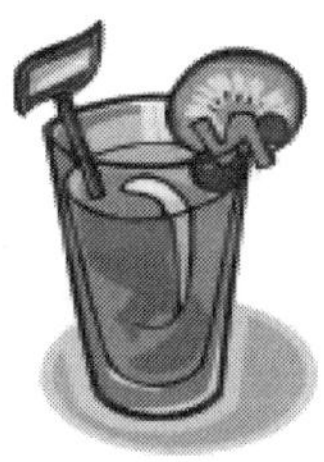

Is alcohol also a drug?
Beverage alcohol, or ethanol, is a powerful and toxic drug disguised as a social beverage. You can "dress up" alcohol with mixers, fruits, fancy glassware, little umbrellas, swizzle sticks, and cute names, but the fact remains that alcohol is a dangerous, addictive drug.

Where is alcohol found?
Besides the obvious – alcoholic beverages – alcohol can be found in other places. These unsuspected sources of alcohol have derailed more than one person's attempts to quit. Alcohol is found in mouthwash (Listerine has 26.9% alcohol[7]), medications such as Nyquil (25%, or 1/4 ounce per dose), and cough syrup. The alcohol in mouthwash, if used for years, can contribute to the development of mouth cancer.

What is alcoholism?
Alcohol is addictive, due in part to allergy; however, it is not as addictive as tobacco, as it is possible to be a nonaddicted occasional drinker. The line between nonaddicted and addicted is not clear cut. Alcoholics Anonymous has a checklist to determine whether alcohol is a free choice or a problem for you.

There are several different patterns of alcoholism, most of which are not stereotypical, but all of which are alcoholism – the person who gets drunk every day (the stereotype), the sneaky drunk who keeps hidden bottles, the person who drinks alcohol every day but is functional and not visibly drunk, or the person who is sober all week and goes on a drunken weekend bender.

Most alcoholics don't accept that they are alcoholics as long as they are still drinking alcohol. They are attempting to judge their degree of impairment or addiction with a mind that is itself impaired.

What are some effects of alcohol?

Although it may initially appear to be a stimulant, alcohol is actually a depressant drug. Seemingly positive subjective effects include euphoria and relaxation of inhibitions. Negative effects include irrational and violent behavior, dizziness, lack of coordination, poor reflexes, and nausea and vomiting. Driving ability is impaired, but so is the ability to judge the degree of impairment, a dangerous and sometimes fatal combination.

Whether or not one is addicted, alcohol is toxic. The amount of toxic effect depends on the amount of alcohol consumed and the length of time that it has been used. The body will detoxify alcohol at a rate of one ounce every 60 to 90 minutes but although the drug is gone the toxic effects linger and are cumulative. These long-term effects include[8]:

- Cell death, especially in the brain.
- Hepatitis and cirrhosis of the liver (dry or scarred liver); also fatty liver.
- Cancers of the liver, mouth, larynx, pharynx, and esophagus. Beer, especially, is linked to higher cancer rates. This is likely due to the fermenting yeast in beer being similar to fermenting cancer cells.
- Cardiovascular disease, stroke, hypertension
- Gastritis, pancreatitis
- Fetal alcohol syndrome in babies whose mothers are heavy alcohol users – low birth weight, learning difficulties, facial and cranial deformities.
- Depression, anxiety, impaired memory and amnesia, blackouts
- Irrational, aggressive and violent behavior.

Habitual use of alcohol contributes to nutritional deficiencies. B vitamins, especially vitamin B1, are often depleted, as are minerals. Alcohol dilutes, dissolves, and takes nutrients out of the body. Since alcohol is an oil solvent (and is used as such industrially), it can carry out fatty acids and the oil-soluble vitamins A, D, E, and K as well. In addition, the typical alcoholic does not eat properly.

Alcohol interacts with a wide variety of other drugs, especially other depressants, sometimes with fatal results.

Patient profile

One patient, a 55 year old man who had been drinking alcohol nearly all of his adult life, developed autoimmune problems, arthritis, gallbladder problems, and liver damage. He was put on a program to keep his dry liver moist, including cod liver oil, oil soluble vitamins A, D, E and K, a liver detoxification protocol, and amino acids and protein powder. His health has returned.

How can I stop drinking alcohol?

Recovery from alcohol use or abuse depends on the extent of alcohol use. A light or moderate non-addicted user may only need to realize the dangers involved, make up his or her mind to give it up, and do so with minimal discomfort. An alcoholic can make use of Alcoholics Anonymous or other programs and support groups.

Before therapy can begin, however, the body must be physically detoxified of alcohol, a process sometimes called drying out, which may require hospitalization and medication. After drying out, the body should be fully detoxified, including getting rid of the fungus overgrowth which is commonly found in those who use alcohol. Alcohol craving can continue if the fungus is not eliminated, since the fungus wants to be fed.

Those in alcohol recovery are often addicted to sugar. After a typical Alcoholics Anonymous meeting, members can often be found in the back of the room with a cup of heavily sugared coffee and a couple of donuts. Sugar cravings will continue until fungus or bacteria are eliminated. Also, alcohol is made from sugar, yeast (a fungus), moisture, and warmth, conditions that exist in the body of a sugar-eating recovering alcoholic. Such a person will be making alcohol in his/her body, a phenomenon called the auto-brewery syndrome or a dry drunk. The fungus, sugar craving, and alcohol craving will keep each other going, and the cycle should be broken via a yeast-free diet to increase the chances of success.

Quitting isn't easy, but it is much easier when the body is detoxified of fungus. Fungus clearing protocols, including the Detoxification diet, are discussed in Part 4. A sober, drug-free life is worth it!

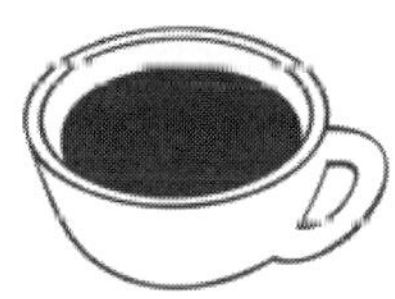

Caffeine

Caffeine can't be a drug, can it?

Coffee is the most commonly used drug in the United States[9], used primarily for its stimulant effects. A cup of coffee or its equivalent in the morning makes the user feel more alert, with improved concentration and greater energy. In actuality, the habitual caffeine user is simply canceling out the withdrawal symptoms of lethargy, brain fog, and headache to attain the state that would be normal if the person were not a caffeine user. Caffeine pushes the adrenal glands to produce more adrenaline, raising energy short term but depleting the adrenals and lowering overall energy over the long term.

Caffeine is addictive, with increasing tolerance and withdrawal symptoms. Unlike addiction to the other drugs, however, caffeine addiction is not disabling (in fact, caffeine can be "abling" in the short term), and a person can drink several cups of coffee a day for years with no readily apparent ill effects. However, caffeine use can cause fungus growth, constricted arteries, constipation, and faster blood clotting which can in turn lead to stroke, heart attack, or phlebitis. Other effects of caffeine are mentioned in Part 2.

Where is caffeine found?
Coffee, tea, and colas are the best-known sources of caffeine, but there are many others. The amount of caffeine in coffee depends on the method of preparation and brewing time.

Other caffeine sources include:

- Dr. Pepper and Mountain Dew sodas, as well as some other kinds of soda
- Energy drinks, which are becoming increasingly popular
- Some pain medications, since caffeine boosts the effectiveness of painkillers
- Caffeine pills such as NoDoz and Vivarin
- Some cold remedies such as Dristan and Triaminicin
- Some weight control aids
- Herbs including Ma Huang, kola nut, and guarana
- Green tea
- Some specialty bottled waters

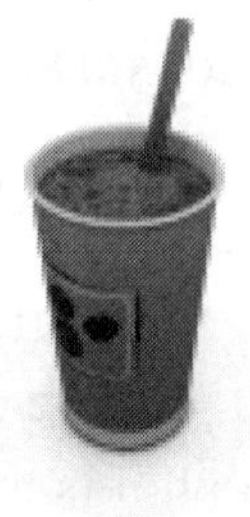

Read labels – most products will usually list caffeine on their labels if it is added. However, if the caffeine is a natural constituent, such as with green tea, it may not be listed.

What are the adverse effects of caffeine?
Symptoms of usage, especially large amounts or long-term use, may be so subtle as to go nearly unnoticed, or may be quite uncomfortable. Many people don't think of caffeine as a drug and so may not make the connection between caffeine intake and symptoms, which include:

- CNS stimulation – irritability, nervousness, insomnia, headaches, ears ringing. Habitual caffeine use, when discontinued, can lead to a withdrawal headache.

- Gastrointestinal – nausea, diarrhea, stomach pain

- Cardiovascular stimulation – palpitations, high blood pressure, heart attack
- Cancer – A caffeine intake of over 3 cups of coffee per day is associated with higher cancer rates.[10] It can damage cellular DNA and interfere with its repair, and sets up a fermenting environment, preferred by cancer cells.
- Miscarriage and infertility
- Bone loss as described in the Bone and Joint Problems chapter.
- Cystic breast lumps

Withdrawal symptoms include headache, irritability, lethargy, drowsiness and yawning, inability to concentrate, depression, restlessness, caffeinated beverage cravings, and runny nose. As with other stimulants, Newton's Law – "What goes up must come down" – is in effect here. Withdrawing slowly often works for those who would like to quit without withdrawal symptoms.

Caffeine may be one of the safer drugs and milder addictions, but like all recreational drugs it still has no place in the body of someone who is working towards better health.

Food-Related Toxins

What's in Your Food Besides Food?

Food keeps us alive, but there are components in most commercially available food that can damage health. These components fall into several categories:

- Food components that are, by their nature, toxic or harmful to health, such as sugar and corn syrup, yeast, and trans fats
- Foods to which the individual may be sensitive or allergic
- Food additives, both intentional and unintentional

Foods in the first two categories, those that are most likely to cause health problems and sensitivities, are covered in detail in the chapter on Detoxification Diet in Part 4. Some additives, such as pesticides, caffeine, antibiotics, and sugar are discussed elsewhere in this book. This chapter is primarily about the rest of the food additives, how they can be harmful, and where they are found and how to avoid them. More healthful alternatives are given where relevant. You may choose to use this information to eat optimally healthfully, or you may use it to make upgrades or tradeoffs; the important thing is that it will be an informed choice.

Many if not most illnesses, including those discussed in Part 2, have excessive chemical intake as a major contributor. Since most of what we take into our bodies is through ingestion – eating or drinking – chemicals in food can be a significant source of chemically caused illness, and this is one of the most controllable factors in total chemical exposure. The first line of defense in protecting yourself from food-related toxins is to be well informed about the various additives, including those not mentioned on the product label.

What are food additives?
Food additives are substances that do not occur naturally in foods. Thousands of chemicals are deliberately added to our food supply, many of which are not legal for use in other countries such as Canada and parts of Europe.

These food additives can be added intentionally, semi-intentionally, or unintentionally.

- Intentional additives include flavors, colors, preservatives, and texturizers which are intended to be in the finished product.
- Semi-intentional additives include antibiotics given to cattle, and pesticides used on the grain they – and we – eat. The term semi-intentional refers to ad-

ditives that are added deliberately at some point in processing, although it is not intended that they be in the finished product.

- Unintentional additives include substances such as mercury in fish, and chlorine and other toxins in water used for processing of many foods.

Why are additives used?
The bottom line for the food producer or manufacturer is profit – making as much money as possible in as little time as possible. To this end, those involved with food production and sale – farmers, processors, shippers – use whatever methods they can, within legal limits (usually). These methods include:

- Using hormones and antibiotics to more quickly fatten a steer to market weight
- Using preservatives to extend shelf life of food, since wasted food is wasted money
- Coloring oranges, waxing apples, and bleaching flour for consumer eye appeal
- Using pesticides on produce and grain to minimize losses and blemishes from pests
- Raising vegetables for good shipping qualities to minimize expensive losses
- Using cheaper or synthetic ingredients to decrease product cost
- Developing and using artificial sweeteners and imitation oils to meet consumer demand for lower calorie products

How harmful are chemical additives?
Much of what we ingest with our food was never intended by our bodies for consumption. The FDA sets allowable limits of food additives and pesticides with the apparent and erroneous assumption that we will have no additional source of that chemical, or any other chemicals that can interact synergistically to create greater harm. Since no agency can guarantee that any individual is getting a less than harmful total dose of chemicals, it is up to each person to monitor and minimize her or his own intake.

Deciphering labels and watching for deception
Media attention and public awareness about our food supply have been steadily increasing. However, food manufacturers want to sell as much food as possible, and if the government regulations designed to protect us can be fudged or circumvented, they often are, in order to increase product appeal to an increasingly aware consumer audience. Thus product labels can be designed to fool the consumers as much as to enlighten them. It is important to know what is and isn't listed and what the listings mean.

Government labeling regulations state that certain information must be printed on the product label or container, and that the information must be accurate. Other information which we might find useful in order to protect ourselves from harmful ingredients need not be on the label.

Ingredients must be listed in descending order by weight. Only intentional additives need to be listed, and only if they are added to the end product rather than to an intermediate product. For example, a loaf of bread may list flour as the first, or most plentiful, ingredient. The chlorine dioxide used to bleach the flour need not be listed, nor does the pesticide that was added to the grain. Another effect of the rule about descending order by weight is that some manufacturers split up certain ingredients so they aren't as prominent. For example, if sugar of some sort would be the first or second ingredient, and might thus deter some customers, a mix of different kinds of sugar – sucrose, dextrose, maltose, corn syrup – is used, so that no one of them predominates and they can all be listed farther down on the ingredients list.

Flavors and spices can be grouped together and simply called "artificial and natural flavors" or "spices" without elaboration. Even so-called natural flavors may not be very natural after the processing and extraction process.

The government has minimum standards of identity for certain foods, such as mayonnaise, ice cream, catsup, margarine, and milk. Mayonnaise, for example, must contain a minimum amount of whole egg, and ice cream must contain a minimum amount of butterfat. These ingredients do not need to be listed on the label, since they are implied by the name "mayonnaise" or "ice cream." If a product resembles another product for which standards of identity have been set, but does not itself meet these standards, it must be called "imitation" or by another name, frozen dairy dessert, ice milk, sandwich spread, process cheese food, and whipped topping.

Manufacturers must comply with these regulations, but they must also tempt consumers to buy their products. This conflict of interest can lead many of them into packaging practices that are, to put it euphemistically, creative. For example, if a product has a commonly accepted word in its name such as fruit, milk, cream, cheese, meat, or crab, the product must contain a certain minimum percentage of these foods. One way around this regulation is to put the word "flavored" after the word, as in "fruit flavored," and the word "flavored" might be in relatively tiny type. Another common dodge is to use an alternative spelling; for example, fruit, cheese, and crab are legally defined, but froot, cheez, and krab are not. Manufacturers can therefore lure consumers with nonfoods that sound like foods, save money by using unnatural ingredients, and avoid gov-government agency penalties.

FRUIT
flavored
DRINK

What do organic and natural mean?

Other words that are commonly used in these health-conscious times are "organic" and "natural." The term "natural" is used to mean something made by nature, even though that may have been many processing steps ago, so the word has little or no legal or practical meaning.

Organic, on the other hand, has a legal meaning, and farms that are certified organic must undergo rigorous and expensive testing, the cost of which is passed on to consumers.

There are several categories of growing methods, from least to most healthful:

- Conventional
- Unsprayed or transitional
- Commercial organic
- Homegrown organic

Conventional foods are those with all allowed additives. Unsprayed or transitional foods are often sold at farmers' markets, and – assuming the seller is honest, since there is no government oversight – may be the same as organic but without the expensive label for whatever reason.

One might think that organic food is organic food, regardless of where grown, but that isn't the case. Commercial organic food is grown for the purpose of making money, and is defined more by what *isn't* used, such as chemical pesticides and fertilizers. They are grown in chemically clean soil, but that's about it. Homegrown organic foods, where the grower is more concerned with health than with containing costs, is often grown in soil that is enriched by years of composting. Such food is likely to be as different from commercial organic in taste and healthfulness as commercial organic is from conventional. Growing your own or shopping at farmers' markets would be the best alternatives.

What additives are in animal foods?

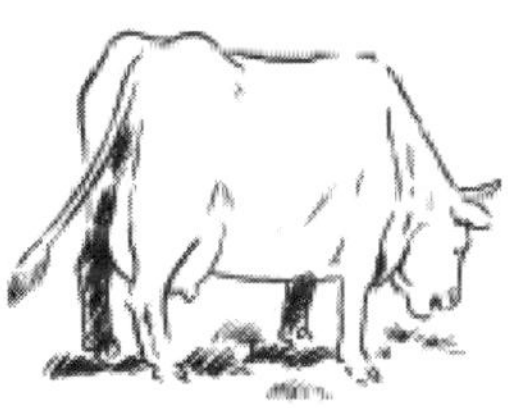

Naturally raised animals, grazing outside on their naturally intended diet, are the healthiest and the most healthful for us, but cattle raising has changed drastically in the name of profit. The ideal beef steer, milk cow, calf, pig, lamb, or chicken is one that stands in one place, usually not voluntarily, and eats around the clock, reaching marketable weight in half the time it would take naturally. Sick or dying cattle cut into profits. To this end, i.e. making money quickly, many drugs and toxins are introduced

Cattle are fed pesticide treated grain, and additional pesticides are often given to treat the parasitic infections that the weakened animals can't fight off themselves. The pesticides can be so concentrated that the animals' excrement will not attract flies.

Antibiotics are used routinely to prevent and treat infections. Since antibiotics kill the beneficial bacteria that keep our yeast under control, the epidemic of recurrent yeast infections may be related to the eating of meat containing antibiotics as well as to the rise in the eating of sugars.

Cattle are given tranquilizers to keep them from wanting to do anything but eat. If you feel sleepy after eating a heavy meat-containing meal, this may have something to do with it, although tryptophans – amino acids naturally found in meat – and the difficulty digesting the protein of large animals can also play a part in post-meal sleepiness.

Growth hormones are sometimes used to cause the animal to grow much faster than nature intended. Parents and doctors throughout the country have noticed that the physical changes of puberty are occurring a year or two earlier on average than in the previous generation, a situation that has been the case over the past few generations. Hormones are given to cattle and chickens to increase their growth rate so they mature and reach marketable weight faster. The resultant meat, milk, chicken, and eggs are consumed in large quantities by children. There may well be a connection between the growth hormones given to food animals and the earlier maturation of our younger generations, as well as a link to the epidemic of obesity in children and adults. If these hormones produce growth, faster maturity, and the accumulation of fat in farm animals, it is reasonable to assume that they would do the same in people.

We are ingesting all these drugs with our steak. Conditions are similar in the mass producing and marketing of other animal products – milk and milk products, lamb, pork, eggs, and chicken.

What about grass-fed meat or free-range chickens?
Meat in itself can be a healthful product, but the additives are so harmful that meat as we know it can be hazardous to health. The best meats are those which have been naturally raised, free to roam and fed pesticide-free food. Some health food store brands and mail order companies can provide such animal products, but it pays to do your homework and not to assume that health food store products are always healthier than commercial alternatives.

There has been more awareness of and concern for how our animals are raised, for reasons of both our health and their humane treatment. A number of buzzwords have been designed to attract these aware consumers: free range, grass fed, cage free, and so forth. Meat from such sources may well be better than the standard feedlot fare, but it still pays to do your research. As with other labeling that has the conflicting goals of informing consumers and catering to their growing awareness, yet wanting to maximize profit, those definitions can be fudged. For example, chickens that are crammed into huge dark coops and let outside for a few minutes a day can be called free range, although the term deliberately and misleadingly calls to mind happy chickens pecking in the dirt all day. Most cattle are grass fed – partially – and then fattened up on grain towards the end of their unnaturally short lives, so the label grass fed might not mean much.

The least healthy animal products are processed meats such as lunch meats, hot dogs, bacon, and some sausage. Ground beef, unless it is very lean, has a very high fat content, in part to keep the cost down, and many chemicals and pesticides are concentrated in fat, making ground beef considerably more toxic than non-ground beef. The high exposed surface area in ground beef also makes it an excellent breeding ground for harmful microorganisms.

Organ meats such as liver and kidney are quite nutritious, but keep in mind that these organs exist for the filtering out of toxins. Unless such meats are from very chemically clean animals, you might be getting a high concentration of the toxins that the animal is trying to remove from its body. Therefore, the source for such meats should be even more scrupulously clean than for muscle meats.

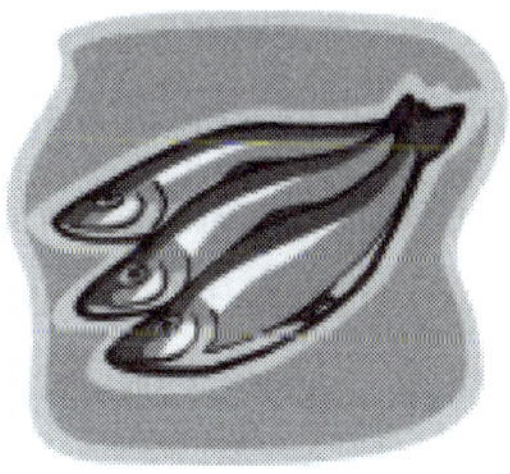

Many varieties of fish are available, and the pollution levels within the fish can vary both by variety and by location. So far there is no definitive answer to the question of which is better, farmed or wild-caught; both have their advantages and disadvantages, both to health and to the environment.

The worst dairy products are those high in fat, such as butter, cheese, and ice cream. Chemicals tend to concentrate in the animals' fat and are excreted in the milk, particularly the fatty cream. Margarine, although not an animal product, is even more toxic than butter and is thus a poor substitute. However, some fat is necessary to fully utilize nutrients in dairy products, so skim milk products have their down side.

So aren't plant foods healthier?

If you have chosen not to eat animal products, you are not home free. Produce and grains are nearly always sprayed with pesticides, unless they are certified organic. Some of the pesticide residues can be removed by washing or by peeling off the vitamin-rich skin, or by washing the produce in a weak bleach solution, hydrogen peroxide, or vegetable washes sold in health food stores. Pesticides, however, are absorbed through the plant roots and permeate the cells of the fruits, vegetables, and grain. Water and air pollution are also absorbed into these plants.

Different types of produce tend to be more or less safe. Grapes, apples, peaches and spinach tend to have higher pesticide and toxic residues than most other produce. Some of the safest produce includes oranges, bananas, asparagus, watermelon, pineapple and cauliflower.[1] Produce with thick skin that is removed before eating is least likely to be contaminated. Organic or home-grown produce is free of most of these toxins; one way to save both money and health would be to shop for organic alternatives to only the most toxic commercial produce.

Plant foods contain many nutritious elements; one that is germane to this book is fiber, which is plentiful in most produce yet nearly missing in animal and processed foods. Fiber helps to undo some of the damage caused by pesticides and other toxins, dietary and otherwise. Fiber binds to toxic chemicals to remove them rapidly from your body, and can also keep them from being absorbed through the intestine into the bloodstream and then into your cells. Fiber exerts a physical action that can be simplistically compared to a whisk broom; it also exerts a chemical action similar to that of a carbon water filter by binding to toxins. Whole grains such as brown rice, whole wheat, quinoa, and millet, especially if organically grown, are good sources of fiber.

INTENTIONAL ADDITIVES

The many types of intentional additives include the following:

Preservatives may be used to prevent the formation of toxic breakdown products such as aflatoxins from the mold on peanuts and potatoes, and to keep out insect pests. In this case they have a beneficial effect which outweighs the hazards. Unfortunately, preservatives are often used for the comparatively frivolous purpose of maintaining a fresh appearance. Harmful preservatives include[2-4]:

- Sodium sulfite — Used in salad bars, dried fruit, fish. High allergic potential
- Calcium propionate — Used in baked goods and processed foods
- Sodium nitrate, nitrite — Used in cured meats. Can form cancerous nitrosamines
- BHA and BHT — Used in baked goods, cereals, oils, potato chips.

Sodium nitrite and potassium nitrite, used mostly in cured and processed meats, are used to keep the color of processed meats reddish rather than the grey color caused by oxidation, add to the flavor, and inhibit the growth of some microorganisms. Nitrates and nitrites can form nitrosamines, which are highly carcinogenic in the body. Nitrates also come from chemical fertilizers, and harmful levels of nitrates are more likely to be found in produce that has been fertilized and in water contaminated by runoff. A diet rich in the antioxidant vitamins C (ascorbate) and E (tocopherol) has a protective effect.

Preservatives that are beneficial or at least not harmful include:

- Ascorbic acid, ascorbate — Used in fruits and acid foods. This is vitamin C.
- Citric acid — Used in acidic foods, fruits. Safer than most.
- Tocopherols — Vitamin E – harmless, beneficial.
- EDTA — Chelating agent to remove minerals that may cause deterioration or discoloration.

- Benzoic acid — Used in beverages, baked goods, ice cream.
- Sodium benzoate — Margarine, soft drinks

A warning, though – sodium benzoate can combine with ascorbic acid (vitamin C) to form the toxic solvent benzene in the body. Both of these can be found together in some sodas and other products.

Antioxidants are a class of preservative. They are used to prevent changes due to oxidation, or oxygen. Examples of these changes are the browning of potatoes, carrot juice, or fruit such as apples and bananas.

BHA and BHT, used in convenience foods since 1947, are used to prevent food from changing color or flavor or becoming rancid. They have been associated with learning and behavioral disorders and cancer. BHA combined with nitrites, under acidic conditions simulating those in the stomach, can form highly toxic compounds with carcinogenic potential. This sort of reactivity is a warning to those who rely on animal studies in which only one additive or chemical is tested at a time – the safe threshold quantity is probably much lower when multiple chemicals are present, as they usually are. TBHQ and propyl gallate are preservatives that are also suspected carcinogens.

Sulfites are a class of antioxidants and preservatives that also include sulfur dioxide, sodium sulfite, sodium bisulfite, sodium metabisulfite, and potassium bisulfite, and are sometimes listed on the label as sulfiting agents. Sulfites used to be used to keep salad bar items fresh, but due to severe allergic reactions that killed several restaurant patrons they are now rarely used for this purpose. Sulfites in amounts over 10ppm, which has been judged an amount sufficient to cause problems in sensitive individuals, must be listed on food labels. However, there is a loophole: if, for example, manufacturers use sulfited dried fruits in baked goods, but do not add sulfites directly to the product, they do not have to put sulfites on the label.

Recommended antioxidants and preservatives with little or no known toxicity include:

- Alpha tocopherol — Vitamin E
- Ascorbic acid, sodium ascorbate — Vitamin C
- Calcium and sodium propionate — Used to inhibit mold
- Erythorbic acid — Used in meat products, baked goods, beverages
- Fumaric acid — Used in baked goods; from plant source
- Lecithin — Used especially in fat-containing products
- Potassium sorbate — Mold inhibitor
- Sodium benzoate — Allergic potential, but otherwise relatively safe

Stabilizers and thickeners are used to keep foods such as salad dressing from separating, and to improve "mouthfeel" (a self-explanatory food industry term). Although they are not necessary, they are for the most part relatively harmless. Most of these are safe and natural products derived from seaweeds, gums, lecithin, pectin, and cellulose. Examples of relatively safe products are:

- Alginate — From seaweed, to thicken salad dressing and ice cream
- Calcium/sodium stearyl lactate — Used to strengthen bread dough
- Casein, sodium caseinate — Complete protein derived from milk
- Furcelleran — Stabilizer and emulsifier from seaweed
- Gelatin — Food thickener and stabilizer; of animal origin
- Glycerin, glycerol — Used in candies
- Guar gum — Stabilizer and thickener in beverages
- Gum arabic — Stabilizer, prevents sugar crystallization
- Gum tragacanth — Thickener and stabilizer
- Lecithin — Emulsifier, antioxidant, prevents ingredient separation
- Sorbitan monostearate — Emulsifier, defoaming and flavor dispersing agent

Bleaches whiten food, or remove color so that artificial color will look better. Bleaches are primarily used on flour, oils, margarine, and fruits. Chemicals used include calcium bromate, potassium bromide, chlorine dioxide, and nitrogen peroxide, which are toxic. The use of these products is especially unacceptable considering the purely cosmetic benefit gained combined with the products' toxicity.

Humectants, also call humefactants, keep food moist by absorbing and retaining water. They are used mainly in baked goods, cake mixes, meats, and marshmallows. Humectants include:

- Polyphosphates — Injected or rubbed into meat
- Propylene glycol — Used in your car in larger amounts as antifreeze; toxic
- Glycerol, glycerine — Used in toaster foods, marshmallows, flaked coconut
- Mannitol, sorbitol — Also used as sweeteners. Not beneficial, but less harmful than other humectants and sweeteners.

Waxes are used to give a shiny coating to jelly beans and other candies, and to both shine (for consumer appeal) and preserve fruits and vegetables such as apples, cucumbers, and peppers. Most of these waxes are petroleum derivatives such as paraffin, carnauba, and petroleum naphtha, and differ from the wax on your car only in quantity. Fungicides, some of which have been associated with the development of cancer, are often added to the waxes. Fruits and vegetables most likely to be waxed include[1]:

- Apples
- Citrus fruits
- Avocados
- Melons
- Cucumbers
- Peppers

- Squashes, pumpkins
- Eggplant
- Sweet potatoes

Anticaking agents are used to prevent caking in powdered foods and table salt. Almost any additive with aluminum and/or silicate in the name, such as sodium aluminosilicate, calcium silicate, or silicon dioxide, is likely to be an anticaking agent. Silica is basically sand, and aluminum is a toxic metal in salt form which has been linked to Alzheimer's disease.

Artificial colors are used to impart, enhance, or disguise colors of foods. Artificial colors can be divided into two categories – naturally derived and chemically created. Chemical colors usually go by names such as FD&C (Food, Drug, and Cosmetic) Red (or blue or yellow) Number such-and-such. Each number has a different formula, and these are periodically taken off the market and replaced as cancer-causing potential or other risk is discovered. Some of these colors are listed individually on labels due to their high allergic potential, while others are lumped together as "artificial colors."

Food dyes are stored in the lymph nodes, essentially forever. For example, if you eat beets or take riboflavin (vitamin B2), your urine may temporarily and harmlessly turn red or bright yellow as your body eliminates the natural coloring agent. However, if you eat an artificially dyed food, your urine usually does not change color. This means the dyes are not being excreted and are thus retained in the body, which does not know what to do with them.

Allergic reactions to tartrazine, also known as yellow dye #5, have been reported as early as the 1940s, so yellow #5 and #6 are now required to be listed separately on labels. Many people who are sensitive to aspirin or salicylates are also sensitive to these two colors. Symptoms of ingestion include facial swelling, tissue swelling (edema), stuffy nose, or asthma attacks. A number of other food colors have been linked to the development of cancer.

Naturally derived colors of plant or animal origin are generally safe, and include:

- Beta carotene — Vitamin A precursor, found in carrots. Orange-yellow color.
- Caramel — From cooked sugar, gives brownish color and characteristic flavor
- Beet juice — Reddish color
- Riboflavin — Yellowish color and nutrient (vitamin B2)
- Saffron — Bright yellow-orange
- Chlorophyll — From green plants. Green color
- Ferrous gluconate — Also a good source of iron
- Cochineal — From ground-up beetle; sounds gross, but harmless
- Turmeric — In curry; beneficial; yellow-orange color
- Annatto — yellow-orange coloring from achiote seed

Artificial flavors – At least 1700 natural and artificial flavoring agents are used in food.[1] Artificial flavors are usually made by analyzing a real food flavor (such as vanilla, lemon, or ham) to determine the combination of chemicals that produce the flavor, then reproducing the primary one(s) in the lab.

MSG enhances flavor by stimulating your taste buds – in other words, it doesn't change the food, it changes *you*. Unlike the other additives, which incidentally have an effect on the body, MSG has such an effect by design. MSG can cause many symptoms, including:

- Flushing
- Rashes
- Fatigue
- Joint pain
- Anxiety
- Irregular heartbeat
- Nausea
- Asthma
- Hunger soon after eating
- Chest tightness
- Worsening of migraines
- Fatal anaphylactic shock in those who are very sensitive

Many people are cleared of a variety of symptoms when MSG is removed from their diet.

If you have problems with MSG (which may or may not be listed on the package label), other compounds which are similar to or contain MSG should be avoided as well:

- Sodium or calcium caseinate
- Hydrolyzed or textured vegetable protein
- Autolyzed yeast
- MSG may be part of "flavoring" or "natural flavoring"

Artificial sweeteners are, for the most part, neurotoxic, and have been discussed in conjunction with several health ailments in Part 2.

What are trans fats, and why are they so bad for me?

Trans fats have been in the news over the past few years. Most people at this point know that trans fats are harmful, but don't know much beyond that. The news about trans fats started making headlines in the early to mid 2000s; prior to that very few people had heard of them. Interestingly, however, the Toxic Twins books, written by the authors of this book and published in 1996, contained considerable information about trans fats, well ahead of the curve.

Trans fats and cis fats are two different shapes of a fatty acid molecule, The cis form is what is necessary to build body tissues, nerve cell sheathing, and cell walls, and to help with detoxification. The trans form tries to perform cis functions in body systems but is unable to do so, and additionally blocks the cis fatty acids from being able to do their job. Trans fats are created when oils are heated, as in food processing. Cis oils turn into trans readily, but the converse is not true. Within the past few years trans fat information has been included on the labels of many foods.

An example of the conversion of cis to trans oils occurs on the outside of an oil bottle. When salad oil drips down the side of the oil bottle and is not wiped up, and is exposed to air, it becomes sticky rather than oily, i.e. trans rather than cis, and is very difficult to wash off. Trans fatty acids are sticky and less easily dissolved in the body as well.

Heating up or frying with oils in home cooking will also change cis oils to trans. Ironically, as saturated (solid) fats have gained a bad reputation, some restaurants have announced that they now fry with vegetable oils rather than solid shortening or lard, implying that this is healthier for you. As the vegetable oil is heated, it converts to the trans form. This occurs even in home cooking, where it can take up to a half hour to fry some foods, but in restaurants or manufacturing plants that fry snack foods such as chips, the oil may be kept at a destructive high temperature for days. The longer the oil is heated, the more conversion takes place. For this reason, you are actually better off cooking or frying with solid shortening than with oil.

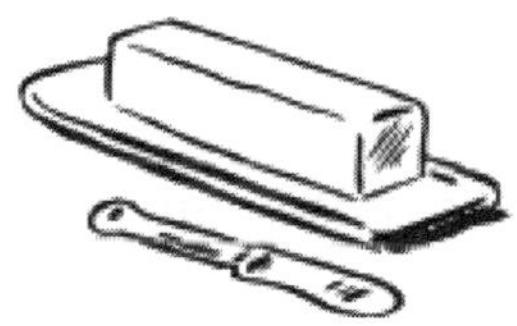

Margarine has been the prime example of trans fat, because oils are hydrogenated to form a solid. With all the publicity about trans fats, some margarine manufacturers claim that their new product has no trans fats. Even if this is true, it remains that margarine is an artificial product, and your body has no idea what to do with it other than store it in your fat cells.

Nutrient enrichment is a good thing, right?

Nutrients are added to enrich or fortify foods. "Enriched" refers to the few synthetic vitamins added, for example to flour, to replace the many natural nutrients removed in processing. People are often misled into believing that such foods are actually healthful, and may be less likely to work at getting proper nutrition as a result.

"Fortified" refers to nutrients added to products where they would not be found normally, for example orange juice with added calcium. Fortification is done primarily to appeal to the health-conscious consumer.

What about the advice to avoid ingredients I can't pronounce?

Advice about which food ingredients are safe and which to avoid has been summed up as: if you can't pronounce it, or don't know what it is, don't eat it. This is sound advice, but only up to a point. The shortness and familiarity of simple, commonly used words such as sugar and flour shouldn't blind people to the fact that these should ideally not be eaten. On the other hand, ingredients such as cyanocobalamin and pyridoxine hydrochloride can sound like a scary chemical brew, but they are simply B vitamins.

What kinds of semi-intentional additives are there?
Pesticides, antibiotics, and hormones, all semi-intentional, are discussed in the Chemicals chapter, the Drugs chapter, and earlier in this chapter respectively.

One class of semi-intentional additives is plasticizers and other materials that leach into the food product from plastic wraps and containers, Styrofoam containers, and milk and juice cartons. There has been little regulation of food packaging with respect to chemicals that could leach into food. There are variables that complicate an analysis of the problem – the different types of containers and chemicals, the types of food stored or cooked (acidic foods can leach certain chemicals, fatty foods can leach others), maximum cooking temperatures, length of storage in the container, and how the food is cooked (oven or microwave). Benzene, toluene, and xylene are among the toxic and carcinogenic chemicals found in some food packaging that can migrate into food when heated. Some plastics may be safe to microwave in, especially hard plastics and those labeled microwave-safe. Less safe to use are flexible plastic containers such as margarine tubs and Styrofoam containers. The food can become hot enough to melt the plastic where it touches the food.

What are some of the unintentional additives?
Metals, discussed in the next chapter, are often found in foods. Metals are both toxic in themselves and work against our optimum health by blocking the actions of minerals with the same chemical valence, or outer electron shell of the molecule. For example, toxic ionic mercury, if present, can take the place of necessary zinc or iron in biochemical reactions. The flip side of this metal-mineral antagonism is the good news: an adequate intake of minerals such as iron and calcium can be protective against the toxic effects of metals.

Some food ingredients contain metals directly:

- Baked goods can contain sodium **aluminum** silicate or aluminum hydroxide for leavening, and aluminum compounds prevent caking in some commercial salt.
- The solder line in "tin" cans used to be lead, and may still be lead in imported food cans. **Lead** pipes and soldered joints are still found in old plumbing, and the lead can be leached out into household water which is then used for drinking and cooking.
- Although **mercury** dental fillings are the most significant mercury source for most Americans, there are food sources of mercury, most notably large fish and some insecticide-sprayed produce.
- **Cadmium** is sometimes taken in by fish which live in polluted water, and by food animals. Cadmium is a component of vehicle tires and brakes, which

slough off tiny particles of cadmium as the vehicle is driven. Cattle feedlots and farms which produce grain for both people and cattle, and which are near well-traveled roads, may thus have significant amounts of cadmium in the soil, air and water. This toxic metal is then passed on in the meat and produce to the people who ingest them.

- **Arsenic** is most often found in seafood and kelp, wine, and in store-bought grains due to insecticide or rodenticide contamination.

What other kinds of pollutants are there?
Pollutants in water, discussed in the chapter on Water Pollution, may be deliberately added to the water or their presence may be inadvertent. Since all produce and food animals are routinely given water, these pollutants end up in the food you eat.

Parasites and microorganisms, which have their own chapter in this section, can contaminate meat and produce. These can be transmitted by fruit pickers and handlers, who are rarely tested for parasites. If you eat out, eat only cooked foods. Foods containing a lot of garlic or cayenne have a protective effect.

Radiation in food is a subject that encompasses fallout from nuclear accidents such as that at Chernobyl decades ago, and radon, a naturally occurring radioactive substance found in the ground and in the groundwater in certain parts of the world. Both forms of radiation can contaminate crops, which then enters our bodies either directly or through the intermediate step of consuming food animals. Radiation can cause a number of adverse health effects, including mutagenic effects and cancers, birth defects, and immune system malfunctions.

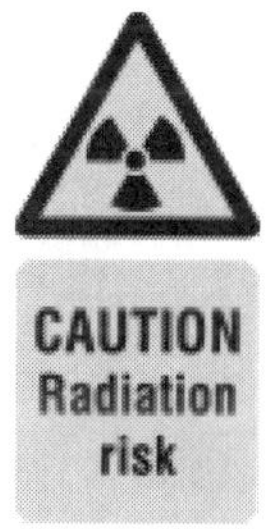

Another aspect of radiation concerns the effect of deliberate irradiation of food, and it has been the cause of some controversy. Proponents say that irradiating food kills bacteria, molds, and parasites, which is true. It allows foods that otherwise need refrigeration or freezing to be kept on the shelf rather than in the refrigerator or freezer, and it increases shelf life for many types of foods, including fresh fruits, vegetables, meats, herbs and spices. Proponents also give the assurance that irradiation leaves no residue on the food, nor does it make the food radioactive. However, there is another side to the story. The frequencies involved are, of necessity, sufficient to kill and mutate cells (bacteria and parasites are cells, as are once-live foods such as vegetables and meat), and it is not known what taking these damaged cells and the resulting enzyme-free dead food into our bodies will do over time. Long term human toxicity studies have not been done, and cancer can take decades to develop.

Metals

What are metals?

To a chemist, a metal is anything in the left-hand two-thirds of the periodic table, classified as such based on the way these elements combine with other materials. Necessary minerals are also in this category, but too much can be toxic. Copper, for example, is a necessary mineral, crucial for enzymatic and other body reactions, but too much is poisonous. Although the lay person might think of a metal as a recognizable shiny substance, the ionic, or salt, form of the metal is the one that is a problem, since metals in this form can combine with body tissues to do damage.

How do metals do their damage?

Metals do their damage in one or more of these ways:

Fight for site – Ions with the same electron valence, or charge (such as +2), can substitute for each other in the chemical reactions which allow the body to function properly. For example, toxic ionic mercury or cadmium, if present, can take the place of necessary zinc or iron in biochemical reactions.

Charge – Two or more dissimilar metals in an electrically conductive medium called an electrolyte form a type of battery. Body fluids such as saliva or blood act as an electrolyte, and metals in the mouth from fillings, crowns, and root canal posts complete the battery, causing what can be called the Battery Effect. Once the dissimilar metals form an anode and cathode, corrosion takes place as on the poles of a car battery and leaches into the mouth. The water-soluble toxic metal salts formed as corrosion products then enter the rest of the body. The charge can also adversely affect the nervous system and the heart, both of which are electrical in nature.

Antibiotic – Mercury, in particular, has an antibiotic (anti-life) effect. Metal salts, in fact, used to be commonly used as pesticides in agriculture, and mercury and other salts were used as antibiotics before more modern antibiotics were developed. Mercury in the mouth kills beneficial bacteria in the body that keep yeast under control.

Stealing substances – Iron transports oxygen to sites where it is needed in the body. If mercury substitutes for iron, oxygen will not be transported to as great an extent. Mercury will bind to the oxygen to form an oxide of mercury, which, unlike oxygen, is not useful to the body. Sulfur and selenium, essential materials, are "stolen" in similar ways.

Genetic – Nickel, in particular, adversely affects RNA, which is part of the process of cell duplication. Improper cell duplication leads to cell mutations which can then lead to cancer and birth defects.

Clog detox pathways – Metallothionein is a natural sulfur containing substance in the body that clears heavy metals. A greater metal burden than the body is able to bear will clog this detox pathway. Mercury in the body can thus interfere with the removal of aluminum, and a buildup of both mercury and aluminum has been linked to Alzheimer's disease.

Free radicals involve an atom with an unpaired electron (an odd number of electrons in the outer shell). The unpaired electron wants to find a mate, and will rip an electron from the nearest atom it finds, creating a new free radical in a chain reaction. These free radicals can sclerose (harden) arteries or cause cancer.

Allergy – The immune system recognizes the body's own tissues as self and leaves them alone, while attacking anything non-self. Metal may bind with the protein in the body's tissues, causing the immune system to see these tissues as unfamiliar non-self. The immune system's resulting attack on parts of the body is known as autoimmune disease, which may also have causes other than metals.

Where are toxic metals found?
Metals can be found in a number of places, some of which are obvious and some less so.

- Amalgam fillings — mercury, silver
- Dental crowns, artificial joints — nickel
- Cooking utensils — iron, aluminum, stainless steel with nickel, copper
- Old paint — lead, mercury
- Antiperspirants — aluminum
- Inexpensive earrings — nickel (in stainless steel)
- Some glazed pottery — lead
- Cigarettes — cadmium, nickel, arsenic
- Batteries — lead, cadmium, nickel
- Auto exhaust — lead, platinum, cadmium, aluminum
- Insecticides — arsenic, mercury
- Metronidazole (antifungal drug) — arsenic

What are some of the most significant toxic metals?
Mercury and nickel are two of the most toxic metals. They are also the ones most likely to be found in the bodies of people of industrialized countries. The majority of people have mercury amalgam fillings in their mouths, at least in the US, and millions of people also have nickel in their mouths in the form of stainless steel crowns, root canal posts, and braces. Other metals like-

ly to cause problems are lead, cadmium, copper, aluminum, and arsenic. The focus in this chapter is on the most likely suspects, primarily mercury and other dental sources.

If metal poisoning is one of your health problems, the chapter on Metal Detoxification in Part 4 can explain how to remove metals from your body.

Mercury

The role of mercury in the development of a number of diseases and ailments is discussed in Part 2. One source of mercury is some large fish, although seafood also has selenium and sulfur, which provide a protective effect by binding the mercury to limit its ability to enter into damaging reactions. Historically, there have been other sources of mercury, such as thimerosal, the preservative in vaccines, as well as pesticides and medicines, but these have been phased out or replaced as the dangers of mercury become known. Today, by far the largest source of mercury is metal dental fillings, although awareness of their harmfulness is growing.

Why is mercury so toxic?

Mercury in all forms is particularly dangerous because it is so easily absorbed into the body, due in part to its being liquid. Metallic and organic mercury especially are very volatile, meaning they enter the air rapidly from the liquid state and are then inhaled. For this reason, a mercury spill from a broken thermometer or spilled fungicide should never be vacuumed up unless exhausted to the outside, as this would disperse the mercury into the air to be readily inhaled. Mercury is also easily absorbed through skin, lung tissue, and, if ingested, stomach and intestinal tissue. Chelators, discussed in the Metal Detoxification chapter in Part 4, can pull mercury out of these tissues.

Methylmercury, 100 times more toxic than elemental mercury, is formed in our mouths by a bacterium called streptococcus mutans, which is in everyone's mouths.[1] Methylmercury is detoxified in the body to the comparatively less toxic elemental mercury, but if this mercury is not eliminated, the mercury will remethylate back to methylmercury in a never ending cycle.[2]

How can I tell whether I have mercury fillings?

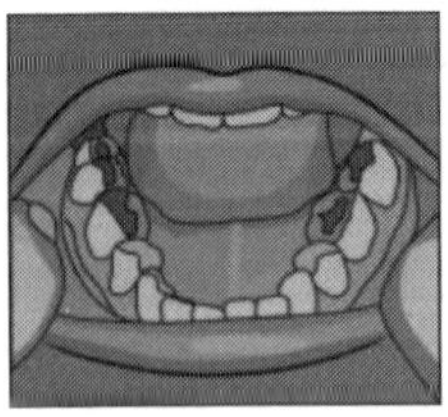

Mercury fillings are the dark dental fillings in the teeth, as compared with composite fillings which are tooth-colored. Mercury fillings range in color from shiny or dull silver to black; they start out silvery and then oxidize to black over time. Release of mercury from the fillings into the body is highest when they are new and silvery.

The terms silver fillings and amalgam fillings are also used; these are synonymous with mercury fillings. These fillings contain about 30-35% silver, 15% tin or tin and copper, a trace of zinc, and a full 50-54% of mercury[3], although the exact composition can vary between manufacturers.

Since mercury is the greatest component of amalgam fillings by weight regardless of manufacturer, they should more accurately be called mercury fillings rather than silver, even though silver sounds nicer and makes a good euphemism.

How is mercury absorbed from fillings?

Mercury is absorbed from our fillings in several ways:

- **Lungs** – Volatile mercury, vaporized from the surface of the fillings, is inhaled, and from there passes into the blood.
- **Nose** – Some of this vapor enters the nasal pharynx in the nose and is absorbed by the nerve fibers there that lead directly to the brain. For this reason, this is the preferred route for ingestion of cocaine and snuff. Inhaled mercury reaches the brain just as quickly.
- **Roots** – Mercury is forced by expansion down through the tooth root, into the bones and gums and from there into the bloodstream. This is particularly true of teeth with crowns, as mercury expands and contracts with heat and cold (remember what thermometers contained, and why). With crowns over the fillings the expanding mercury has nowhere to go but toward the root. The strongest battery-driven migration is for nickel/stainless steel caps and posts.
- **Stomach** – Broken bits of fillings and minute amounts of corrosion products are worked loose through chewing and then swallowed. Expansion and contraction of the filling from eating hot and cold foods can crack teeth over time, releasing more mercury bits to be swallowed. The mercury is then absorbed from the stomach into the bloodstream.
- **Gums** – Mercury is absorbed through the gums and mucous membranes of the mouth. It then enters the bloodstream through the capillaries in these tissues.

Mercury is transported and absorbed primarily through the blood, lymph, and nerve axons, and migrates throughout the body.

Mercury is released continuously even when one is at rest. An even greater amount of mercury is released during placement or removal of fillings and when chewing and swallowing.

What kinds of symptoms does mercury cause?

Symptoms of mercury toxicity are many and varied, since mercury can both reach and affect nearly every cell in the body. Systemic (overall) effects can occur for this reason; some of these are discussed in more detail in Part 2. The particular symptoms you experience first depend on your own genetic weakest links and on other toxic suppressors. These symptoms may include the following[4]:

- **Behavioral** – depression, mood swings, inability to concentrate, forgetfulness, sleep disturbances, irritability
- **Central nervous system** – light and sound sensitivity, headaches, tremors and muscle twitches, numbness and tingling of extremities, dizziness, hearing or vision difficulty, MS. Mercury is one of the substances that can cross the blood-brain barrier, and so it tends to accumulate in the brain.
- **Detoxification systems** – By overloading the detoxification pathways, other toxins such as aluminum are eliminated less efficiently.
- **Cardiovascular** – abnormal heartbeat and blood pressure, pressure and pain in chest, damaged blood vessels
- **Blood** – Mercury binds to hemoglobin in the red blood cells, reducing oxygen carrying capacity.
- **Digestive** – constipation or diarrhea, digestion problems, colitis, loss of appetite, ulcers, bloating and gas, loss of smell and taste due to zinc displacement
- **Endocrine** – thyroid dysfunction, decreased libido
- **Energy** – Chronic fatigue, drowsiness, muscle weakness
- **Immune system** – allergies, asthma, multiple chemical sensitivity, swollen glands, susceptibility to colds and infection
- **Joints and muscles** – arthritis, fibromyalgia, leg and muscle cramps, lupus
- **Kidney problems**, frequent night urination, kidney stones
- **Oral cavity** – bad breath, bleeding gums, canker sores, bone loss, increased salivation (due to battery effect), metallic taste, periodontal (gum and jawbone) disease, purple-black gum pigment near fillings (sometimes called mercury tattoo), leukoplakia (an oral precancerous condition)
- **Reproductive** – infertility, miscarriage, premature birth
- **Skin** – acne, itching, skin flushing, rough skin, rashes; pimples on skin over fillings

What is the dispute about mercury?

Mercury's poisonous nature is not in dispute. The American Dental Association (ADA) admits mercury comes out of amalgam, reversing its previous position that it does not. However, their official position, as is the case with tobacco companies, is that their primary product, in this case mercury, has not been proven to be harmful. As in the case with the seemingly arbitrary assigning of drugs into categories of legal and illegal, decisions that appear to be about public health are really about politics and powerful lobbies – political science rather than science. Dentists are trained in ADA-accredited schools, and in some states are even prevented from telling patients about the toxicity of mercury, so it is ultimately up to the consumers to gather their own data and protect their own interests.

What can sheep tell us about mercury toxicity?

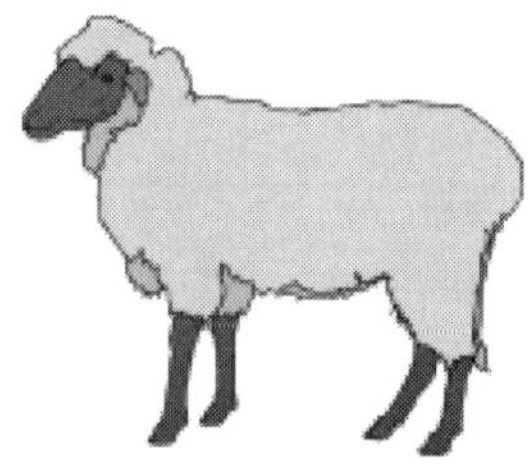

In an experiment done at the University of Calgary in Canada[5], sheep had amalgam fillings placed in their mouths. After 29 days, tests were run on the sheep and their tissues to determine whether and where the mercury had migrated in the body. Keep in mind that fillings leach mercury into our bodies for far longer than 29 days.

Large amounts of mercury were found in the kidneys, liver, feces, stomach, tooth bone, and gums. The highest amounts were shown in the kidneys, but comparatively little was found in the urine, which is where many doctors look. This means that the mercury concentrates in the kidneys and is not released into the urine; i.e. doesn't come out of you. Since the kidneys filter out all kinds of toxins for excretion as urine, the fact that mercury is concentrated there indicates that this detoxification pathway can be blocked by the mercury and will not work as well as it should in removing other toxins. Since the kidneys are involved in electrolyte balancing, blocking the kidney may cause electrolyte imbalance in the body, particularly of potassium, sodium, magnesium, and calcium. Large amounts in the stomach indicate that mercury is indeed ingested from fillings during chewing. Mercury is also found in the fetus and placenta, indicating that, contrary to prior belief, the fetus absorbs a substantial amount of this toxin before birth.

Should metal fillings be removed?

In the large majority of cases, metal fillings should be removed; only then can the accumulation of mercury in the body start to be reversed. However, it is crucial that they be removed properly; otherwise, more mercury can enter the body. The chapter on Metal Detoxification in Part 4 includes detailed guidelines for safe mercury removal, as well as information about chelating out the mercury and other metals from the body afterwards.

What kind of improvement is expected after removal?

Nobody can make any guarantees about the amount, type, or timing of improvement after amalgam removal. Some patients, especially those with a mercury sensitivity or electrical charges, report a dramatic and almost immediate (within one day) improvement. Some report an improvement so slow and slight that it was only noticed several months later upon looking back. Some report no improvement at all, or improvement in only some of their symptoms. This may be due in part to the fact that, although mercury is out of the mouth, it may take some time to get it out of the body. Removing the fillings is like turning off the faucet. Now you still have to drain the tub through chelation.

Many patients and both authors feel strongly enough about mercury toxicity that they have had their amalgam fillings removed and replaced. Most patients and both authors experienced noticeable improvement after removal.

What are some statistics for improvement?

In one study[6], 762 patients who had their mercury fillings removed filled out a report detailing a wide variety of symptoms present before amalgam removal, and then evaluated whether each symptom improved after removal. Each symptom experienced by each patient was looked at separately. 3792 symptoms were reported by the 762 patients. Of these 3792 symptoms,

- 758, or 20%, were reported cured after amalgam removal
- 2812, or 74%, improved noticeably
- 188, or 5%, stayed the same six months after removal
- 34, or 0.9%, reported a worsening of the symptom

This improvement is convincing evidence of the toxicity of mercury fillings. It also provides cause for optimism for those who are considering amalgam removal. Some symptoms showed an especially impressive improvement:

Symptom	Improved or cured
Depression	100% (of 181)
Fatigue	95%
Allergies	88.7%
Headaches	95%
Memory loss	93.5%
Multiple sclerosis	78.5%

What should metal fillings be replaced with?

Plastic composites and porcelain are suitable replacements. It is important that the fillings used be biocompatible: not harmful in general, and not something that the individual might be sensitive to. To minimize sensitivity reactions, there are various types of testing of dental materials.

Nickel

What is another of the most harmful metals?

Nickel is one of the most common severe metal toxicities in humans in industrialized societies. Like mercury, the primary source of poisoning is right in your own mouth. Although trace amounts of nickel are needed to enable the enzyme system to run properly, nickel has no other known use in the human body.

What kinds of harmful reactions can nickel cause?

Allergies – Nickel is the most potent allergen of all the trace elements, accounting for more contact dermatitis and other allergic reactions than all other metals combined. Up to 33% of women and 17% of men are allergic to nickel. A sign of nickel allergy is the development of hot, red, itchy earlobes soon after putting on inexpensive earrings, which are usually made of nickel-containing stainless steel, although lack of a noticeable reaction does not mean that one is not allergic. People wearing cheap earrings can actually develop nickel allergy by being sensitized to a metal they might not otherwise come in contact with. If you have a reaction to earrings in addition to having root-canalled teeth and/or other allergies and health problems, nickel is likely a problem for you.

Most allergic symptoms from nickel in the mouth are systemic, not oral. These symptoms include eczema, asthma, autoimmune disease such as lupus or arthritis, headaches, and mucus in the throat. Itchy anus is often caused by nickel irritating the lining of the intestinal and anal mucosa as it is excreted. The itching and soreness is essentially the same reaction as sensitive individuals have on their earlobes from inexpensive earrings. Nickel can cause an anaphylactic reaction, an acute (sudden) allergic response in which the body's systems are overwhelmed by a massive histamine reaction that can be fatal within minutes.

Carcinogenicity – The cancer causing potential of nickel is so well known that laboratory scientists who want to study cancer in animals will often inject the animals with a nickel solution to reliably cause cancer. Intestinal, oral, and breast cancer are often caused by nickel.

> **Patient profile**
> One patient, a nurse, got braces at age 26. A sharp end of the braces poked her repeatedly in the side of her mouth. A cancerous tumor developed at the site of irritation and quickly enlarged to the size of a melon. She was dead from cancer at age 28, only two years after she got the braces. Information learned from this nurse's condition was used to save the life of another patient in a similar situation.

Immune system effects – Nickel can decrease the effectiveness of the immune system, which can result in infection and cancer. Nickel can cause or at least contribute to autoimmune disorders such as lupus, arthritis, ulcers, endometriosis, and digestive system inflammations.

Other effects – Other symptoms caused by nickel and its compounds include[7]:

- Chronic fatigue, which usually has multiple causes; malaise
- Digestive system difficulties such as nausea, diarrhea, colitis, ulcers, and poor digestion
- CNS stimulation leading to muscle tremors, and paralysis

- Dizziness, insomnia, irritability, muscle weakness
- Meningeal contraction from nickel irritation can cause headache and head pressure, low back and neck pain, and light sensitivity.
- Cirrhosis of the liver
- Low blood pressure, with dizziness on arising and lack of energy
- Nasal polyps from root canals in the top front teeth
- Bipolar disorder, also known as manic-depressive illness, can be caused by the nickel in dental braces; depression
- Both nickel and mercury suppress iron, copper, and cobalt (found in vitamin B12), leading to anemia.
- Nickel can block calcium channels in the heart, lowering magnesium levels and leading to heart arrhythmias.
- Seizures from electrical charges or allergy – one patient who was given a nickel dental retainer developed epileptic seizures within three weeks, which stopped when the retainer was removed.
- Urinary tract infections, endometriosis
- Arthritis

Patient profiles

A 20 year old male had a wire dental retainer made from nickel / stainless steel. For five years, he had ulcers, digestive problems, mucus in his throat, and recurrent lung infections. He had the wire taken out and dealt with fungus problems caused by the antibiotics the doctors had given him for the presumed lung infections. The health problems, caused initially by nickel allergy, cleared up.

Another 20-year-old patient with a wire dental retainer was experiencing seizures of unknown cause. He was on Dilantin, an anticonvulsant medication. As soon as he had the retainer taken out and was chelated for metals, the seizures, throat mucus, low energy and attention problems cleared.

Where else is nickel found, and how does it get into the body?

The primary sources of nickel are dental, dietary, and industrial. Nickel is commonly used in dental work to make crowns, and as components of orthodontic braces and root-canal posts. Dietary sources include[8]:

- tea
- cabbage, legumes

- herring, oysters
- buckwheat, oats, unrefined grains
- refined and processed food, especially those with hydrogenated fats and oils

Nickel is used as a catalyst in the hydrogenation of vegetable oils, including margarine production. Stainless steel is used in grinding grains, unless stone ground, and the nickel in the stainless steel may contaminate the ground grain.

Industrial and other sources include fossil fuel emissions, batteries, stainless steel, nickel plating, some cosmetics, super-phosphate fertilizers, tobacco smoke, and "white gold" metal. Stainless steel cookware may transmit some nickel to foods, particularly acidic ones which can cause metal leaching. Frequent handling of coins, especially – not surprisingly – nickels, can cause sensitization to the metal.

Cadmium

How is cadmium like mercury?

Cadmium is in the same group in the periodic table as mercury and zinc. Like mercury, cadmium blocks the usage of the essential mineral zinc in the body. Zinc is needed for the immune system, and lower zinc levels correlate to lowered immune function. Cadmium, having a +2 charge, also interferes with other +2 minerals such as iron (needed in blood) and calcium (needed in bones).

Where is cadmium found?

Cadmium is found in:

- Cigarette smoke
- Paints
- Metal plating
- Galvanized pipes
- Batteries (nickel-cadmium)
- Fish from polluted water
- Particles from auto tires and brakes
- Dental amalgam

What happens when you are exposed to cadmium?

Cadmium tends to accumulate until the threshold of resistance is overcome, and can then strike with apparent suddenness. One of the first symptoms of cadmium overexposure is high blood pressure. With higher exposure, likely due to cadmium's effect on aldosterone, the kidneys and liver are damaged and the blood pressure then falls. The higher blood pressure puts strain on the heart, which can lead to an apparently sudden heart attack.

Cadmium poisoning can also contribute to:

- Abdominal pain, anorexia, weight loss and vomiting due to cadmium replacing zinc
- Antibody suppression and immune dysfunction

- Sore joints can be caused by the suppression of potassium by cadmium.
- Decreased fertility from decreased progesterone and testosterone production
- Lung disease, slow healing, acne, anemia
- Decreased body temperature is a symptom of decreased thyroid function, which can result when cadmium blocks the copper that, along with iodine, promotes proper thyroid function.

How can zinc supplementation help?

Cadmium displaces zinc in the body, but the converse is also true. Zinc, taken orally, displaces cadmium and can stop and even reverse symptoms of cadmium poisoning. When cadmium causes leg arteries to narrow with resulting poor circulation and pain, zinc can reverse the spasms in the minor arteries and thus alleviate the symptoms.

Another example of the zinc-cadmium relationship is the symptom of anosmia, or lack of smell. Anosmia is attributed to zinc deficiency but could just as well be caused by an unbalanced excess of cadmium or mercury. Since cigarette smoke is a significant source of cadmium, it is not surprising that smokers lose their sense of taste and smell and their appetite. People who quit smoking will usually get their sense of taste back even without taking zinc supplements because more zinc in the body is now available for use without cadmium fighting for zinc's biochemical sites.

Aluminum

What is the correlation between aluminum and Alzheimer's disease?

High concentrations of aluminum have been found in the brains of Alzheimer's victims, likely due to the mercury blocking the metallothionein detox pathway and the filters (liver and kidneys) that remove aluminum.

What other problems can be caused by aluminum?

Bone loss may be due to interference with calcium and magnesium. There is a possible correlation between aluminum and multiple sclerosis (MS). Aluminum lowers the amount of the phosphate group in the body, leading to muscle aches and weakness.

Where is aluminum found?

Aluminum can be found in[9]:

- Soft drink cans
- commercial salt
- foil
- food cooked in aluminum cookware
- antacids
- antidiarrheal preparations
- buffered aspirin
- antiperspirants
- food additives such as sodium aluminum phosphate

What can help in aluminum detoxification?

Chelation can help to remove aluminum from the system, as it helps to remove other metals. Zinc supplementation has been shown to slow the accumulation of toxic aluminum in the brain.[10,11]

Secondary Suppressors – Microorganisms

What is a parasite?

A parasite is a living microorganism that stays alive through dependence on the body of an animal, called the host, often to the detriment of the host. Once you are infected, microorganisms can stay within your body for decades. Parasites causing today's symptoms may have entered your body in childhood. They will rarely, if ever, go away by themselves, so identification and treatment are vital.

How are these microorganisms opportunistic secondary toxic suppressors?

Microorganisms can be secondary to an overabundance of toxins that have overwhelmed the body's defenses. Just as flies and buzzards are attracted to rotting meat, organisms are attracted to a sick body that can no longer fight them off. However, microorganisms can also be a primary problem; some infections can overwhelm even a healthy body. If the infection or infestation is secondary, upstream thinking states that the primary causes must be dealt with before the infection can be brought under control for good.

The condition of the host is more important than the organism, which explains why only a few of the people exposed to someone with a cold will end up getting it. To treat parasites effectively, first change the environment in which they best live and thrive.

What are the major types of parasites?

Types of parasites discussed in this chapter include:

- **Protozoa** and **amoebas** such as entamoeba histolytica and giardia
- **Worms** such as pinworm or roundworm.
- **Bacteria** such as streptococcus (strep throat), helicobacter pylori (ulcers), klebsiella, and borrelia (Lyme disease)
- **Viruses** such as flu virus, HIV, herpes, Epstein-Barr virus, cytomegalovirus
- **Mycoplasmas**, which are very tiny organisms.
- **Fungi** such as yeast, which are plants.

These microorganisms range in size from single celled protozoa, to viruses which are even smaller, to roundworms several feet long.

Parasites are often plural

Once the stage is set for a parasite infestation, other parasites often follow or co-exist. For example, blastocystis hominis is normally found with either entamoeba histolytica or giardia, which tend to be found together, as are giardia and roundworm. A more complete solution to the parasite problem involves treating the "go-withs" as well as the diagnosed parasite. Fungus/yeast often follows parasite infestation and may also follow parasite treatment, as the treatment may kill the protective bacteria which keep the yeast under control. It is therefore wise to treat for yeast after treating parasites.

What are some indications that you may have a parasite infestation?
While some symptoms are specific to a particular type of parasite, some general symptoms, especially in combination, can be attributed to parasite infestation:

- Fatigue
- Stiffness and pain
- Arthritis
- Widespread allergies
- Low-grade fever
- Autoimmune disease
- Chronic anemia
- Itchy ears or anus
- Light sensitivity
- Dark under-eye circles
- Nail biting
- Headaches, neck and back aches
- Weight loss
- Thyroid and other gland problems
- Diarrhea or constipation, constant or alternating
- Elevated eosinophils (white blood cells)
- Chronic viral infections, frequent colds
- Irritable bowel symptoms (gas, intestinal pain, bloating)

Nail biting and nose picking may be caused by parasites, which use these routes to reinfest your body.

Why is symptom suppression not a good idea?
Symptom suppression, as opposed to going after the parasites themselves or boosting the immune system, often does more harm than good. Most symptoms of colds, flu, or other infection happen for a reason driven by immune system responses, with the ultimate goal of triumphing over the invaders. Body temperature is usually raised to better fight the invaders. Taking aspirin or a similar medication will lower the fever, reduce the body aches, and make you feel better in the short term, but will thwart one of the immune system's ways to make you feel better in the long run; it is better not to suppress the fever. Mucus production and diarrhea are the body's way of flushing out the microorganisms and their waste products, so it is best not to interfere with these either.

How do parasites enter the body?
Whether or not you have parasites, it is important to know how they enter the body and how this entry can be prevented.

Water – Parasites, especially giardia and roundworm, can be ingested from contaminated water, including that used to wash produce which is then eaten raw.

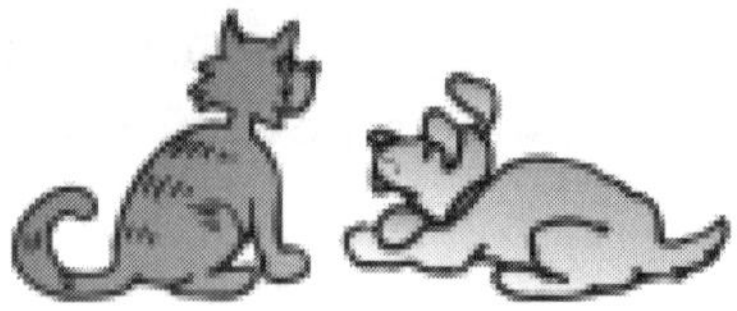

Pets – Animals harbor parasites that can be transmitted to humans. Wash your hands after petting an animal, changing your cat's litterbox, or cleaning up after your dog. Keep your pets wormed and vaccinated.

Meat – Some parasites can be transmitted through raw or incompletely cooked meat and fish.

Produce – People who pick and handle fruit can pass on infection. Produce should always be washed thoroughly before eating, especially if it can't be peeled. A few drops of food grade hydrogen peroxide (preferred) or chlorine bleach (if not allergic) in a dishpan full of wash water has a microbe-killing effect.

Sex – Disease can also be spread through any sexual practices in which body fluids are exchanged. Scrupulous hygiene is important, as is testing of any potential partner.

Babies and young children – Day-care centers are notorious for parasite epidemics, such as giardia and pinworms, since there are a lot of baby diapers and hand-to-mouth contact in that age group. Wash your hands and your child's hands frequently.

Restaurants – One of the unknowns you face when eating in a restaurant or at a salad bar is the personal hygiene habits of the workers. If you eat out, eat only cooked foods.

Insects – Many parasitic diseases can be transmitted by fleas, houseflies, mosquitoes, and ticks, which are called disease vectors.

Soil – Animal parasites can enter the soil through fecal and other contact. Wear gloves when gardening and/or scrub your hands and nails afterward.

What are other ways to protect against parasites?

Preventive measures other than avoiding the above sources include:

- **Washing** your hands regularly, especially after using the toilet, petting animals, gardening or changing diapers.
- **Clenzology** makes an iodine-based hand and face wash kit; iodine kills parasites.
- **Resistance** – Keep your immune system in good shape. Avoid sugar and mucus-producers such as dairy products, as parasites don't like clean intestines.
- **Stool testing** for parasites, done on a regular basis, perhaps once a year.

How can you be tested for parasites?

Stool samples are often used for testing. In some cases, such as pinworms, the small wiggling white worms can be seen by the untrained eye. Stool samples are usually examined microscopically by a professional for the parasites themselves or for their eggs. Be aware that most parasites lay eggs, or enter the bowel, only at certain times in their lives, and are thus not always detectable. If you have a negative test, you may not be free of parasites; if parasites are still suspected, repeat the test at least once at a later date or do a different type of test for confirmation.

Tape applied to and then removed from the unwashed anus upon awakening will pick up pinworm eggs, which can be detected microscopically on the tape.

ELISA testing – This is a noninvasive laboratory test which can diagnose giardia and possibly other parasites.

IgG and IgM antibody testing can be done for giardia and entamoeba histolytica. Antibodies are also found in saliva.

Kinesiology, or muscle testing, is sometimes used to detect signs of parasites.

EAV (computer) testing can pick up signs of parasites as well.

String – A method to detect upper gastrointestinal parasites involves swallowing a capsule attached to a string, one end of which is left outside the mouth. The string is withdrawn through the mouth after a few hours and examined microscopically.[1]

Endoscopy – This is an invasive procedure in which intestinal tissue is extracted by way of the mouth. It is a very accurate test for some parasites, but they can usually be detected using less drastic measures.[1] Duodenal intubation and biopsy are other invasive procedures which are effective but drastic.[2]

What are some treatments for parasites?

Treatment options and protocols, some of which are discussed in Part 4, include the following:

Allopathic drugs, such as vermifuges for worms or Metronidazole for amoebic infection, can be used; these are available by prescription only. Alinia, although it is primarily antiprotozoal, can be effective on other types of microbes as well. These may or may not do the job, but they have the potential for serious side effects.

Botanicals and natural remedies work with the body in partnership against the parasites. They are much less likely than allopathic drugs to cause side effects. Paragon (Integris) and AP Mag are both herbal antiparasitic preparations. Black walnut, cayenne, garlic, artemisia annua and wormwood are also useful. Citrus seed extracts such as Citricidal, Nutricidal, or AgriSept brand are active against viruses, protozoa, bacteria and yeast. It may be necessary to take it for up to several months, which is possible because it is nontoxic and rarely allergenic.

Immune system strengthening through a variety of methods such as detoxification. This is always useful but will often not do the job by itself. Gamma globulin and cyclic AMP by injection also strengthen the immune system, and is especially effective with viruses.

Liver/gallbladder flush, discussed in Part 4, gets parasites out of the gallbladder in addition to other benefits.

Protozoa and amoebas

Protozoa are single-celled animals that are slightly larger than bacteria. Most protozoa are found in the digestive tract, particularly the bowel, causing diarrhea and general ill health in the short run, but, if untreated, can migrate to vital organs such as the lungs, brain, and liver, causing chronic problems.

Giardia lamblia is the most common parasite found in humans in the United States. The disease caused by the parasite, giardiasis, is not fatal but can be very disabling. It is passed through fecal-oral contamination from contaminated drinking water or produce, anal/oral sex practices, or cleaning up after infected pets.

Chronic giardial symptoms include:

- Fatigue
- Allergies
- Gallbladder problems
- Headaches and other pain
- Foul smelling stools
- Depression
- Autoimmune diseases
- Gastrointestinal problems
- Flu-like feelings
- Loose and then hard stools

Entamoeba histolytica is the most deadly of the parasites; unlike giardia, it can cause death if untreated. As with giardia, entamoeba is passed by fecal-oral contact. The acute form is dysentery; more commonly the disease develops slowly, with intermittent diarrhea, cramps, vomiting, and general malaise. Chronic fatigue, fibromyalgia, and multiple chemical or food allergies can result from this infestation.

Toxoplasmosis is most commonly transmitted to humans from cat feces via handling infected litterbox material or soil or the cats themselves. The central nervous system and brain, blood, and lymph nodes can be affected, causing confusion, headaches, dizziness, swollen glands, and malaise. The greatest danger in toxoplasmosis occurs when a pregnant woman contracts the disease, since problems can be transmitted to her child.

Trichomonas, one of the most common protozoan parasites in the United States, is best known as a gynecological, and usually sexually transmitted, disease. A vaginal discharge with a very unpleasant odor is the most common female symptom. The protozoa are identified directly from vaginal smears or cultures. Metronidazole is the drug most often used for treatment, taken for 5-10 days, although it contains arsenic and has its own negative effects.

Blastocystis hominis lives in the digestive tract and has been implicated in cases of acute and chronic diarrhea and gastroenteritis. When B. hominis or cryptosporidium are present, other organisms such as E. histolytica, giardia, or roundworms are often also present. These other organisms may be wholly or partially responsible for symptoms attributed to B. hominis.

The organism is present in small quantities in up to one-fifth of hospitalized patients, but is associated with diarrhea only in heavily infested patients. Other typical symptoms are[3]:

- Osteoarthritis – B. hominis has been found in affected joints such as kneecaps
- Abdominal pain and gas, nausea and vomiting
- Low-grade fever and chills, general malaise
- Colitis

Cryptosporidium is found especially in those who are immunodeficient, such as AIDS patients. Its first symptom is profuse, watery diarrhea that can deplete vital minerals.

Worms

What symptoms can be caused by worms?

Worm infestation can cause symptoms as diverse as asthma and bronchitis, ear infections, appendicitis, bedwetting, diarrhea, allergic symptoms, and appetite loss. Many species of worms migrate through different organs as part of their life cycle, compounding the damage they cause.

Worm eggs are passed in the feces of humans and animals and can be found in soil. Hygiene, especially careful and frequent washing of the hands and nails, is the best preventive measure.

The most common types of worms in the United States are:

- Pinworms
- Tapeworms

- Roundworms
- Threadworms
- Whipworms
- Hookworms
- Trichinosis
- Flukes

Roundworms (ascaris) are the most prevalent worm infestation worldwide and are perhaps the most powerful cause of allergies and hypersensitivity. Roundworms can grow up to 18 inches long and can lay up to 200,000 eggs per day. Testing is usually done by identifying the characteristically shaped eggs in the feces.

Roundworms can cause a number of symptoms:

- Malnutrition, as roundworms consume much of the liquid contents of the intestine.
- Allergic responses to metabolites produced by the worms include rashes, asthma, and insomnia.
- Abdominal pains and nausea are not uncommon.
- Clusters of worms can knot up sufficiently to block the intestine, and some cases of appendicitis are caused by roundworms in the appendix; roundworm medication rather than surgery is sometimes sufficient and certainly safer.
- Roundworms can wander into the pancreatic and bile ducts, the esophagus, the trachea, or even the Eustachian tubes of the ears, causing extensive damage.[4] Persistent or recurring childhood ear infections may be due in part to roundworm infestation.
- Roundworms often inhabit the upper respiratory area, and are responsible for many cases of asthma and bronchitis.
- Roundworm eggs can cause a tooth abscess; roundworms lay eggs at the base of the tooth.

Pinworm is the most common worm infestation in the United States. As many as 50% of children have this worm infection at some time. Transmission is fecal to oral from unwashed hands or contaminated food. The worms are easily visible on the surface of the feces as ¼ to ½ -inch white, moving, threadlike worms. They migrate to the anus at night to lay their eggs in a sticky chemical that causes intense anal itching. Since children tend to scratch where it itches and then to suck their fingers, bite their nails, and pick their noses, they keep the infestation going, for years if untreated.

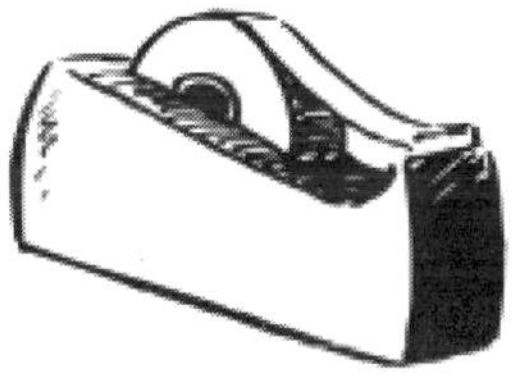

Testing is simple and accurate. The worms can be identified visually in the stool, as can the eggs with the aid of a microscope. A piece of tape applied to the unwashed anus upon awakening will pick up eggs and even whole worms.

Tapeworms are spread via the fecal to oral route, and from eating undercooked meat. They are generally flat, long, and segmented. While they primarily infest the intestines, some species or their cysts can infiltrate almost any part of the body. The broad tapeworm of humans absorbs so much vitamin B12 from the intestine that the host can develop pernicious anemia.[5]

Testing is done by checking the stool for eggs and segments. In treatment, the head must be killed or the tapeworm will be able to regenerate.

Trichinosis is caused by the trichinella worm, which is most commonly transmitted to humans by eating undercooked pork and sausage. Most commercial sources of pork are safe, however. It attacks the muscle, including that of the heart. Symptoms are varied and vague, and include muscular pain and heart damage, and can lead to death if untreated. The most accurate, although drastic, diagnostic method is muscle biopsy.

Flukes are among the most common and abundant of parasitic worms, infesting the liver, intestines, blood, and lungs. They are contracted by swimming or wading in infested water. Flukes vary considerably in size, shape, and part of the body that is preferentially infested; i.e. where they develop into adults and deposit their eggs. If a person is heavily infested, liver flukes can cause sharp, hard to diagnose pain in the area of the liver.

Bacteria

Bacteria are one-celled animals that can originate both inside and outside the body. Over 99% of all bacteria in the body are beneficial, and less than 1% are disease-producing. Antibiotics, which can be either prescribed or inadvertent (mercury from fillings, chlorine in water), thus kill about 100 times more beneficial bacteria than bad ones.

Bacteria enter the body in a number of different ways – through the skin, breathing, eating, or sexual transmission, or from root-canalled teeth.

Most disease symptoms come from toxic waste products of bacteria which can interfere with metabolic processes or destroy body tissues. Bacteria can also incapacitate the immune system to a certain extent, thus ensuring their own continued survival. This explains how many bacterial infections can become chronic, and how one infection can follow another once the immune system is weakened.

Many bacteria are anaerobic, which means oxygen-hating. Keeping the blood well-oxygenated, as with deep breathing or aerobic exercise, will discourage the growth of anaerobic bacteria.

Campylobacter and helicobacter are spiral-shaped bacteria which are found in the intestinal tract of humans and animals. Infection is usually contracted through contaminated food or water. Campylobacter has been found to be present in up to 90% of chickens sold in supermarkets. Acute food poisoning symptoms include vomiting, chills, and abdominal pain. Long-term symptoms include arthritis, pericarditis (inflammation of the heart lining), and neurological disorders. The disease can be fatal to the very young, the old, and those with weakened immune systems.

Helicobacter pylori may cause up to 80% of stomach ulcers and nearly all duodenal ulcers. The bacterium is thought to burrow through and digest the layer of mucus that protects the stomach and duodenum from gastric acid. In one study, only 5-25% of ulcer patients treated with antibiotics had a relapse the following year, as compared with a 75-90% relapse rate in those treated only with ulcer drugs[6]; until recently ulcers were believed to be caused by stress. Helicobacter pylori is also implicated in stomach cancer. Some allergic symptoms such as hives can be caused by helicobacter, as well; the probable mechanism of action is a suppression of hydrochloric acid by the bacteria, leading to poor protein digestion and the development or worsening of food allergies.

> **Patient profile**
> A man from Australia came to the clinic with ulcers which he was treating unsuccessfully with antacids. H. pylori treatment was instituted, as well as eliminating dental metals (mercury in amalgam fillings acts as an antibiotic and kills beneficial bacteria which keep infectious organisms under control), cleared his associated candida, and implanted the beneficial bacteria acidophilus and bifidus. This regimen cleared up the ulcer cause and therefore the ulcer symptoms.

Campylobacter and helicobacter are detected by a blood culture or a saliva test.

Lyme disease is one of the most prevalent parasitic diseases in the United States. It is caused by a spiral-shaped bacteria (spirochete) called Borrelia burgdorferi. The vector is the deer tick, a tiny black tick not much larger than a pinhead.

Disease symptoms show up in at least two stages. The tick will inject the spirochetes (bacteria) 24 hours to 4 days after biting, which allows plenty of time to locate and remove it. Once infected, the first sign is a small red bump where the person was bitten, often followed shortly by a ring-like or bull's-eye rash around the bite site, which can be two or more inches in diameter. There may also be flu-like symptoms, which disappear within a few days. The disease is easily treated with antibiotics at this stage; the ringlike rash, although often not present or noticed, is characteristic enough to be diagnostic.

If untreated, there may be no symptoms for years, and then serious symptoms, difficult to treat, set in. A wide variety of symptoms affect nearly every organ system, and diagnosis is difficult unless the patient remembers the tick bite and bull's-eye rash. These symptoms, which can be chronic and disabling, include:

- Arthritis, one of the most common effects
- Nervous system disorders, multiple sclerosis-like symptoms
- Psychological disorders, dementia, memory loss
- Heart rhythm abnormalities, heart damage
- Fatigue
- Joint pain and swelling, especially the knees
- Miscarriage and birth defects
- Jaw pain, facial paralysis (Bell's palsy)
- Headache, neck pain
- Occurrence or worsening of allergies

Minimize insect contact by avoiding woods and tall grassy areas, wearing long sleeves and pants, checking yourself for ticks after being in wooded areas, and checking your pets for ticks.

Escherichia coli (E. coli) is the organism most frequently associated with diarrhea in travelers to less-developed countries; it can account for 30-70% of cases of the "tourist trots." It surfaces in the news periodically as a particular food is contaminated. Some strains of the bacteria can be fatal.

E. coli are normally found in the digestive tract and do not cause trouble unless host resistance is lowered or the intestinal wall becomes diseased. Once they enter the bloodstream, they start causing problems. Coliform bacteria can then cause such diseases as

- Pyelonephritis — a kidney infection
- Cystitis — urinary tract infection; e.coli is the most common cause
- Cholecystitis — gallbladder infection
- Abscesses — local infections, usually of the skin
- Peritonitis — infection of the peritoneum, or abdominal lining
- Meningitis — infection of the meninges of the brain
- Gallstones

Chlamydia, now the most widespread sexually transmitted disease, is caused by a bacterium, chlamydia trachomatis. Chlamydia begins as an infection of the cervix, and from there may spread to the uterus and fallopian tubes. It can cause or contribute to infertility, ectopic (tubal) pregnancies, and miscarriage, as well as endometriosis. Many infected women and some men experience no symptoms at all other than conception problems. Symptoms include:

- Vaginal discharge – copious cloudy, sticky discharge with little or no odor or itching
- Lower abdominal pain in women
- Painful urination
- Bleeding between periods
- A dripping discharge from the penis, similar to that of gonorrhea

Once diagnosed, antibiotic treatment is fairly simple, especially in the early stages. A ten-day course of an antibiotic such as doxycycline or tetracycline will kill the bacteria. Advanced cases can result in irreversible scarring.

Viruses

Unlike other microorganisms, viruses are not self-containing, or even technically alive. A virus is essentially an extremely tiny packet of genetic information surrounded by a protein covering. They must hijack cells to carry out their intended purpose: replicating themselves.

Many types of viruses infect humans. They are very specific in the types of cells they attach to, and will not affect other cells, tissues, or organs. Viruses enter the body through the same routes as bacteria, including respiration or ingestion.

The susceptibility of a person to infection depends primarily on the state of the immune system, which in turn depends on the presence or absence of toxic suppressors, the presence of pathogenic bacteria, or low levels of protective bacteria, copper, lysine, and gamma globulin. The environment is more important than the presence of the virus in determining whether viral infection will develop.

Prevention involves blocking the spread of infection by washing hands, covering sneezes, and carefully disposing of used tissues in the case of rhinoviruses (cold viruses), or by practicing abstinence or monogamy to help prevent the spread of the HIV or herpes viruses. Using an iodine based hand and face wash such as Clenzology can help prevent the spread of infection, as iodine has a viricidal (virus-killing) effect like chlorine.

Viruses cause their damage in several ways:

- They can cause destruction of the cell or its function, for example polio's attack on the nerve cells, producing permanent paralysis. Damage is confined to the part of the body actually infected.
- Viruses can stimulate an autoimmune attack.
- They can cause hyperplasia, or a buildup of cells, as in skin or genital warts (papilloma).
- They can cause DNA mutations which lead to uncontrolled cell growth, or cancer, in combination with other stressors and immune system suppression.
- They can weaken the immune system so that other, more dangerous viruses and bacteria can gain a foothold and do their damage. An example is pneumonia following a cold.

Since each virus has a specific shape, the immune system will attack it, usually successfully, once the immune system recognizes the invader and produces antibodies against it. For this reason, a viral disease is rarely contracted more than once. Flu and cold viruses mutate often enough that a different cold or flu can be caught months later.

A comprehensive blood test can show a number of indicators that viral disease is present, although they are not diagnostic in themselves. The more of these that show up in the blood, the greater the likelihood that viruses have gone out of control.

- Low uric acid
- High bilirubin
- High albumin / globulin (A/G) ratio, above 2.0
- High lymphocytes, white cells that fight viral infection
- High monocytes, another white blood cell type
- Lowered total white blood cell count

How are viruses treated?

There is no true allopathic treatment for most viral diseases, if what is meant by treatment is a drug or agent that will selectively kill viruses in the body. Antibiotics are useless against viruses and can cause harm of their own, but they are sometimes misprescribed for a viral infection through ignorance, or as a preventive measure against the bacterial infections that sometimes follow viral infections.

"Treatments" for viruses are therefore of three types:

- One type aims for symptom suppression, such as antihistamines, cold capsules, fever reducers, or cough drops. These suppress the immune system's effectiveness and can make things worse in the long run.
- The second type treats the opportunistic infections, often bacterial, that may occur once the virus has weakened the immune system.
- The most effective measures for both prevention and cure are any ways in which immune system function is enhanced. Stronger and more numerous antibodies will then mount an attack on the viruses.

Some substances which support the immune system in fighting viruses include:

- Copper and the amino acid lysine which form copper lysinate
- Injected gamma globulin and cyclic AMP (adenosine monophosphate)
- Bio-Ag, which is humic and fulvic acid in liquid format
- Livit-I, an herb that both supports the liver and goes after viruses
- Vitamin C IV with minerals and HCl
- Oxygenation methods such as hydrogen peroxide, ozone, or Dioxychlor (chlorine dioxide)
- Hyperthermia, in which the blood is heated outside the body and reinfused
- Rife and other frequency generators
- Germanium and Coenzyme Q10
- Antioxidants such as vitamins A, E, and C; bioflavonoids like pycnogenol, grape seed, quercetin, rutin; selenium. These control free radical damage and inflammation
- Transfer factor, which tells the immune system what to attack and programs the immune system to work normally.
- Alpha interferon
- Personalized vaccination, in which a vaccine is made from viral material from your own body.
- Colloidal silver, used only during viral infection and not as a daily supplement
- Garlic is shown to protect against viruses and to enhance the production of antibodies. It should be eaten raw or as an extract, as it loses much of its medicinal value when cooked.

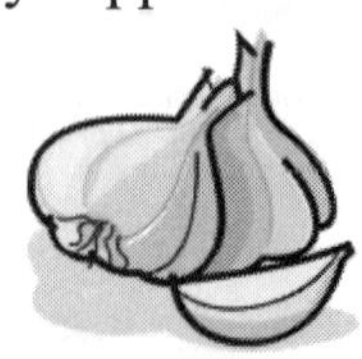

Herpes simplex I is said to cause cold sores and other mouth lesions, while the more dangerous herpes simplex II causes genital sores. Genital herpes typically causes a severe initial outbreak of symptoms – painful genital blisters, swollen glands, and flu-like symptoms – followed in most but not all cases by less-severe outbreaks. Stress and the consequent immune system depression usually precipitates an outbreak. Herpes is considered to be infectious only when the blisters are present and are shedding virus particles. Since herpes II is sexually transmitted, sex should be avoided during outbreaks. Condoms provide some but not total protection, since viruses are so small.

Acyclovir (Zovirax) is often given to treat the initial outbreak, although it is not recommended for continued use or for subsequent outbreaks. L-lysine, an amino acid, may have potential in inhibiting the growth of the herpes virus. Copper lysinate helps to boost the immune system, as copper is depleted by fighting infection. Arginine, found in nuts, acts against lysine and should be restricted.

Herpes zoster, the chickenpox virus, can reappear decades later as shingles, a very painful rash that follows a nerve trunk on one side of the body. Acyclovir during the first 2-3 days, gamma globulin / cyclic AMP injection, and lysine along with copper to form copper lysinate are recommended. Dr. Dworkin, who experienced firsthand the overnight reversal of her viral shingles following a GG/c-AMP injection, calls it "an immune system in a syringe."

Cytomegalovirus (CMV) is also a herpes virus, with which most of the adult population is latently infected. It can cause a syndrome similar to mononucleosis, and can also be involved in hepatitis. This is usually a problem only in immunocompromised patients. CMV is one of the leading serious infections of pregnancy, causing miscarriage, prematurity, fetal malformations, and fetal death. CMV can destroy the cells of the pancreas and limit their ability to produce insulin, and so has been implicated in playing a triggering role in diabetes.[7] CMV can also cause blindness by directly attacking the optic nerve.

Mononucleosis (sometimes called mono) is an acute infectious viral disease caused by the Epstein Barr Virus (EBV), which causes sore throat, enlarged and tender lymph nodes and spleen, mild fever, and fatigue. It usually affects children and young adults up to age 30. The immune system is adversely affected by mononucleosis, leading to opportunistic infections.

A characteristic change in lymphocytes, a particular type of white blood cell, can be seen under the microscope and makes the diagnosis. As with most viral diseases, there is no known external agent which will kill the mononucleosis virus directly.

Epstein-Barr virus (EBV) is best known as the virus that causes mononucleosis. It used to be considered a major cause of chronic fatigue, but is now one of many possibilities; the most likely theory is that the many toxic suppressors described in this book cause both the chronic fatigue symptoms and the EBV infection through immune suppression.

Hepatitis refers to inflammation of the liver, and can be caused by several agents, viral and otherwise. Early symptoms of hepatitis B infection resemble those of the flu. The hepatitis B virus targets liver cells, and swelling and tenderness of the liver and spleen, jaundice (yellow skin and eyes), and darkened urine can result.[8] Intolerance to food, alcohol, and medications may develop, as the liver, primarily involved in detoxification, is unable to function fully. Most people recover in two to twelve weeks, although some do not recover fully and these symptoms become chronic.

Treatment usually involves letting the disease run its course, because allopathic medication will tax the liver and often do more harm than good. Liquid liver and silymarin (milk thistle) are also recommended for liver support.

Genital warts, also called condyloma, are caused by the human papilloma virus (HPV). The virus is highly contagious, and is spread by sexual contact, so a condom can help in prevention. Genital warts are twice as prevalent as the more highly publicized genital herpes. Unlike herpes, genital warts are painless and may not even be noticed, so they are not taken nearly as seriously as they should be. A number of research studies have linked HPV to an increased incidence of cervical cancer in women. About 30% of HPV warts will progress to dysplasia, a stage of precancerous cell changes, within five years of infection.[9]

Fungi and yeast

Fungi and yeast are organisms in the plant kingdom, varying in size from single-celled organisms to mushrooms. The fungi that are most important medically are microscopic, such as yeast. A general indication of fungus infection is allergy to dust, grass, cigarette smoke, and mildew.

Fungus diseases (mycoses) in humans are characterized by both amount of penetration and by seriousness, ranging from skin infections to systemic problems that can affect the entire body. However, if you have the infection on the outside, there's a pretty good chance it's on the inside too.

Fungal infections include:

- Ringworm — Fungus, not a worm
- Jock itch — Red, scaling, itchy areas in groin
- Athlete's foot — Itching, scaling lesions between toes
- Onychomycosis — Thickened, crumbly, whitish nails
- Coccidioidomycosis — Very infectious, starts in lungs, can spread through body

Fungi prefer an alkaline environment, and fungi and bacteria set up an alkaline condition in a vicious cycle. Carbonated beverages alkalinize the gut, promoting fungal growth. Sugars and simple carbohydrates such as white flour products provide food for the fungus, causing it to proliferate. Diabetes or a blood sugar problem can contribute to fungus growth, for more sugar, their food, would be in the blood.

Mold and fungus can be present around the house, especially in moist climates, and can be a major trigger for fatigue. To deal with this, it is first necessary to have a major professional cleaning of the mold or even a change of residence or climate.

The most common manifestation of fungus is yeast overgrowth. Localized manifestations, which can indicate a systemic problem, include vaginal yeast infections, thrush in the mouth, skin infections, and nail infections. Symptoms of systemic yeast overgrowth include:

- Chronic fatigue, or fatigue in mid-afternoon or after meals
- Depression, brain fog, poor concentration, irritability
- Hyperactivity and learning disabilities in children
- Loss of sexual desire, dry vaginal area
- Immune impairment, autoimmune disorders
- Headaches, stiff neck and back, joint pains
- Constipation, diarrhea, or alternating
- Bladder infections, vaginitis
- Sunlight sensitivity, light hurts eyes
- An overall feeling of not being well (malaise)
- A reaction or aversion to perfumes, dust, cut grass, tobacco smoke
- Hypersensitivity to foods, chemicals, molds, pollen, perfume, tobacco smoke
- Food cravings, especially for sweets (including fruit), cheese, bread, vinegar, alcoholic and carbonated beverages, pickles, or mushrooms
- Bloat and gas, since yeast produces gas and thus bloat, like the gas bubbles that cause the rising of bread

A number of conditions predispose a person to get candidiasis, an overgrowth of yeast:

- Antibiotics, including mercury, kill the beneficial bacteria that keep the yeast under control.
- Birth control pills change the vaginal lining to make it more hospitable to yeasts. Progesterone also causes the release of yeast-feeding sugar into the bloodstream.

- Cortisone, prednisone, and other steroid drugs suppress the immune system, thus letting yeast overgrow.
- Suppressed immune system function, whether caused by the presence of allergens, toxins, other stressors, or immunosuppressive drugs.
- Living in a damp, moldy environment.
- Diabetes or a diet high in sugar, including fruit and juices – both conditions raise the blood sugar level, and yeast feeds on sugar.
- Poor diet – yeast-feeding foods are listed in the Detoxification Diet chapter.

To tell whether you have a fermentation (yeast) problem, test your urine pH as described in the Assessments chapter. The optimal pH is 6.0, and a pH of 7.0 or higher generally means fermentation, which in turn points to yeast and bacteria.

What can be done to control yeast?

- Diet to control yeast is detailed in the Detoxification Diet chapter in Part 4.
- Certain medications, such as Nystatin, Diflucan, and Nizoral, act as fungicides in the body and can be useful for severe infections. The yeast will probably come back unless the primary problem is remedied and the protective bacteria reestablished.
- Acidophilus capsules or plain unsweetened yogurt repopulate the good bacteria in the gut.
- Garlic (e.g. Kyolic brand), whole or in capsules, to create an inhospitable environment for yeast.
- Mycopril 680 (caprylic acid) is useful but is only effective while being used.
- Aloe vera gel or powder is also useful for controlling yeast in the mouth and intestinal tract.
- Dioxychlor, hydrogen peroxide, or ozone oxygenate the blood, making it inhospitable for fungi and yeast.
- The herbs myrrh, black walnut, taheebo, pau de arco, melaleuca (tea tree oil)
- Grapefruit seed extract, Citricidal, Nutricidal, AgriSept
- Aqua Flora is a homeopathic liquid preparation to treat yeast infections in two phases.

- Boric acid powder suppositories (not boric acid crystals) and tea tree oil suppositories have been successful in treating yeast infections.
- Any measures to build up the immune system as discussed elsewhere in this book can be of benefit.
- Recommended nutritional supplements for the direct treatment of candida through the building of immune function include B vitamins, vitamin A, C and E, antioxidants such as selenium, calcium and zinc, and essential fatty acids.

How critical is the problem of mold?

Mold – and not just the better-publicized black mold – is implicated in a startling number of ailments. Molds give off biotoxins that can cause nervous system problems, cognitive deficits, severe fatigue, and other debilitating symptoms.[10]

Mold and fungus can suppress neutrophils, the white blood cells which control bacteria such as Lyme and the bacteria that cause abscesses and arthritis. Beta glucan stops the neutralizing of neutrophils. NSC100 is a supplement that is a good source of beta glucan.

Mycoplasmas

Mycoplasmas, the least well-known of the microorganisms, are smaller than bacteria but larger than viruses. Mycoplasmas cause a number of diseases in animals; in humans, the respiratory and genitourinary systems are most affected. Mycoplasmas are associated with AIDS due to the compromised immune function.

Diagnosis is made from cell culture, or from observing a rising antibody titer.[11] Doxycycline is one of the few antibiotics that are effective against mycoplasmas.

Part 4
Solutions
Types of Detoxification

General Discussion of Types of Detoxification

What are the detoxification organs and pathways?

The body has a number of detoxification organs and pathways, each of which has a somewhat different function and way of operating. As mentioned previously, toxins are eliminated in two steps: from the storage depots such as fat, muscle, and liver into the bloodstream or colon, and from there out of the body. The organs of detoxification help to remove toxins from the body into the bloodstream, while the elimination pathways remove the waste from the body entirely. In some cases the organs of detoxification and elimination are the same.

The organs of detoxification are:

- Liver – metabolizes toxins to breakdown products that are flushed out of the body
- Kidneys – filter out toxins that are then urinated out
- Lungs – removes some toxins, especially gaseous ones, from the blood as it passes through the lungs
- Bowels – dump dietary toxins as well as those from the liver
- Lymph – store and move out toxins

The organs of elimination are:

- Colon – through feces
- Skin – through sweat
- Lungs – through breathing
- Bladder – through urine

There are biochemical detoxification pathways in addition to the physical organs, including metallothionein, which detoxifies metals; cytochrome P450, which detoxifies chemicals; and glutathione, which also detoxifies chemicals. These are the major ones, but dozens of biochemical reactions in the body help to detoxify harmful substances.

The detoxification organs and biochemical pathways work remarkably well, but they can be overwhelmed by having to deal with more than they can handle. Any help we can give them in the form of detoxification and avoidance of toxins will help them to perform more efficiently.

What is the best type of detoxification?

There is no one best type of detoxification. The best one for you depends on what you are trying to detoxify, what facilities are available, and financial and personal preferences and constraints. These decisions are the focus of this chapter.

How are practitioner-assisted and do-it-yourself detoxification modalities differentiated?

When this book was first conceived, we were thinking in terms of having a do-it-yourself (DIY) section and a practitioner-assisted (PA) section, given that some people have the geographical and financial access to knowledgeable practitioners, and some do not, or they prefer to go it alone, or they are looking to optimize health in general rather than to deal with a specific illness. This DIY/ PA approach was soon abandoned, since these two are not distinct categories and there is much overlap. Even the protocols that are most do-it-yourself, such as a detox diet, are more useful when a practitioner can oversee the process and interpret your reactions. At the other end of the spectrum, even those modalities such as safe removal of dental mercury, clearly not a do-it-yourself project, have a DIY component in that it is important for the patient to be well-informed as to procedures and about how to choose dentists with an understanding of how their work affects the whole body.

To this end, the detoxification modalities have been arranged by type. Where relevant, both practitioner-assisted and DIY versions are given; the PA version is almost always superior, but the DIY version will certainly work, although the DIY version will often be slower and less effective, and over time may end up costing even more than the practitioner version. The biggest risk is electrolyte loss, dehydration, and the lack of supervision of marginal patients who may run into problems.

What detox approaches work best for a person's personality and situation?

There are a number of personal factors to consider when choosing a detoxification modality. Since personalities, finances, and personal preferences differ, it is wise to look at these personal factors to determine what type of detox would work best for you.

Level of commitment – We would all like to see ourselves as committed to getting healthier, but let's make a realistic assessment of this. Some types of detox are difficult and require a firm long-term commitment, while others are easier and even a little bit would help. Some people are committed to doing whatever it takes to get to the root cause, while others prefer the "just give me a pill" approach. If you want the quick and easy solution, it is good to recognize this without self-judgment and choose accordingly, or you may not stick with the chosen program.

Timeline and tolerance – Some people find that their motivation is highest at the beginning of a new protocol, and would prefer to dive right in, while others would rather ease into it. By way of analogy, one person prefers to just dive into the cold water and get it over with, while others slip in inch by inch at the shallow end, both minimizing and prolonging the discomfort. It's best to know your preferred approach and choose a treatment plan that is compatible with it.

Energy level - Can you follow a complex or difficult protocol?

Aversions and phobias – If you have aversions or phobias that could affect your ability to follow a protocol, it is good to look at these before you start. For example, those with MS or other conditions might be very heat sensitive, and sauna might not be the best choice for them without support, or should only be undertaken with practitioner support. A person with a severe needle phobia would probably find IV chelation to be too stressful, although in some cases it is necessary anyway. Some people can't swallow pills without considerable difficulty if at all, and a supplement-heavy regimen is not likely to be adhered to for long. With this said, though, sometimes it is necessary to bite the bullet and do what needs to be done regardless of aversions. Other times there is a choice of approaches and a realistic assessment would help in choosing the right one.

Financial considerations – There is a huge difference in the cost of various types of detox, from almost no additional cost in the case of the detox diet (other than supplements) or liver/ gallbladder flush to thousands of dollars in the case of a full sauna program. If a specialized treatment facility is involved, this adds considerably to the cost, especially if travel and overnight stays are necessary. Figure out what you can afford and are comfortable with spending. A good bit of financial prioritizing lies in how sick you are and how badly you need detox. Even a small expense can be a hardship if all you are looking for is a tune-up – although it might well still be worth the expense – but if you are so sick that your quality of life is quite low or your life itself it threatened, any expense that could get you well would be worth it.

Access to progressive healthcare – Although it is almost always best to have the support of a knowledgeable practitioner, not everyone has access to such a person or facility, so this will affect your decision making.

Relationship to practitioner – If you work with a practitioner, what is your preferred relation ship with that person? Do you want a doctor who tells you what to do and when so you don't need to make decisions, or do you prefer someone who is in partnership with you to work towards your mutual goal, your health? Is it important that you be compatible with the person emotionally, or is that irrelevant as long as s/he knows how to help you?

What type(s) of detox would be most beneficial particular to root cause?

Different types of detoxification are best for different types of toxic loads. For example, the detox diet is best for dietary toxins, food allergies, and yeast overgrowth. Sauna is best for chemicals but is also good for metals, while chelation is best for metals. The following chart sums up which detox modalities are best for which types of toxins; detailed discussion is in the chapters that follow in this section.

Best detox protocols for toxin types

Detox protocol	**Protocol addresses:**						
	Chemicals	Metals	Dietary toxins	Allergies	Yeast	Microorganisms	Low nutrients
Detox diet			**X**	**X**	**X**	x	**X**
Sauna	**X**	x					
Lymph massage and exercises	**X**	x	x				
Chelation		**X**					
Colonics and enemas	**X**		**X**				
Liver / gallbladder flush	**X**	x					
Skin cleansing	**X**						
Parasite cleanses				**X**	**X**	**X**	
Allergy desensitization, NAET				**X**	x	x	**X**
Nutritional support		x					**X**

X = major benefit
x = minor benefit

Detoxification Diet

The Detoxification Diet Itself

The detoxification diet can also be called an elimination diet or cleansing diet. It is intended to be short-term, eight days in this case.

Although nutrition is addressed on this diet, the primary purpose is detoxification, and nutrition seems secondary. If you feed microorganisms or take in toxins or allergens, you can sabotage your whole detox. This program focuses more on what is eliminated from the diet rather than what is eaten, although both are important.

What is a detox diet?

A detox diet:

- Eliminates foods and additives that can be harmful in a number of ways.
- Helps to eliminate toxins, both dietary and non-dietary, from the body.
- Provides optimal nutrition so the body can utilize its own detoxification capabilities to the greatest extent possible.

Should I do the diet as a do-it-yourself project?

Although the diet can usually be done without practitioner input and is presented here as a do-it-yourself treatment, it is recommended that you work with a knowledgeable health professional. People with ulcers, Crohn's disease, brittle (hard to control) diabetes, hypoglycemia, or anorexia should only be doing such a diet under medical supervision. Call the Center for Advanced Medicine, 760-632-9042 or toll-free 888-244-4420, if you are uncertain as to whether you can do the diet on your own, given your particular health concerns.

Realistically, though, consider that this diet is likely healthier than the standard American diet you may have been consuming, and for which, ironically, nobody recommends that you get medical guidance. If you follow the protocol and are aware of and deal with any symptoms, chances are you will benefit and experience few if any adverse effects.

If there is an apparent contradiction between instructions here and recommendations by your practitioner, follow your practitioner's advice as it should be tailored to your particular health situation.

Do not make any adjustments to prescription medication unless directed to do so by a medical doctor. Be aware that dosages of some medications such as insulin or blood pressure medication may need adjustment downward as the underlying condition may be improved by the detox. Physician monitoring is recommended.

Why start with a detox diet?

The detox diet is one detoxification modality that is recommended as a starting point for nearly everyone for several reasons:

Ease – Of all the do-it-yourself procedures, dietary detoxification is the easiest and cheapest, as well as being nearly risk-free. The diet asks only an eight-day commitment, although it can be modified after the first detox into a four-day form.

Success – Over 60% of the patients at the Center for Advanced Medicine, where such a diet is routinely administered and monitored, show at least some improvement in their symptoms from the eight-day detox diet alone.

Potential for dramatic improvement – Once toxic dietary components are removed from your diet, as outlined in this chapter, dramatic improvement is often quite noticeable, to the extent that such components have been a part of your particular symptomatology.

For example, certain vegetables belonging to the nightshade family can contribute to arthritis and aching joints in susceptible individuals. If you don't have arthritis, or if your arthritis doesn't stem from nightshade sensitivity, eliminating nightshades will make little if any difference. However, if you have a nightshade-sensitive form of arthritis, eliminating these foods can make a noticeable difference in mobility and pain, other than that caused by actual tissue destruction.

Since one of the easiest treatments has potential to lead to substantial improvement, it makes sense to start with this diet.

Cost – Although supplements will need to be purchased, costly junk food and processed foods will be eliminated, so the overall increase in your food budget should be minor, or food costs may even decrease since junk food, now eliminated, can be expensive.

Food is a major factor – Most toxins enter the body in tiny amounts that accumulate over time in our fat, lymph, and gastrointestinal tract, in many cases parts per million or even parts per billion. However, food-related toxins, such as sugar or trans fats, enter the body by the forkful or even the cupful. Even toxins found in smaller amounts, such as hormones and pesticides, can be forced into the body with every meal. It follows that food-related toxicity is contributory to many if not most ailments, and that detoxification from these substances is a good first step.

The only step? – If improvement on the detox diet is substantial, it may be the only detox needed. More often, however, other things are going on and more detoxification and other work would be needed. You are the best judge of whether the detox diet results make it sufficient for your needs.

Why do a detoxification diet?

Nearly any symptoms are an indication for going on the detoxification diet because it meets a number of needs so completely. The detoxification diet has a number of purposes:

Providing clues – The reactions to the diet can be indicative of where your problems may be based, such as the small or large intestine, or what they may be due to, such as allergies, fungus or parasites. Certain symptoms that you have hopefully for the last time, or the improvement or temporary worsening of symptoms, can provide you, or your practitioner, with valuable clues as to what may be the root causes of your health problems. Even lack of response to the diet is useful in that it gives the important clue that the primary problem or problems are likely not dietary, and that other detoxification avenues should be pursued. Since a positive response to the diet can mean a prior problem with gastrointestinal microorganisms or allergens, a lack of response to the diet can also mean that these are not your problems either.

Relieving allergies – An allergen is something, dietary or otherwise, that an individual has sensitivity to that most people do not, or greater sensitivity to relative to most other people. The body interprets something that is not in itself a toxin, for example cat hair or shellfish, as being toxic, and reacts accordingly.

Allergies take many forms other than obvious sniffles or rashes, and such symptoms as the following may be due to allergens:

- Fatigue
- Difficulty sleeping
- Irritability
- Indigestion, gas, and bloating, colitis
- Difficulty concentrating, brain fog, ADD, ADHD, bipolar disorder, autism
- Any pain, any -itis (meaning inflammation) such as arthritis or diverticulitis
- Head, neck or backaches, tight neck, head pressure, or any ache or pain
- Urinary tract infections
- Mood swings, depression, anger, anxiety
- Autoimmune problems such as MS, rheumatoid arthritis, or lupus

The diet involves the use of food and supplements that are least likely to cause allergic reactions. Eliminating these allergens from the diet often causes a dramatic alleviation of symptoms.

Reducing microorganisms – Many people have problems with microorganisms (parasites) such as entamoeba histolytica, helicobacter pylori, which is implicated in ulcers, or yeast (candida), which can cause a variety of symptoms. This diet may reduce the population of these parasites both by removing much of their food supply, such as sugars, and by setting up a hostile environment for these microbes, as well as for viruses and mycoplasmas.

Relieving cravings – Pure aloe vera in supplement form, such as Aloe Vera 7000 swished in the mouth for two minutes and then swallowed after each meal, can help to control microorganisms such as yeast and pathogenic bacteria in the mouth and alimentary tract, thus avoiding upper respiratory tract infections and alleviating cravings for sweets. You may find that it tastes unpleasant or bitter at first. This is from microbe dieoff, and after continued use the taste will improve, itself an indicator that the microbe population has lessened. The use of healthful oils such as fish and flax oils can relieve the craving for fatty foods by providing the cells with the fatty acids they need. Taking more Life Solubles (Integris), or protein such as Only Whey, a hydrolyzed/predigested form of whey, or Ultra Balance / Ultra Clear protein powder, or Ultra Meal, Essential 7 (E7) or Goatein, as needed can also reduce cravings. Sources of these supplements are listed towards the back of this book.

How can a detox diet help with non-dietary toxins?

In addition to the benefits listed above, the detox diet helps to deal with environmental and other non-dietary toxins in the following ways:

Reducing the burden on the body – By reducing the amount of food-related toxins, allergens, fungus and parasites in the large and small intestines that the body has to contend with, your body is freed up to deal with other toxins such as chemicals and metals more efficiently.

A person who has allergies to non-food items such as cat hair or pollen, or the nickel in root canals and some other dental work such as metal crowns and bridges, might well find that these allergies are at least partially alleviated by the detox diet. Once food-related reactivity is lessened, the body can better deal with non-food allergens since it is less overwhelmed. This is also the case with secondary allergy caused by the waste products of microorganisms.

Nutrition – All components of the diet, both foods and supplements, are healthful and provide all of the needed nutritional elements. Supplements provide concentrated predigested nutrients, especially protein. Although the food intake seems limited, the nutrient content is higher overall than most people are used to consuming. It is important to feed the cells without feeding the microorganisms.

Colon cleansing – The reduction of food intake, the use of non-mucus-forming foods, and the use of oils and a fiber supplement help to clean out the colon.

Cleansing of the rest of the digestive system, the lymph system, and the blood capillaries is accomplished through the use of enzymes.

Removal of toxins – We emphasize plenty of water and beneficial oils, which, among other helpful effects, help to carry water-soluble and oil-soluble toxins out of the body.

What is involved in the diet?

The diet is eight days long. During the first four days, you eat certain vegetables along with non-hydrogenated oils such as olive and flax, and supplements. This is primarily to clean out your system, since it takes 3-4 days for previously consumed foods to exit the body. On the second four days you add in non-gluten or low-gluten grains. The specifics are spelled out in this chapter, along with the rationale behind each step. Rotating the foods eaten lowers the possibility of an allergic response, as discussed in greater detail later in this chapter.

Although the diet can usually be done without practitioner input and is presented here as a do-it-yourself treatment, you may be working with a knowledgeable health professional, which is recommended. If there is an apparent contradiction between instructions here and recommendations by your practitioner, follow your practitioner's advice as it should be tailored to your particular health situation.

Any specific food allergies or sensitivities that you are aware of should guide your food choices.

What not to do before the detox

If you know you're going to start the detox diet in a few days, it is human nature to want to have one last binge, a hearty meal complete with wine, a last weekend of freedom. Don't do it. The purpose of the detox diet is to detox from past excesses and to emerge from the experience as clean inside as possible. If you deliberately precede the detox diet with more unhealthy food and beverages, the diet will mostly be coping with the results of that binge, and you will have less overall improvement. In addition, there would be an increased likelihood of withdrawal symptoms from sugar, alcohol, and/or caffeine. The goal here is to purge the long-accumulated toxins, not just the previous weekend's excesses.

The Detox Diary

As mentioned, there are a wide variety of symptoms that may or may not be experienced. Some of these symptoms can indicate allergy, yeast or other microorganisms in the small intestine or large intestine, or other root causes of your symptoms. Symptoms that come on after the first day could point to possible different problems than symptoms that come on after, say, the third day. Even if you have no apparent reaction to the diet, this in itself is useful information – the primary problem is not likely located in the intestines, or is probably not food sensitivity or microorganisms. Therefore, it is important to document your symptoms, and when they occur, for you (or your practitioner) to interpret.

Sample Detox Diary

Day	Urine pH	Tem-perature	# Stools	Foods eaten	Symptoms experienced
1					
2					
3					
4					
5					
6					
7					
8					

Urine pH is taken during the first morning urination after sunrise. # Stools refers to the number of stools per day.

Temperature is taken under the arm first thing on awakening, using a mercury rather than a digital thermometer (preferred), or use a digital thermometer under the tongue if a mercury thermometer is not available. The temperature under the arm should be no less than 97; if it is lower, it could indicate thyroid suppression that can be due to high toxicity. A temperature that climbs up into the normal range after being on the detox diet is an indicator that the detox is working as it should.

Symptoms to watch out for include, but are not limited to: fatigue, dizziness, nausea, vomiting, constipation, diarrhea, appetite loss, indigestion, urinary problems, insomnia, anxiety, depression, difficulty concentrating, irritability, headache, and neck or back ache.

Since it is an elimination diet, what is eliminated, and why?
Foods that are most likely to cause trouble in one way or another are eliminated.

Allergy – Foods that are most likely to be allergenic in the general population are eliminated:

- **Wheat**; both the wheat protein and the gluten that is part of the grain can cause problems
- **Gluten** grains, including wheat, barley, and rye. Spelt and kamut are related to wheat and also contain gluten.
- **Dairy** products are a commonly allergenic. Additionally, many people are lactose intolerant, which is not a true allergy but can manifest in bloating, cramping, and gas. Dairy is also mucus forming, which accounts for the sniffles and throat-clearing that many people experience from it. The dairy category includes milk, cheese, and yogurt. Some people are more tolerant of dairy products from goats or sheep rather than cows, but for the purposes of this protocol all dairy from whatever source is eliminated. Whey, a milk product, rarely causes problems if hydrolyzed.
- **Soy**, including edamame (whole soybeans), tofu, soy protein powders, and soy beverages.
- **Nuts**, which are hard to digest and may contain mold, especially peanuts and pistachios, in addition to being allergenic; peanuts can contain highly toxic aflatoxins.
- **Corn**, including corn syrup which is in many processed foods, including quite a few that you might not suspect – read the labels.
- **Citrus** fruits: oranges, grapefruit, lemons, and limes. However, in most cases unless there is a major allergy, a small amount of lemon juice is allowed with oil as a flavor enhancer, as it is least likely to cause problems.
- **Eggs**
- **Tomatoes**

Yeast – Certain foods feed yeast or contain yeast or yeast-related substances such as fungi and molds. Yeast can cause all kinds of problems in the body, from fatigue to foggy thinking to athlete's foot. Foods that contain or feed yeast include:

- Breads, rolls, pretzels
- Mushrooms, which are fungi related to yeast
- Fermented foods such as tempeh and miso. Although some fermented foods are products of beneficial bacterial fermentation rather than yeast fermentation, they may not be entirely benign, and may contain yeast as well.
- Foods preserved in brine and/or vinegar, such as pickles and olives
- Nuts, which can contain mold, especially peanuts and pistachios.
- Vinegar, also found in most mayonnaise, salad dressing, ketchup, and prepared mustard
- Sugar – see below
- Brewer's yeast, sometimes used as a food supplement, is a good source of B vitamins. However, it is still yeast, although of a different type than baking yeast, and it is best to avoid it since there would likely be cross-reactivity.

Sugars can feed yeast and are often allergenic. In addition, sugar is toxic in itself and can be a huge stressor to the body. Since sugar is being increasingly recognized as a villain, manufacturers often list sugar on their labels in less-well-recognized forms, or split the sweetening among several different sugars so no one sugar appears at the top of the ingredients list. A good rule to follow is "Do not eat if it tastes sweet." Sugars and sugar-containing foods include:

Do not eat if it tastes sweet

- The obvious: candy, cookies, ice cream, cake, and sodas, as well as sugar added to coffee or tea.
- Anything with any -ose listed in the ingredients, such as fructose, dextrose, or maltose. Some people believe that fructose, since it's found in fruit, is "natural" and thus relatively harmless. However, after processing, one has a white granular powder or syrup that is as concentrated and damaging as sucrose (table sugar).
- Any fruit. This is especially the case with dried fruits, which concentrates the sugars, and with fruit juices.
- Any kind of juice other than lemon. Even vegetable juice is a bad idea, since natural sugars become too concentrated without fiber to buffer them or chew-

ing to tell the stomach to prepare for digestion, and internal fermentation and bloating can result.

- Honey, syrup, molasses, maple syrup, agave syrup. Some of these are arguably less harmful than sucrose or corn syrup, but for the purposes of this detox they should be eliminated altogether.
- Anything sweetened with corn syrup, sometimes called high-fructose corn syrup. This is found in a surprising number of commercial products, including those not thought of as sweet such as salad dressings and pasta sauces.
- Sweet vegetables such as tomatoes, peas, corn, carrots, beets, bell peppers (especially red, the sweetest kind), sweet potatoes and yams, and winter (orange, thick-skinned) squash.
- Stevia, a natural sweetener, is less harmful than most of the others. However, it should be avoided in the beginning until urinary pH (see Assessment chapter) stabilizes. A good rule to follow is: if it tastes sweet, spit it out.

Nightshade vegetables can contribute to arthritis symptoms in susceptible individuals:

- Tomatoes. As an interesting aside, tomatoes were considered to be poisonous at one time because of their association with and inclusion in the biological group deadly nightshade. Perhaps this theory was not as wrong as was later thought.

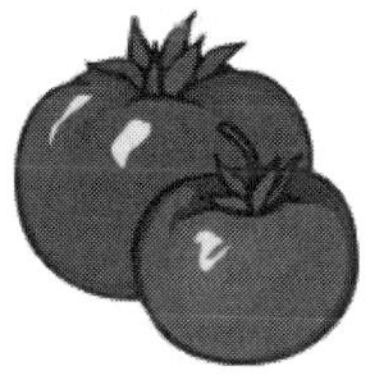

- Potatoes. In addition to their inclusion in the nightshade family, potatoes contain toxic solanine, especially in green spots on the skin.
- Peppers, which include bell peppers, chilies and other spicy peppers
- Eggplant
- Tobacco, while not a food, is also in the nightshade family. But of course you're not *smoking* while doing a detox diet, are you?

Legumes can be hard to digest. They can ferment in the intestinal tract, causing bloating and gas:

- Lentils, beans, peas
- Some nuts such as peanuts are also considered to be legumes

Meats can be hard to digest and sometimes allergenic:

- Beef
- Pork
- Lamb
- Chicken

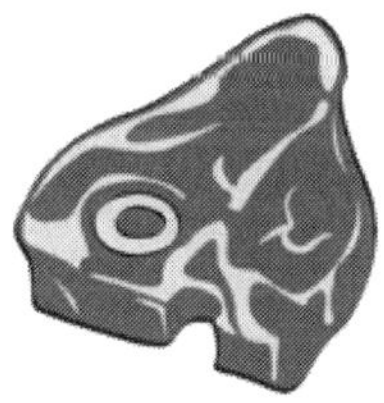

- Fish
- Shellfish, especially, have allergenic potential

Lamb, chicken, and fish are less difficult to digest than beef and pork, due to their size and protein complexity, but are not on the detox diet, since we want the enzymes that are taken to digest allergens, microbes, and waste food protein, not meat protein. Some studies have implicated meat, as well as dairy products, in the formation of some cancers.

Toxic drugs that are consumed as beverages:

- Alcohol, including milder forms such as wine and beer
- Coffee, including decaffeinated, and caffeine-containing tea

Other toxins

- Carbonated drinks, including carbonated water, make the bowels more alkaline, a condition favored by yeast and other microorganisms. A more alkaline digestive tract leads to less hydrochloric acid (HCl) for digestion, and food will then putrefy and ferment rather than digesting. Another consideration is that carbon dioxide, used to make carbonated beverages, is a waste product to the body that is expelled by the lungs; it doesn't make sense to breathe it out and then drink it in.
- Saccharin, aspartame, any artificial sweetener. Splenda and stevia can be used once the urinary pH (described in the Assessment chapter) stabilizes at 6 for at least a week.
- Unhealthy oils – fried foods, partially hydrogenated oils, margarine
- Food additives – colors, flavors, preservatives

So what's left? What foods are eaten on the detox diet?

In general:

Days 1-4: Allowed vegetables, oils, seasonings, and supplements

Days 5-8: Same as days 1-4, plus add in allowed non-gluten grains (rotate grains)

It is imperative that you eat vegetables all 8 days and grains every day from days 5-8 even if you are not hungry – and, amazingly, you may not be all that hungry, especially if you eat as much E7 supplement as you need, and swish Aloe 7000 in water for two minutes and swallow to alleviate sweets cravings.

There is no limitation on quantities eaten, when or how often during the day a particular food is eaten, or how the permitted foods are combined, which is another thing that will help keep hunger at bay.

The foods that can be eaten include:

- **Vegetables**: All green vegetables can be eaten, except peppers (nightshade), peas (sweet), edamame soybeans (allergenic), and lima beans (starchy, gas-producing). Vegetables can be raw or cooked, and can be eaten separately or together. They should be eaten in their natural fiber-filled form, not juiced. Sprouts are fine. Permitted vegetables other than green ones include onions, garlic, cauliflower, and red cabbage, and any other non-sweet vegetables.
- **Oils**: Oils are necessary nutrients, and they aid in cleansing the colon and removing toxins, especially oil soluble toxins, from the body. Organic cold-pressed or expeller-pressed oils are best, because oils extracted with heat or chemicals can contain trans fats, solvents, or other toxins. They must not be cooked, so frying foods is not permitted. The most healthful oils are olive, flax, sesame, sunflower, safflower, and coconut; avoid canola. If cancer is present, limit yourself to fish oils and olive oil, since some other oils are high in omega-6 fatty acids which can be converted to arachidonic acid, which feeds fast growing cells.
- **Grains**: The non-gluten grains buckwheat (which is not related to wheat despite the name), brown rice or wild rice, and millet, or low-gluten grains amaranth and quinoa, are added in on days 4-8. Grains should be cooked only until chewy, not crunchy and not soft or soggy; they ferment quickly if overcooked, and undercooked grains can lead to allergy. They must be cooked fresh at each meal or they can ferment. Eat one grain a day starting with the grains you eat the least and also starting with the non-gluten grains to avoid reactivity. An example of a well-chosen order would be millet on the first day, then buckwheat, rice, quinoa, and amaranth on subsequent days. Rinse quinoa twice before eating.
- **Seasonings**: Real Salt, Celtic salt, or sea salt can be used, but not commercial salt, which can contain toxic aluminum and dextrose (sugar). Kona Gold (Integris), which contains vital minerals, can taste like a slightly sweet salt when the capsule is opened and it can be used as a condiment. Lemon and lime juice are the only fruit allowed; they can be used as a condiment. It is best to have it fresh squeezed if possible because it can ferment, and bottled lemon juice contains undesirable preservatives. Some herb seasonings and teas can contain mold, which is allergenic and puts off toxins. Permitted seasonings include celery salt, dill weed, marjoram, cayenne pepper (not black pepper), garlic, onions, dry mustard (avoid prepared mustard, which contains vinegar), and cinnamon.

- **Teas** – Most non-sweet herbal teas, such as spearmint, desert herb, red raspberry herb, and Pau de Arco are okay.
- **Supplements** – These are discussed later in this chapter and in the Supporters section.

Only pure foods should be eaten, organic if possible to avoid pesticides and other chemicals as well as to provide greater nutritional value. It is important to use foods without additives, artificial colors, or preservatives to the greatest extent possible. It is best to prepare vegetables and grains in purified or bottled water, not tap water which can introduce chlorine, fluoride, and other contaminants.

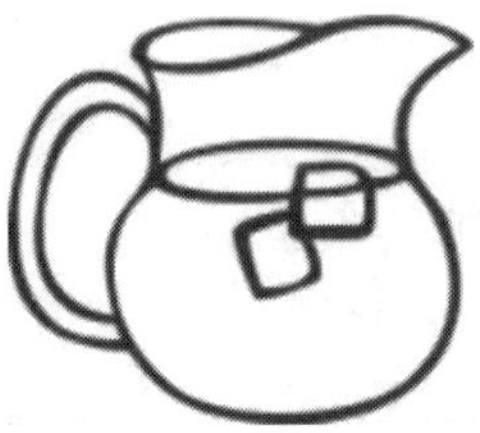

Why is water so important in detoxification?
Do not skimp on this life-giving fluid. Water dissolves and helps to carry water-soluble toxins out of the body. It also promotes sweating and urination, through which toxins are eliminated. In addition, dehydration slows down metabolism.[1]

Drink a lot of water (purified, spring, or bottled, not tap water) to help flush toxins from the body. A minimum of eight cups a day, or ½ ounce for each pound of body weight, is recommended in addition to water for powder supplements. Distilled water is fine for detoxification, but not for long term use because it contains no minerals and can deplete the body's minerals.

What are some water myths and confusion?
There has been some confusion regarding what exactly is counted as water. Some practitioners only count water that is drunk as water itself, and they say that herb teas, the water in vegetables, soups, and so on does not count. Let's look at that one. Many people go years and even decades without actually drinking water as such, preferring other beverages, and, although a person will die after only three days without water, such people are alive and at least somewhat well, so obviously water from other sources does count. However, still aim for the amount recommended above, and include water in other forms as best you can in your calculations.

Another myth about water that is in some books and teachings is that thirst only kicks in once the person is already dehydrated, so therefore one should drink before becoming thirsty. Let's think about that one as well: assuming that the body is designed correctly, such a mechanism would not be in the body's best interests. The body's thirst mechanism, like its hunger mechanism, kicks in when the supply is running low, not when there is imminent danger of dehydration (or starvation, in the case of hunger). This mechanism can be compared to the gas tank light that comes on when there is about an eighth of a tank of gas left, rather than when it is empty, at which point the problem would be obvious and the light would be useless.

What about hunger?

Some people are concerned that their hunger and their sugar and food cravings will keep them from following the diet, or that adherence to the diet will require a great deal of willpower and difficulty. Many people on this diet program – perhaps most of them – are pleasantly surprised and even amazed to find that food cravings and desires for binge eating typically dissipate rapidly on what would seem to be a very limited diet within a few days. Causes of cravings and ravenous hunger, such as yeast, nutrient deficiencies, and allergies, are all addressed by the elimination of troublesome foods and the taking of supplements.

Much hunger and craving comes from poor nutrition; insufficient nutrients cause the body to need and want more regardless of the high number of calories consumed. Strong hunger that isn't the result of lack of food is typically the sign of a malnourished, toxic, out-of-balance body, and this unproductive hunger should ease within days of starting this diet, which includes the taking of E7, Aloe 7000, and Cleanzyme.

Although willpower may be needed for the first couple of days, hunger often practically disappears after that, leading to the surprising advice to be sure to eat enough. One thing that this eight-day diet detox does is reset the body's desire thermostat. After a junk-food diet, bland vegetables sound pretty boring and restrictive, but after only four days on this first phase, one's taste tends to shift dramatically. Even a non-sweet vegetable such as cabbage has its own natural sweetness when it's not drowned out by heavily sweetened foods, and a level of seasoning formerly enjoyed may now seem too salty, too spicy, too sweet, too much. After the first four days, adding in grains can feel like a remarkably tasty and awaited treat rather than a limitation. You may find that the foods on the diet, which were previously uninteresting, take on unexpected flavors and sweetness as your system is cleaned out.

It is not uncommon for the first grains introduced on day 5 to taste wonderful after four days of only vegetables. Once your system is cleaned out, food desires are more likely to reflect actual nutritional need to be heeded rather than unhealthy cravings to be battled.

What about sugar and other cravings?

People with a sugar addiction often worry about sugar cravings torpedoing their good intentions.

First off, just as general hunger tends to ease, so do sugar cravings. After just a few days of not feeding either their allergic sugar addiction or their yeast-in-residence, sugar cravings often ease. At worst, you may need to exercise willpower in order to avoid sugar, but this shouldn't last, and sugar will likely seem unappealing after just a few days after removal from the diet and the taking of E7 and Aloe 7000, as amazing as this may seem.

Sugar cravings are also kept at bay with the Aloe 7000 supplement that goes along with this protocol. Aloe helps to control yeast and pathogenic bacteria in the mouth and digestive tract, which would in turn reduce cravings for sugar, yeast's food, as well as help to clear upper respiratory infections.

When you first start using the aloe, you may find the taste to be quite unpleasant. This is not necessarily the taste of the aloe, but rather the taste of aloe reacting with fungus. Once the fungus is mostly gone, the taste of the aloe typically goes from unpleasant to neutral. This is a good measure of the initial amount of fungus and of the improvement after only a few days on aloe and the detox diet.

Cravings for fatty or fried foods often come from lack of beneficial oils. The oil supplement that is part of this program addresses this, and fatty food cravings are rare on this diet for this reason.

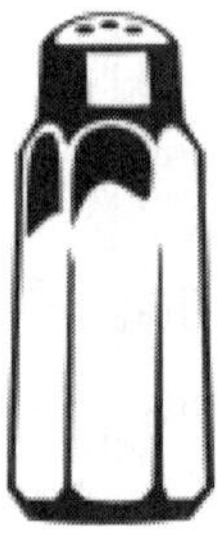

Although healthful forms of salt are allowed on this diet, provided that you don't need to limit salt for health reasons, it is recommended that you use a minimal amount of salt, if any – a maximum of 1½ tsp per day from all sources – to let the true food flavors come through. As long as you're retraining your palate, you might as well work on this at the same time. You may find that your desire for your former preferred level of saltiness will soon shift for the lower and better.

What supplements should be taken during the detox?

The vegetables, grains, and oils, while nutritionally useful, do not provide protein and some nutrients. Supplements are used to keep this detox period as nutritionally rich as possible. It is important that the supplements be pure and as free from additives as possible. The recommended supplements are:

- **Essential 7** (E7), which provides the seven basic nutrient groups: Protein, digestive enzymes, vitamins (coenzymes), minerals (cofactors) and trace minerals, fiber, fatty acids, antioxidants, and lactobacilli (beneficial bacteria to aid digestion). All of these ingredients are natural and organic.
- **Cleanzyme** – One capsule of this should be taken every waking hour. Enzymes help with digestion when taken with meals and with other metabolic processes when taken away from meals; this dosage schedule covers both. Enzymes also help to "digest" certain microorganisms, which are protein. Cleanzyme should be taken after meals if you have ulcer or acid reflux.
- **Kona Gold** is an important source of minerals, and two should be taken before each meal. The capsules can be opened and the contents used as a slightly salty seasoning, if desired. The contents of the opened capsule can also be placed under the tongue for more rapid sublingual absorption.

- **Aloe 7000** – Mix one part aloe to two parts water; swish in the mouth for two minutes and swallow. Aloe helps to control yeast and pathogenic bacteria in the mouth and digestive tract and therefore helps control sugar cravings.
- **SoZo** – Take one capsule per day away from food (one hour before and two hours after eating) and other supplements. Many people who take SoZo report improved sleep and energy as well as relief of pain and stiffness.
- **AdvaClear** supports the production of cytochrome P450, a natural detoxifier of chemicals.
- **MetalloClear** contains metallothionein, which helps to detoxify metals.
- **Paragon** – This is a parasite cleanse, and two should be taken before each meal. Parasites are so common that this has become a routine part of the detox protocol. If you plan to travel abroad, take two Paragon before each meal as a good preventative measure.

Manufacturers and suppliers for these supplements are given at the end of this chapter, and the supplements can be ordered from the Center for Advanced Medicine, 760-632-9042 or toll-free 888-244-4420.

What can I expect during and after the detox?
Some people – not all – experience a temporary worsening of symptoms, usually on days 1 or 3 and lasting up to three days. You may want to keep this in mind when planning your detox diet so as not to interfere with a busy schedule. Friday is a good day to start for someone with a typical Monday-to-Friday work schedule. The worsening of symptoms, if it happens at all, is usually a good sign that the program is doing its work, and you should soon feel better.

When microorganisms die off, they release toxins that can cause symptoms. A detox causes the release of larger quantities of toxins than usual, often resulting in symptom worsening. If you are giving up coffee, withdrawal-type symptoms such as headache and fatigue are possible.

Some flu-like symptoms that are not uncommon on a detox can include:

Headache	Fatigue	Weakness	Dizziness
Nausea	Achiness	Loss of appetite	Constipation
Sleeplessness	Diarrhea	Depression	Brain fog

Some people do not feel worse on the detox diet. In fact, many if not most people, whether or not their symptoms worsened initially, feel significantly better than when they started by about day 4 of the program.

What about weight loss?

Many if not most people who do the detox diet lose weight. They may lose a few pounds due to taking in fewer calories, but there is more to it than this. People who are retaining a lot of water to dilute toxins or allergens may lose quite a bit of this excess water as toxins and allergens are eliminated. Although water weight loss is often derided as not being real weight loss, if you are holding water to dilute toxins, losing this excess, as well as losing cellulite, is real indeed, and an indication of the success of the detox.

If you don't want to lose weight or would like to gain weight, you may lose weight at first, but this is not cause for alarm. You will probably put the weight back on after the detox. Since one of the secondary goals of the detox diet is to normalize digestion, as well as to finally absorb the food you eat, improved food utilization may result in needed weight gain and even weight redistribution.

> **Patient profile**
>
> One patient was of normal weight before the detox, about 126 pounds. However, it was distributed unevenly: she had a slight upper body and a substantial rear and thighs, the result of toxin storage. After eight days on the diet she lost ten pounds and was then 116 pounds; her body, although thin, was better proportioned. Within a month or so she was back up to 126 pounds, but the weight was more evenly distributed and balanced than before, a visible indicator of the benefit of the detox diet.

If rapid weight loss occurs on the detox, chemicals or pesticides that are stored in your fat, lymph, and water and elsewhere in your body can be released into the bloodstream, which may cause some of the previously listed symptoms. This is actually good news, as the toxins are closer to being released from the body. Other detoxification steps in this book can help facilitate this release.

What can be done if I don't feel well during the detox?

Symptoms are due to two major categories of causes: unavoidable and avoidable. If this diet, or any detox procedure, causes toxins to enter the bloodstream as it opens the capillaries and releases toxins from the cells and lymph, this is a good and necessary (unavoidable) prelude to getting rid of them altogether, but their presence can cause discomfort, or more discomfort than you started out with. Stick with the detox – this is important – and manage the symptoms as best you can with the following suggestions.

Nutrient depletion or imbalance can occur, and these are avoidable discomforts. Simply identifying the deficient nutrient, usually a mineral, and adding it to your protocol can help ease the symptoms. Symptoms and recommendations regarding the major minerals are listed in the Mineral Balancing chapter. Kona Gold contains most of the needed minerals and a few additional capsules of this might take care of the problem without needing to identify the particular mineral deficiency.

Headaches, nausea in the first few days is sometimes due to detoxification or withdrawal from caffeine. Ginger root capsules (1-2 for symptomatic relief) can help. Epsom salt baths (1 cup Epsom salts in a tub of very warm water) can also alleviate symptoms. An ice bag on the back of the neck can also help with headache.

Vomiting can deplete sodium from the upper GI tract. Take a capsule of Kona Gold or 1 teaspoon of mineral salt /Real Salt in a glass of water.

Nausea, vomiting – Stop taking all supplements except enzymes, and reduce enzyme intake to one tablet every three hours. Take Kona Gold to remedy a possible salt deficiency, which can contribute to nausea. If the nausea or vomiting is really severe, which is quite rare, especially if the detox is supervised, take salted chicken to stop the detox entirely. The enzymes will stop digesting the yeast and will digest the chicken, stopping the detox, and the salt will help with nausea and vomiting.

Fatigue, shakiness, and brain fog can be hypoglycemic symptoms. Take more Life Solubles or Essential 7 protein powder as needed, up to 10 scoops per day.

Backache, headache, flu symptoms, bad breath, coated tongue, gas and bloating, skin problems, trouble concentrating, and fatigue may be due to the release of toxins into the bloodstream prior to elimination. This is also called a healing crisis and these symptoms are actually a good sign. Most of the time the worse you feel the first three days, the better you will feel by the end of the detox. They should be at their worst for no more than 3 days and then improve. Sun Chlorella can help with these symptoms.

Diarrhea or loose stools and frequent urination can cause depletion of minerals from the lower GI tract. Take potassium and calcium on an empty stomach, or Ultra Flora IB. Avoid taking too much magnesium.

Other recommendations – Rest when needed, and keep your environment as stress-free as possible. Check your first morning urine pH as described in the Assessment chapter.

How can I interpret detox diet symptoms?

As mentioned earlier in this chapter, it is important to keep track of what is eaten, and how you feel, on each day, in the form of a Detox Diary.

If you don't feel substantially different after doing the detox, the problem is likely not food allergy or is not located in the gastrointestinal tract. It may be dental, structural, microbial, or due to airborne toxins or allergens. It's time to go on to the next, non-dietary, detoxification phases.

If you improve noticeably during or just after the detox, it is quite likely that food allergy or sensitivity, food toxicity, or gastrointestinal and digestive problems are major players in your health challenges. Further treatment can be tailored by your practitioner accordingly.

Adjunctive therapies

Other therapies can be done in addition to the detox diet. These therapies complement the diet and increase detoxification. Such therapies, both DIY and practitioner, include the following, most of which are discussed later in this book section:

- Colonics or enemas clean out the lower GI tract and alleviate toxic symptoms. Other types of colonic cleanses are also valuable, such as Super Aloe 450.
- Liver/gallbladder flush is indicated for nausea after eating fatty foods, tightness between the shoulder blades (the trapezius muscles on either side of the neck are related to gallbladder function due to referred pain), stiff neck, or head pressure.
- Lymphatic exercises and lymphatic massage help eliminate toxins.
- Mineral IVs replace lost minerals, often indicated for weakness or if oral minerals are poorly absorbed.
- Allergy desensitization, such as NAET, can reduce reactivity.

Colonics or enemas during and/or just after a dietary detox are much more thorough than diet or colonics alone. The detox diet helps to dump the toxins into the bloodstream; from there they go to the colon where they can exit on their own, but providing assistance is really helpful. People who have colonics just after a detox, whether dietary or via a liver flush (in this book section), are often delightfully surprised by how much comes out, compared with the same colonic on its own. It's wonderfully gratifying to see everything from gallstones to the bright orange-yellow of pesticides exiting, never to return.

How long does the diet last?

The diet lasts for eight days. It is not necessary or advisable to continue on the diet for longer than this unless individually recommended, as it is both nutritionally and psychologically limited for long-term use. However, it is a good idea to limit or eliminate most of the undesirable foods listed previously, especially sugars, yeast-feeders (sweets, alcohol, vinegar, and yeast), and allergens (dairy, wheat, corn, soy, and peanuts), even after the diet has ended. The Maintenance diet is discussed in the next chapter.

Detox diet summary chart

Category	Can eat	Avoid
Green vegetables	All except peas, lima beans, peppers	Peas, lima beans, green peppers
Other vegetables	Thin-skinned squash, cauliflower, onion, garlic, avocado	Carrots, thick-skinned squash, potatoes, tomatoes, eggplant, bell peppers, mushrooms, yams
Grains	Millet, buckwheat, amaranth, quinoa, teff, brown rice, wild rice	Wheat, barley, oats, spelt, kamut. Also bread, pasta, granola
Fruits	None	All fruits and their juices
Juices	None	Any juices, even vegetable
Meats	None	All meats
Beans and legumes	None	All beans and legumes
Dairy	None	All dairy
Eggs	None (allergenic)	Eggs
Nuts	None	All nuts
Oils	Olive oil, flax, fish oil, coconut oil, safflower, sunflower	Fried foods, heated oils, canola oil, butter, margarine
Condiments	None except seasonings	All condiments (most contain vinegar and/or corn syrup) – vinegar, catsup, mayonnaise
Seasonings	Sea salt, cayenne, celery seed, dill, garlic, marjoram, dry mustard, cinnamon, thyme, basil, oregano, parsley, cilantro, ginger	Black pepper, commercial salt
Beverages	Filtered water, non-sweet herbal teas	Soda, juice, coffee, milk, black and green tea, alcohol
Sweeteners	None	Sugar in any form, maple and other syrups, corn syrup, honey, artificial sweeteners

Maintenance diet

After the detox diet – what then?

One benefit of the detox diet is to clean out the system enough that you can introduce foods, one at a time, and actually be able to tell whether you're having a problem with that particular food. This concept is similar to being able to tell whether a violin is out of tune when it is being played solo, but when the out-of-tune violin is part of an entire orchestra it's much harder to tell where the problem is. Similarly, if you feel crummy overall, you would have no idea which food or foods – or other factors – are causing the problems, and isolating them in a cleaned-out system helps with this process. Adding foods back one at a time, rotating them every five days, can help you find and eliminate foods to which you may be sensitive.

Assuming that you feel much better after the detox, the usual case, it is a good idea to add in new foods one at a time so a return or worsening of symptoms, if any, can be noticed and correlated with a particular food, which can then be avoided. Once a new food is introduced, the symptoms that you are looking for are, for the most part, the symptoms that were bothering you before, which could be fatigue, brain fog, headaches, joint pains, gas, and bloating.

If you are working with a practitioner, it is a good idea to schedule an appointment for about day 4 to day 9, just before or after completing the diet, so you can be guided as to follow-up.

What is the best diet for after-detox maintenance?

Ideally the diet should consist of:

- 30% protein
- 40% grains
- 30% vegetables

In addition, beneficial oils should be part of the diet.

Meats can be added in, although beef is not recommended at first because it is less digestible than others because of the larger and less digestible protein size, which can set up conditions leading to allergies. It is important that meats be from a good source – organic and grass-fed; otherwise you could be ingesting toxic and allergenic substances such as antibiotics, hormones, and pesticides that are often found in commercial meats. Organ meats such as liver and kidneys, especially, must be from a good source; since these organs help to detoxify the animal, commercial organ meats may be especially loaded with toxins.

Fish of most types are recommended for their healthy oils, except that large fish such as tuna and swordfish should be avoided because they can contain toxic mercury.

Eggs should be added with caution, since egg allergy is common. Try an egg by itself to be sure you aren't reacting to it. Now is not the time to get creative with a multi-ingredient omelet, since if you react, you won't know what you are reacting to. Eggs are best soft-boiled or poached, rather than with a hard-cooked yolk, because more cooking makes the protein less digestible.

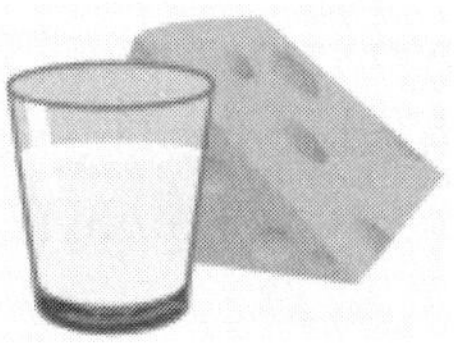

Dairy – Many people can tolerate dairy products, such as cheese, from goats or sheep, but not cows. Most bovine (cow) dairy products sold in stores are both pasteurized and homogenized, which can have adverse health effects. Pasteurization involves heating the milk to a temperature high enough (over 118F) to kill microbes, which also kills enzymes – such as lactase, which helps to digest milk – as well as beneficial bacteria such as lactobacillus. Pasteurized milk doesn't sour, as in the process used to make pleasant-tasting sour cream and buttermilk; rather, it simply rots and putrefies. If it sits in your body, at 98.6 degrees, for several days, it rots in your body as well.

Homogenization breaks up the milk into almost microscopically tiny particles to keep the cream and the skim component permanently blended. However, these smaller particles are more likely to escape into the bloodstream from the intestines, especially if the intestines are unhealthy and overly permeable, setting the stage for dairy allergies and sensitivities.

Yogurt, unsweetened, especially "health food" brands, can sometimes be tolerated by those who have trouble with dairy milk, since they often contain lactase and beneficial acidophilus bacteria to help with its digestion.

Other sources of protein include:

- Beans, lentils, legumes, and dried peas are best if they are soaked first, then drained before cooking in fresh water. The use of enzymes or a product called Beano may reduce gas or discomfort associated with eating beans.
- Nuts, except peanuts or pistachios, can contain toxic mold or, in the case of peanuts, aflatoxins. Almonds are one of the most healthful nuts, and almond milk is a good alternative to dairy milk.
- Seeds such as sunflower and sesame seeds

Vegetables and juices – The sweeter vegetables, listed in and banned from the detox, as well as vegetable juices, contain more sugars than many people can tolerate. However, they also contain many nutrients and enzymes. Should you, then, eat sweet vegetables and drink juices? Whether the detrimental effects of the sugars outweigh the benefits of the enzymes and nutrients does not have a simple one-size-fits-all answer, but can only be answered on an individual basis. Once your system has been cleaned out from the detox diet, try one of the sweeter vegetables or a one-vegetable (not a combination) juice, taken from the detox diet list – carrot juice is too sweet for most people – and see how you feel. Urinary pH testing, described in the Assessment chapter, is another way of monitoring whether you are handling a particular food well.

Wheat grass juice is touted as being very beneficial, and it may well be. However, since it is so concentrated and has a sweet taste, it may be too sweet for many people. As with other foods that are being introduced at this time, proceed cautiously and try it separately and in a small amount to see how you do with it.

For more information

A cookbook is available that may be useful, especially after the detoxification diet is over and other foods are added. The cookbook is the ***Toxic Immune Syndrome Cookbook*** by Dr. Bill Kellas, coauthor of this book. This cookbook explains in more detail what foods are and are not good for a healthy immune system and why. Hundreds of recipes and cooking suggestions liven up a diet that may be more limited than what you have been used to. IMPORTANT – The recipes in this cookbook are not necessarily recommended for the eight-day detox diet itself as most of them contain foods not permitted on the diet. The recipes are more applicable to the follow-up maintenance diet. Read the ingredients list for the recipe carefully to see if the recipe would be suitable.

Maintenance diet summary chart

When foods are added in after the detox diet, proceed cautiously and in small amounts, being mindful of your particular sensitivities. Follow the rotation diet on the next page.

Category	Can eat	Avoid
Green vegetables	All except peas, lima beans, peppers	Peas, lima beans, green peppers
Other vegetables	Thin-skinned squash, cauliflower, onion, garlic, avocado	Carrots, thick-skinned squash, potatoes, tomatoes, eggplant, bell peppers, mushrooms, yams
Grains	Millet, buckwheat, brown rice, wild rice (if gluten sensitive). Add in amaranth, quinoa, teff, barley, rye, or oat groats if not gluten sensitive	Wheat, pasta, granola
Bread	Unleavened, yeast-free and wheat-free breads	Yeasted breads
Fruits	None	All fruits and their juices
Juices	Non-sweet vegetable juices	Fruit juices or sweet vegetable juices
Meats	Turkey, chicken, fish (smaller)	Beef, pork
Dairy	Plain yogurt, butter	Fluid milk, cheese, sweetened yogurt; avoid dairy if you have cancer
Beans and legumes	Beans, lentils, legumes, dried peas (soak before cooking)	Large amounts of beans and legumes
Eggs	Eggs (if not allergic), soft boiled or poached	Eggs (if allergic)
Nuts and seeds	Almonds, pecans, filberts. Sunflower, pumpkin, sesame seeds. Nut and seed butters from these.	Peanuts, pistachios
Oils	Olive oil, flax, fish oil, coconut oil, safflower, sunflower, butter	Fried foods, heated oils, canola oil, margarine
Condiments	None except seasonings	All condiments (most contain vinegar and/or corn syrup) – vinegar, catsup, mayonnaise
Seasonings	Sea salt, cayenne, celery seed, dill, garlic, marjoram, dry mustard, cinnamon, thyme, basil, oregano, parsley, cilantro, ginger	Black pepper, commercial salt
Beverages	Filtered water, non-sweet herbal teas, non-sweet vegetable juices	Soda, sweet juices, coffee, milk, black and green tea, alcohol
Sweeteners	None	Sugar in any form, maple and other syrups, corn syrup, honey, artificial sweeteners

Rotation diet

An adjunctive diet to the detox diet is the rotation diet, which is similar to and utilized during the detox diet but is a good idea afterwards or if not on the detox diet. The principle behind the rotation diet is that allergies to a particular food are more likely to occur if that food is eaten frequently, especially if eaten almost every day. It takes at least 72 hours to clear allergens from your body. Allowing four days between each day of eating a particular food lessens the chance of such allergic reactions.

Following the rotation diet can allow some individuals to eat foods they like that would otherwise cause sensitivity symptoms if one is just mildly sensitive.

As an example of how the rotation diet works, if you eat brown rice on Monday, you can have all the rice you want throughout the day on Monday but not have it again until Friday or later.

An example of food rotation, using meats and fish as well as non-gluten grains, is:

Day 1 - Salmon/Millet
Day 2 - Chicken/Quinoa
Day 3 - Tuna/Amaranth
Day 4 - Turkey/Brown Rice
Day 5 - Mackerel/Buckwheat

Then repeat and rotate in gluten grains (oats, barley, rye) on every fifth day and see how you feel. Watch out for fatigue, mucus (runny or stuffy nose), rashes, aches, gas, headaches, or hunger even after eating.

Bad ideas to stay away from

What kinds of detox diets are not a good idea?

Fasting, either total or juice fasting, has some proponents. It can work for some people, in large part because they are pretty healthy to begin with, or because, by fasting, they are eliminating toxic or allergenic foods. For most people, fasting is too drastic. On the plus side, toxic and allergenic food is eliminated, but on the minus side, little or no nutrition is added, and mineral depletion and the attendant symptoms can easily occur. The detox diet in this book provides the positives of fasting without the negatives.

Fasting can lead to constipation due to lack of fiber or any food that can cause the bowels to move, which is counterproductive as a detox because the bowels are a detox pathway and it makes no sense to stop them up.

Fasting is a stress on the adrenals, and detoxification can cause adrenal stress as well. Some of the symptoms encountered during fasting might well be due to adrenal stress. The adrenal stress of detoxification is a necessary part of the process, but adding in stress from fasting is not particularly useful.

Juicing, also called juice fasting when not accompanied by food, is another bad idea for most people. It can lead to good results for some, in part because a juice diet is an improvement on their previous poor diet, and because some nutrients and enzymes are provided, but it has its down side. Juices, even vegetable juices, are much too sweet for most people to handle, and a diet of juices can cause a hydroponic garden of fungus to flourish. A diet composed wholly or mostly of juice also provides no fiber, leading to constipation as is the case with fasting, and lack of chewing fails to alert the stomach that digestion would be needed and the appropriate enzymes should be secreted.

Cathartics are sometimes mistakenly used as a detox aid. Cathartics are herbs, such as senna, that can overstimulate the colon to eliminate wastes. The theory behind cathartics can be summed up as, "if a little is good, more is better." If better bowel elimination is good, it follows, erroneously, that something that makes for more, and more forceful, bowel elimination is even better. However, cathartics essentially make your colon vomit, which is quite the opposite of supporting the body in optimal natural function. Cathartics can result in diarrhea and depletion of crucial minerals (electrolytes).

High fiber diets, with the aim of increasing detoxification through more bowel action, are a good idea, as long as they are not taken too far. Some people, operating under the "if some is good, more is better," principle, take large amounts of a concentrated fiber such as psyllium or wheat fiber, rather than natural fiber as a component of food. There are several drawbacks to this. For one thing, addition of a large amount of fiber can result in gas, bloating, and intestinal pain from forcing the intestines to work harder, somewhat like suddenly forcing a muscle to do much more work than it's accustomed to. Secondly, roughage can be too rough; taking wheat bran is rather like swallowing a rasp.

Another serious problem with such high fiber supplementation is that if the person taking the fiber doesn't get enough water, the intestines can actually get blocked up by what is essentially a brick of solid fiber. In extreme cases intestinal blockage severe enough to require medical intervention can result. This danger is one of the reasons why sufficient water, about half your weight in ounces (e.g. 64 ounces daily if you weigh 128 pounds), must be taken along with any fiber supplement, and is strongly recommended on this detox diet.

Clay is sometimes used to increase bowel action, and as is the case with high fiber diets, it can cause blockage, especially if you don't consume enough water. As with high fiber diets, clay with too little water can cause what is essentially a brick to form in the intestines, possibly causing blockage.

Drastic diets of many kinds are promoted for both detoxification and weight loss. A drastic diet can be described as one in which there are only a handful of foods, or even just one food. For example, a rice diet, popular a few decades ago, limited the diet to white rice and not much more, and it helped many people to feel better and lose weight. The weight loss was likely due to both elimination of allergens – white rice is rarely allergenic – and to boredom with the limited diet that didn't encourage overeating. Energy gain from such a diet might also be due to the elimination of allergens. Strictly speaking, a diet of one or a few low-allergenic foods will probably have desired detoxification effects, but at the cost of your long-term nutrition and health.

Then what about the detox diet in this book?

You might be thinking that the detox diet described in this chapter fits the definition of "drastic diet" – just vegetables and a few grains. However, there are a couple of important differences. For one thing, the diet is vegetables and grains, *plus* oils, protein, and other supplements. For another, the detox diet is intended to be followed for eight days only, after which other foods are added in; it's not intended as a dietary lifestyle in itself.

Sauna / Hyperthermia

Sauna treatment, also known as hyperthermia (high temperature) treatment, is often used to detoxify from chemicals and metals.

The high, dry heat helps to remove toxins from the storage depots within the body – from the fat and lymph nodes especially, but also from the muscles, liver, and elsewhere. The toxins are then removed from the body via sweat, which is stimulated by the heat, as well as via breathing, the digestive system, and urine.

What are some of the proven benefits of sauna detoxification?
Sauna detoxification has been researched, and benefits of the procedure have been written up in scientific journals.

One of the physical aspects of drug addiction is the accumulation of drug residues in adipose tissues. Such accumulation, released gradually, has the effect of a tiny daily dosage of the drug, prolonging drug cravings and making it more difficult to stay off the drug. Sauna detoxification helps to release drug residue from the fatty tissue. Drug flashbacks and the feeling of being stoned can occur as the fat-soluble components are released into the bloodstream.

Sauna is consistently successful in eliminating toxins that can be stored in fat even from childhood, such as DDE, PCBs and dioxin.[1,2] Pesticides can be eliminated from the body, even if the initial exposure was decades ago. It is not uncommon for someone else to notice the smell of these chemicals coming from the sweat of someone in the sauna.

Chemical hypersensitivity is usually due to a buildup of chemicals in the body that overloads detoxification systems such that even a tiny amount of additional chemical can cause symptoms. Sauna therapy, by reducing the chemical buildup, can contribute greatly to the patients' improvement in their hypersensitive condition.

Viral and other microbial diseases can be helped with sauna, which makes use of the body's own defense against microbes: fever. The heat from the sauna raises the body temperature, which proves to be inhospitable to many microbes.

Fifty patients with peripheral neuropathy / MS with a history of chemical exposure underwent sauna treatment, and all experienced total remission or marked improvement.[2]

Sauna therapy is useful as an adjunctive treatment for cancer. Hyperthermia modifies cell membranes both to protect healthy cells and to make tumor cells more susceptible to chemotherapy and radiation.[3,4]

What is usually the best approach to sauna detoxification?

The best complete sauna program for detoxification is almost always a practitioner-assisted one, monitored by physicians and nurses. However, such programs are in short supply nationwide and tend to be very expensive, much more than $1000 a week and up to $5000 a week – for good reason considering what is involved – with 2-9 weeks typically recommended depending on the level of toxicity. Thus a do-it-yourself (DIY) adaptation of such a program is the most practical for the large majority of readers. Each of the aspects of a professional sauna program is discussed here with suggestions for a DIY adaptation. If a compromise is possible, we recommend a supervised sauna for at least the first week, and then DIY after that if there are no problems. As with all detox programs, check with a knowledgeable practitioner or the Center for Advanced Medicine, 760-632-9042 or 888-244-4420, to determine whether you are a good candidate for a do-it-yourself detox program. The Center for Advanced Medicine has run a successful sauna program for decades, and has a fully equipped sauna with adjunctive therapies available.

Why is a professional sauna program so expensive?

A complete professional sauna program includes a specially equipped sauna, vented to the outside so heating costs are higher and with oxygen pumped in. It also includes at least one evaluation by a medical doctor, follow-up appointments with a nutritionist or other practitioners, nursing staff, supplements, lymphatic massage, colonics, mineral IVs, blood test, allergy treatment, towels, gowns, and shower with filter. Actually, the sauna program at Center for Advanced Medicine is relatively inexpensive compared to similar programs elsewhere, and CAM prices have remained stable for over a decade. CAM subsidizes part of the cost because the program has so much value for patients who can't be helped any other way.

A full sauna program can seem to be quite expensive, but with good reason. It can be justified even financially: A person who was too sick to work but can now earn a living has reaped material benefits beyond the cost of the sauna, in addition to the nonmaterial benefits such as having a life that is worth living.

How much of a commitment is needed for a sauna program?

A sauna program, do-it-yourself or otherwise, is a high-level commitment. However, for someone who has a high level of chemical toxicity, sauna detox can give you your life back, and it is well worth the commitment of time and money. See coauthor Dr. Dworkin's own story at the end of this chapter, in which doing a professional sauna program returned her to a useful life.

A typical professional sauna program – and we are also using this for our do-it-yourself model – is a five day a week program for 2-9 weeks, although 2-3 weeks is more typical. These are full days, which include four to six sauna sessions, multiple showers and clothing changes, lymphatic exercises, blood pressure checks, breaks to take supplements, and adjunctive treatments. The bottom line here is that a sauna detox protocol is a serious commitment, best undertaken when you are ready and able to commit up to a month or two to spending all day on this.

Since, as discussed in the introductory chapter, detoxification is a two-step procedure – toxins go from fat and other storage to the bloodstream, and then from the bloodstream on out – toxins are temporarily dumped into the bloodstream during sauna, and it isn't uncommon to feel worse before feeling better. Minerals, lost in sweat, need balancing, and if this isn't done properly you can feel worse. Heat in itself drains energy, as anyone who has spent time sitting listlessly in front of a fan on a hot sticky summer day can attest. You will probably not feel well enough to work or get much accomplished during this time.

Another way of putting this is: sauna detox is not for someone who intends to just sit in a sauna for brief periods. Doing that will likely not accomplish much, if anything, and if there are toxins coming from the commercial non-detox sauna itself or from other sauna occupants in an unsupervised program, you could end up worse off.

Is there anyone who shouldn't do a do-it-yourself sauna program?

If you are very ill, you should not embark on a sauna detox program without practitioner supervision. If you are very toxic to the extent that you are experiencing alarming symptoms, increasing the amount of toxins in the bloodstream, however temporarily, could push you over the edge into a health crisis. A word of reassurance here: if you are somewhat sick, fatigued, or not up to par, you are likely not so overloaded that there will be any risk. This paragraph is geared towards those who are quite ill, to the extent that the illness itself is dangerous.

People with multiple sclerosis (MS) are often heat intolerant, finding that heat worsens their symptoms. However, since chemicals are often contributory to MS, sauna could be beneficial. However, given the heat-sensitive nature of MS, a person with MS should only do a supervised sauna. MS patients tend to have little fat to store chemicals, so they don't have much room to be able to release chemicals from what fat they have without professional backup.

Lupus is another illness with a high chemical toxicity component. Since lupus is an autoimmune disease, reactivity to chemicals dumped into the bloodstream from detox could worsen it. Those with lupus should do sauna only if supervised.

People with multiple chemical sensitivity (MCS) – also called environmental illness, or EI – are overloaded with toxins and can benefit from sauna detox. However, even the temporary dumping of additional toxins into the bloodstream on their way out of the body can pose a risk. Sauna is highly recommended for someone with MCS but should not be done as a do-it-yourself project, since there is potential for unpleasant reactions and the speed of detox can be controlled by a professional.

If you have any severe symptoms that could be chemically related, it's best to not even consider an unsupervised sauna program. Some people are so toxic that other, milder forms of detox should be employed before even thinking about doing sauna to bring chemical levels down to a more manageable level.

Wait…before you start…
It is preferred, but not required, that you have your metal fillings, if any, removed prior to doing the sauna program. Toxic mercury in metal fillings can enter the body from the fillings after it is detoxified. If you want to drain the bathtub, turn off the faucet first, metaphorically speaking. However, if you need sauna, don't avoid it because you still have metal fillings.

All saunas are not created equal
You can't just go to any sauna, such as that at a health club, and get detoxified; in fact, the use of such facilities can actually add more toxins, such as those from treated wood, gas heat, or the perfumed products used by others in the sauna. Smokers or other very toxic people can outgas materials that you really don't want to absorb into your body.

Some factors in a healthful detoxification sauna include:

- A sauna for detoxification should be made from non-treated wood, since toxic standard wood preservatives can outgas in the heat and enter the body.
- The sauna should be heated with electricity rather than gas, since if gas is used a small amount of gas might enter the sauna. Infrared (IR) and microwave heating are not considered to be safe since both IR and microwaves excite the cell from the inside out. Although the person in the sauna is not actually microwaved, it is best to err on the side of caution when heating the sauna.
- Commercial saunas are typically tightly built to minimize the escape of heated air and thus to minimize heating costs. A detox sauna has as its priority, not saving heating costs, but the regular elimination of air within the sauna that can contain outgassed toxins.
- Discomfort in the sauna can be due in part to the increased need for fresh air – oxygen – combined with a tight seal that reduces fresh air. A good detox sauna has oxygen pumped into it during use.
- The sauna should have a glass door for safety, so someone on the outside can monitor you. The glass door also minimizes claustrophobia, which can add to anxiety and discomfort.

The choice of sauna is likely to be the one over which you would have the least control, but you still have options, assuming you take the DIY route after the first week of supervised sauna. If you have a choice of saunas in your town, such as those in health clubs, see if you can find one that at least makes some health claims, and ask what kind of wood (ideally untreated) and heat (electric) they have, as well as their policies on people wearing synthetic garments or scented products (none allowed). Based on the information in this part of the chapter, you could make the best choice of what is available.

If space and finances permit, small personal saunas are available for purchase and setup in your home. Such saunas differ in their marketing orientation: some market detox and others focus on relaxation, so shop carefully. Such saunas can be as small or as large as you choose; a small one geared to one or two people would be much cheaper to heat than a larger one, and can allow for some needed ventilation without breaking the budget. As mentioned, look for untreated wood and electric heating. An additional advantage of having your own sauna is that you can set your own rules regarding clothing, detergent, personal care products, and other aspects that could make the difference between detoxifying and becoming more toxic.

The sauna temperature should be set so it measures 170-180 degrees on the top shelf, although the temperature is lower at the lower seating level. Although many saunas have a steam option, sauna heat must be dry; damp heat at that temperature can cause scalding without the desirable raising of the core temperature.

What should I wear, and not wear, in the sauna?

To prevent outgassing of toxins, everything that goes into a sauna, including your and others' bodies and clothing, should be as externally chemically clean as possible.

Cotton clothing and towels should be worn and used. Better yet – and this may be an option in some health clubs and certainly in your own sauna – wear just a towel or nothing at all. Clothing traps toxin-containing sweat which could then be reabsorbed, and the less clothing you wear the more comfortable you will be in the heat. If you wear clothing, other natural fibers in addition to cotton can be used: linen, hemp, or silk, or some of the new natural bamboo or birch blends. Women, you are strongly advised not to wear a bra in the sauna. A bra constricts the lymph nodes, which are part of the detoxification system, and bras also contain stretchy plastics that can outgas. Underwire bras are even worse, since they can block lymph drainage. Don't worry about how you look – you're going to be red and sticky and sweaty anyway. Bathing suits, especially women's bathing suits, are almost always made of synthetic material and can outgas, and so are not recommended.

Organic cotton garments should be worn if at all possible. Conventional cotton is one of the most heavily pesticide-treated crops, and heat could cause these pesticides to outgas into the sauna air.

An alternative to organic cotton is to wear cotton garments that have been washed many times over months and years; pesticide residues should be negligible.

Any garments and towels for use in the sauna – and this is a good idea for all your clothing as well – should be washed in detergent that is as natural as possible, and unscented. Most brands sold at natural food stores or Trader Joe's stores would work well. Avoid almost all laundry additives, such as bleach, brighteners, or dryer sheets. Laundry products such as enzyme-based stain removers are fine.

Shoes should not be worn in the sauna, even to quickly step in to check on someone in the sauna or to clean it. Shoes, unless they are strictly for indoor use, can track in oil from the driveway, pesticides from the grass, and other things you don't want to be breathing; also, they are usually not of natural materials and may outgas in the heat.

Soap and shampoo should be unscented, and no creams, lotions, cosmetics, perfumes, or hairspray should be worn. Makeup should not be worn, since it can outgas and also be absorbed through heat-enlarged pores. Deodorants, if used, should be unscented, although it is better not to use any deodorant at all (we know…eewww). Antiperspirants, especially, should not be used, and many commercial deodorants are combined with an antiperspirant. Think about it: the purpose of a sauna is to sweat, and the purpose of an antiperspirant is to prevent sweating; there's no point in cancelling each other out.

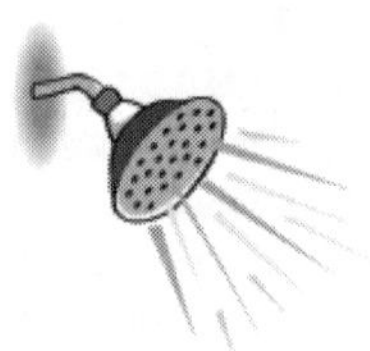

Showers, in addition to not using scented cleansing products, should be done in water that is filtered to remove the chlorine and other chemicals commonly found in tap water. This is especially important during sauna treatment, since lots of showers are involved – several a day – and because your pores would be open from the heat and you could take in more waterborne toxins than usual.

Plan on doing plenty of laundry. You will be using lots of towels. Always sit on a towel so any sweat-borne toxins won't be absorbed into the sauna wood and can be laundered away. Wipe away sweat frequently so it doesn't just get reabsorbed into the body. Change towels and clothing after every shower, which could be three or four in a day.

What about ventilation?

As mentioned, a professional detox sauna ventilates to the outside to get rid of toxins that were in your body, or the bodies of others, so they won't be reabsorbed. Such a sauna may also be pumping in additional oxygen. In a sauna, the need for oxygen increases as the body temperature increases and the body detoxifies, but the typical sauna is tightly sealed for energy efficiency and thus often provides even less oxygen and clean air than a typical room. Oxygen can be pumped in via a tube from an oxygen tank outside. What would be even easier is to simply open the door for a minute or so between sauna sessions (described soon) to provide air exchange, and then the door can be closed to heat the sauna back up again while you are showering or exercising between sessions. This isn't particularly energy efficient, but your goals in a detox sauna are more important than the financial cost of additional heating, or you wouldn't be going to all this trouble and expense in the first place.

There's more to a sauna program than just a sauna

The sauna program includes more than simply sweating in the sauna.

Mineral and other supplements will be needed, since minerals can become unbalanced due to sweating. The Mineral Balancing chapter in the Supporters section gives indications for the use of certain minerals.

Adjunctive therapies include lymphatic (tissue cleansing) exercises and lymphatic massage, and enemas and/or colonics, both described later in this book section. Other therapies in a professional setting include allergy treatments and mineral IVs.

A complete professional sauna program includes the availability of medical personnel to deal with everything from routine blood pressure monitoring to episodes of dizziness. A DIY version advises that someone be nearby to summon help if needed or at least bring minerals, water, or anything else that is wanted or needed. Although almost any responsible adult will do for this purpose, it would be even better to have a nurse, trained person, or someone who is familiar with sauna detox.

Chelation to remove metals from the body is another adjunctive treatment, described in a later chapter in this section. This should only be done after all metal is removed from the mouth, which would ideally have been done in any case before starting sauna.

I have high blood pressure. Or I have low blood pressure.

Blood pressure should be monitored at regular intervals during the sauna or if you feel woozy. If you are prone to unusually high or low blood pressure, it should be checked even more frequently. A number of home blood pressure monitors can be utilized. A person who is prone to high blood pressure might have it go higher from the stress of the heat. A person who tends to have low blood pressure might have it drop low enough for dizziness and even fainting to be a possibility. Salt in water, about a half teaspoon to a glass of water, can help to raise blood pressure if needed, and usually works in about fifteen minutes.

Both high blood pressure, more common in men, and low blood pressure, more common in women, can have toxicity as a contributory factor. You may find your blood pressure improved and brought closer to normal in either case after sauna or other rigorous detox, an often welcome side benefit.

Some of the supplements that are routinely used in sauna programs include niacin, which brings about a flush by increasing circulation; the increased circulation helps to bring toxins to the skin's surface to be eliminated. The niacin flush also brings a feeling of heat, which increases sweating. Other forms of niacin, such as niacinamide, don't have the sometimes uncomfortable flushing effect, but these forms are not useful in sauna. Use niacin with caution if you tend to have low blood pressure because, by dilating the blood vessels, it can lower blood pressure too much. Those with high blood pressure controlled by medication need to be aware that their blood pressure may drop too low and their medication may need to be adjusted to compensate; physician input may be needed here.

But I never sweat

Some people, especially women, report that they just don't sweat, or don't sweat much. Even on a hot day or with strenuous exercise, they just get mildly tacky, and never drip. Such a person typically gets quite red in the face when hot or exerted; interestingly, this redness often disappears around the time the person trains her body to sweat properly. Such a person can go from crimson-faced and sticky to soaking wet and light pink in a few weeks.

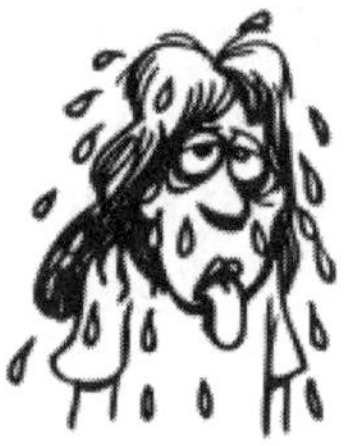

Wait a minute – trains their body to sweat properly? Yes, it can be done, and that is one of the goals of the sauna program. Once you start to sweat in the sauna, this natural mechanism will be activated to work properly as needed. And don't worry – if you already sweat easily you won't sweat more when you don't want to.

Why do some people rarely sweat? This is in part determined by both genetics and gender – women are more likely to have trouble sweating. However, toxicity can cause this particular detox pathway, like the other detox pathways, to overload and jam up and not work properly. Toxicity can be both cause and effect of lack of sweating, in a vicious cycle.

Electrolyte imbalances can also lower the ability to sweat. Too little sodium lowers the ability to sweat; the body suppresses sweating in an attempt to hold onto minerals.

Niacin (not niacinamide), as mentioned, is routinely taken in a sauna program. Its use can speed the journey of toxins to the skin to be eliminated via sweating; it can also increase the amount of sweating itself. Start with a low dosage, maybe 50mg, and increase it until you find the highest level you can comfortably tolerate.

Ginger is a spice that increases sweating, and ginger capsules or a cup of ginger tea can be taken if getting yourself to sweat is a problem. Other spices such as cayenne, which can also be taken in capsule form, can also jumpstart the sweating process. Here's an interesting bit of background regarding spices. You may have noticed that the cuisines of tropical or desert countries and southern states are high in the hot spices: Indian, Thai, Mexican, and Vietnamese food is typically quite spicy, as is much of the food in Louisiana (Cajun), Texas, New Mexico (famous for its chilies), and southern California (nearby Mexican influence). Foods from northern countries or states, such as Canada, England, the Scandinavian countries, or the northern parts of the US, are rarely spicy. This use of hot spices in hot places may seem counterintuitive, since these spices are warming, but they promote sweating, a major cooling mechanism of the body as the water evaporates. Residents of these hot places long ago found that including these hot spices in their cooking makes the heat easier to bear. In addition, hot spices kill parasites which tend to be a problem in these parts of the world. This knowledge, the connection between spices and sweating, is put to use in the sauna program: by increasing sweating, both detoxification and comfort are increased as well. Such spices in capsule or food form can be taken as desired; a few capsules a day are recommended. Cayenne can also increase circulation, and ginger can help ease nausea, so these spices have multiple purposes in a sauna detox.

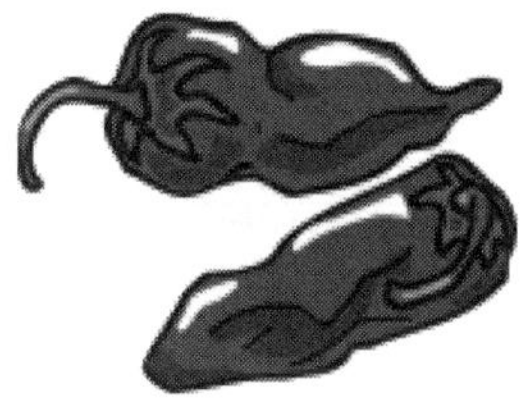

Another note on sweating: People who sweat in non-sauna situations such as heat or exertion might have occasion to taste their sweat, such as by licking their upper lip. As expected, the sweat tastes somewhat salty but not unpleasant. However, those who sweat in the sauna, especially after at least a week of sauna detox, might find that their sweat is strong tasting, acrid, even bitter or metallic. This is the taste of eliminated toxins.

Water water everywhere

Something that is very important in the sauna program is drinking plenty of water, and we mean plenty. More than you need to quench your thirst. More than the 64 ounces or so that are usually recommended in normal, non-sauna conditions. Water is needed to detoxify optimally, and plenty of water along with minerals is needed to promote the most beneficial profuse sweating. Water in large quantities can help to jumpstart sweating in people who rarely sweat.

Can too much water be dangerous? There have been cases in the news where too much water is consumed, causing hyponatremia – literally low levels of salt – and low levels of other minerals due to dilution, to the extent that this can be dangerous. However, this isn't a consideration in the sauna when done as directed. For one thing, you will be monitoring your mineral levels via watching for symptoms as detailed in the mineral balancing discussion in the Supporters section, and checking your blood pressure (too low means to add sodium) and pulse (too high means to add potassium), as well as taking mineral supplements routinely during the program. For another thing, you will be sweating as your body intended so any excess is quickly removed from the body via this mechanism, as well as urinating out both water and toxins. So while in sauna, drink as much as you can comfortably hold, whenever you happen to think about it.

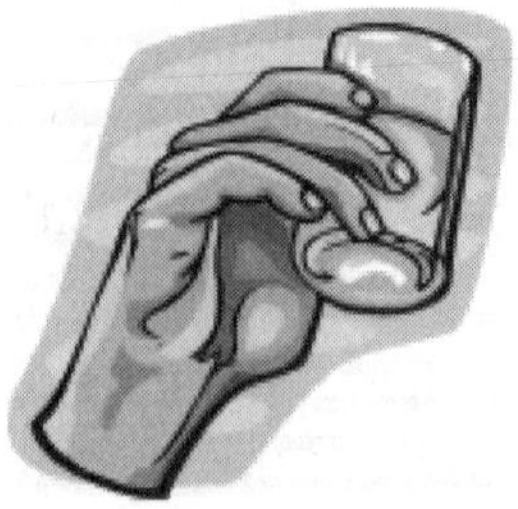

How about too little water? Someone who is trying to lose weight might think that cutting down on water consumption while maximizing sweating is a good way to lose weight. Technically this is true; you could lose enough water to make an impressive difference on the scale, but you would just gain the weight back as soon as you drank enough water, so don't waste your time and endanger your health. Sufficient water is crucial in preventing dehydration, which could easily happen in a hot dry sauna and could be quite dangerous. In addition, the water helps to flush out toxins, which would otherwise be released into the bloodstream with nowhere to go and nothing to do except cause trouble. So drink up.

Minerals, such as those provided by Kona Gold, help the water to enter the cells. When minerals are low and insufficient water gets into the cells, the result is effectively dehydration regardless of how much water is consumed. In addition, the body won't let go of toxins without sufficient minerals; this is why a mineral IV, especially in the first week, is so crucial.

People doing sauna are often surprised that, while they drink much more than usual, they aren't urinating more than usual. The additional water is used by the heat-activated increased metabolism, plus much of is lost in sweat. If you find you are urinating less than usual, increase your water intake. If you are urinating more than usual, you may cut back on the water, but you don't have to.

Keep the water in a glass container, not an outgassing-prone plastic bottle. As lovely as a dripping glass of ice water may sound, water should be room temperature or a bit above. Ice water will indeed be cooling, but keep in mind that you're in the sauna to heat up, and cooling down your insides will be counterproductive. Also, ice water can be a shock to the system and can interfere with digestion.

Speaking of water, you'll be showering several times during the day, and, as mentioned, you should be using a water filter. This shower includes a shampoo (with or without soap), as your scalp will probably sweat profusely as well as the rest of your body. You don't need to dry your hair each time. Soap and shampoo are optional, but if used they must be nontoxic and unscented. Always use a clean towel for each shower and put on clean clothes afterward.

What should I eat during the sauna program?

Sometimes people are so gung-ho about getting all this detoxing done that they may try to do too much too fast. Although the detox diet is a great adjunct to the sauna detox and is recommended before or after it, it isn't a good idea to combine the detox diet and the sauna at the same time. For one thing, the heat will raise the body temperature by design and thus increase metabolism, and the detox diet may not be able to provide enough calories to fuel this. Also, although the body has a limit to how fast it can detox, doing too much at once to detox will increase discomfort as too much is dumped into the bloodstream. It may be hard for your body to handle all this.

So what should you eat? The previous chapter on the detox diet, in particular the discussion of what to eat after the detox, can give some valuable ideas on what to eat. The important thing is this: you're expending considerable effort to detox in the sauna, and so eating anything that puts toxins right back into your body would be less than optimal. In addition, your body is doing some hard work during this time, and needs optimal fuel. Therefore, it's best to have no sugar, processed food, fried food, and so forth. Even if you aren't planning to do the detox diet until after sauna, this is still a good time to upgrade your food choices.

So let's go over the sauna program, step by step

Okay, you've arranged your schedule, you've set up or chosen your sauna – DIY (at your own risk) or professional – and you've got piles of freshly and non-toxically laundered towels and cotton clothes nearby. You have lots of filtered water on hand, as well as plenty of healthy food. You've put a water filter on your shower. You have consulted with your physician and/or healthcare professional if you have blood pressure problems, extreme toxicity, severe illness, or other concerns, and you know you can call this person if problems come up. You'll have a friend nearby or in the sauna with you for an extra level of security, like swimming with a buddy, or you will be in a professional program with trained personnel on hand. You're ready to go!

Keep in mind that this program schedule is only a recommendation, based on a professional detox program.

Here's a typical day, with sample times:

Before 9AM — Shower and dress in clean clothes, if indeed you will be wearing any clothes in the sauna. The sauna should be preheated. You've had a healthy breakfast. Have plenty of water on hand.

8:45 — Take a mineral/electrolyte supplement, such as Kona Gold, as well as protein powder in water. Take ginger if needed. Also take 50-100mg of niacin, enough to bring on a flush but not enough to cause dizziness. This is also a good time to take any other supplements that you would like to take or that have been recommended, such as AdvaClear for an excess of chemicals or MetalloClear to help clear metals.

9:00 — Get into the sauna and sit on a clean towel. Drink water whenever you think of it. Set a timer or keep an eye on a clock (note: keep in mind that timepieces may be adversely affected by heat; most saunas have windows in the door for safety and monitoring, and putting the timer or clock in this window works well). Sit in the sauna for 15 minutes at a time to start.

9:15	Get out of the sauna, and open the door for a minute for ventilation, then close it. Shower, change into clean clothes. Use a clean towel for the shower and for sitting on in the sauna each time. (Yep, plenty of laundry. Don't say we didn't warn you.)
9:30	Do tissue cleansing lymphatic exercises as described later in this book section.
9:45	Get back into the sauna for another 15 minutes, your second session.
10:00	Ventilate sauna, shower and change.
10:15	Take another Kona Gold and some more protein powder. Get back into sauna for a third 15-minute session.
10:30	Ventilate sauna, shower and change.
10:45	Do lymphatic exercises.
11:00	Take a break. Eat some lunch.
Noon	Get into the sauna for a fourth session of 15 minutes.
12:15	Ventilate sauna, shower and change.
12:30	Do your daily protocol – see below.
1:30	Take protein powder and Kona Gold. Get back into the sauna for your fifth and final daily session.
1:45	Ventilate sauna, shower and change.
Rest of day	Rest; you're probably going to need it.

Don't feel that you have to adhere to this timetable precisely. Feel free to take a break, make a phone call, or whatever. Just don't take a break of more than a half hour, preferably no more than twenty minutes, between sauna sessions if you can avoid it, because you don't want your core temperature to cool down too much.

In addition, you should check your blood pressure and pulse at least once per sauna day, or if you feel dizzy or weak. If your pulse is too fast, over about 100 beats per minute, the sauna schedule could be too strenuous for you or you may be low in potassium. If your blood pressure is much higher or lower in the sauna than your baseline (not in sauna) pressure, you may need to slow down in the sauna schedule as well; first try salt if your blood pressure is too low.

Daily protocol: In the early afternoon of each day, assuming a Monday-Friday sauna schedule, do at least one of the adjunctive DIY or practitioner-assisted therapies. Here's a sample schedule:

Monday	Mineral IV (or enema if DIY)
Tuesday	Lymphatic massage

Wednesday	Colonic
Thursday	Lymphatic massage
Friday	Mineral IV

After the first week, the length of time of each sauna session can be lengthened. A suggested schedule for this is 15 minutes per session the first week, 20 minutes the second week, 25 minutes the third, and 30 minutes after that. Sauna sessions should not exceed 30 minutes. Be guided by how you feel: if you feel wiped out at the end of the day, rather than just tired, your sessions could be shortened; if you feel okay or mildly fatigued, you can increase your time ahead of this schedule, which is just a general guideline. If you are in a professional program, your practitioner can monitor your progress and advise you.

How can I expect to feel during the program?
Since toxins may enter and leave the bloodstream in waves, energy, weight, and feelings of well-being or illness can fluctuate daily. Emotional symptoms such as anger or tearfulness may increase temporarily due to increased toxins in the bloodstream. Brain fog is common, again due to temporarily increased bloodstream toxins. You will likely have days, more frequently as the sauna program progresses, in which you have increased energy and a feeling of well-being, although some people don't start feeling better until the program is completed.

Headache is possible due to increased toxins. An ice pack at the back of the neck when you are out of the sauna can help alleviate headaches. Try not to take pharmaceutical pain relievers such as aspirin or acetaminophen, since these are treated by the body as just another toxin to get rid of. An Epsom salt bath helps to relax muscles – the active ingredient is a form of magnesium, which is a muscle relaxant – and also helps to detoxify.

How do I know how long to do the program?
Most people doing sauna do the program for about two weeks. It is best for these weeks to be continuous to keep the detoxification cycle going.

Even practitioner-assisted saunas involve a certain amount of guesswork as to how many weeks you should be doing sauna. If you are a do-it-yourselfer, be guided by the severity of your beginning symptoms, which is a rough gauge of your level of toxicity, and also by your history. If your work history includes being a chemist (as was the case for Dr. Dworkin), working with molten plastics, house painting, or spraying pesticides, figure on a longer term. If you don't have a significant history of chemical exposure, you don't feel all that awful, and you just want a tune-up, a couple of weeks may be sufficient.

Patient profile

One patient, who had been a house painter for forty years, became quite sick as a result of work-related toxin exposure. He gained a lot of weight as his body tried to dilute the toxins with water and fat, he ached all over, and he had diarrhea. He did the sauna detox, lost 50-70 pounds, and felt much better.

Also be guided by how you feel at the end of each week. Typically you will feel worse, and then better, as you go through the weeks of the program. Once you hit "better," you might just finish out that week and see how you're doing after that. Because detox is an inexact science, a week or a few days more or less isn't all that crucial. Other indicators that you are almost finished with sauna detox are:

- No more loose stools, if you have had loose stools during detox
- Blood pressure and pulse are stable, don't fluctuate as much
- Body temperature, taken under the arm in the morning, is stable
- Reactivity to chemicals, if you have had noticeable reactions before, have ceased
- Urine is pH 6 and this reading is pretty stable
- Moods are more stable; aren't as extreme nor do they fluctuate as much

What if I just can't stand any more?

An intensive sauna program like this one can be quite grueling for some people. Sometimes people doing sauna get to the point where they have a very strong aversion to getting back in. Sometimes it feels like you can't stay in for even another minute. This could mean one of several things.

Minerals can become unbalanced while in sauna. Potassium levels can go too low, and if you tend to have the low potassium symptoms listed in the mineral balancing section in the Supporters section, take potassium routinely (a 99mg capsule) during sauna. Anxiety and irritability are a couple of the symptoms of low potassium, and an "I can't take it another minute" feeling, especially if it comes on fairly suddenly, may be due to a low level of potassium; this is even more likely to be the case if the pulse is rapid. Take one or two capsules of potassium – if this doesn't work try magnesium – and see how you do after that; it takes about 15-30 minutes to work.

You may be detoxing too rapidly for your body to be able to comfortably handle. Suspect this if your feelings of aversion are accompanied by feeling much worse than when you started. This can be an indication that you need to shorten your sauna sessions, take fewer sessions per day, or both. See how that works for you.

Part of the problem in many cases is simple boredom. Doing the program with one or more people that you can talk to rather than just watching the clock can make a big difference. Reading in the sauna isn't recommended since most printed material can outgas, but try watching a video through the glass door window. You might be able to listen to an MP3 player in the sauna, but keep the body of the player as close to the floor as possible, where it's cooler.

Sauna isn't an easy program and requires a high level of commitment. Sometimes all you need is a pep talk by yourself or a friend to keep you going. Think about the improved health you are likely to enjoy long term after this short term bit of discomfort. If you've ruled out low potassium, too-rapid detox, or boredom, just grit your teeth and hang on.

Be aware, though, that, the previous few paragraphs notwithstanding, most people find the program to be mildly unpleasant, if that, and they just get through it with no particular problem. In fact, if you've taken time off of work to do the program, this might feel like a vacation.

Patient profile – Dr. Dworkin's sauna success story

I – Dr. Andrea Dworkin – went through the sauna program run by the Center for Advanced Medicine in Encinitas, CA, in 1993. They are still doing this program, as it has been very successful and beneficial for a large number of people. I am one of them, and here is my story.

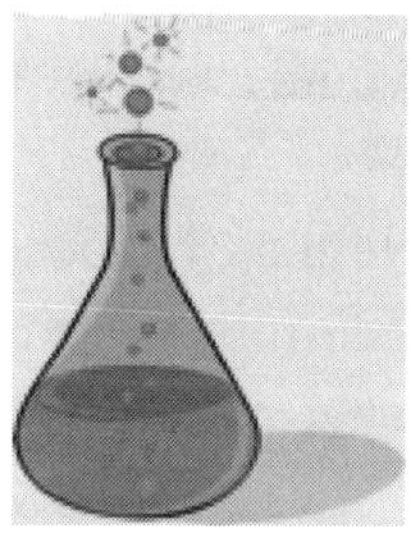

I got my Bachelor's and Master's degrees in chemistry in the 1980s, which of course involved taking many laboratory courses during which I worked with various chemicals. I then worked at several chemist jobs over the years. I got used to the typical laboratory smell and rarely noticed it, but non-chemist friends who would visit would remark on the odor, an indication that I was breathing in significant amounts of toxic solvents and other chemicals for forty hours a week for years.

In early 1992 my career came to a grinding halt. By then I was so fatigued that I took brief naps in the restroom, and put my head on my desk when I thought I wouldn't be observed. I ate lunch quickly and spent the rest of the hour sleeping in my car. In addition, my mind didn't seem to be working right. I got to the point where I, formerly an A student and reader of graduate chemistry and physics texts, could barely follow a popular magazine article, a TV show, or a conversation. I finally quit my job, although I didn't know then that chemicals were the problem, because I simply couldn't do the work anymore.

My health continued to deteriorate even after I quit work. I developed chemical sensitivities so severe that, on one occasion, they nearly killed me when I went into full anaphylactic shock. One whiff of a solvent, paint, glue, cologne, or just about any toxin, and my blood pressure would plummet and I would come close to passing out, a very unpleasant sensation as well as being dangerous. I had to rearrange my life to accommodate these sensitivities; life became about avoidance. By then I had become so fatigued that I couldn't climb a flight of stairs without having to stop and rest halfway up. I could put off a shampoo or load of laundry for days because too much effort was involved, and a day in which I was able to do these things was a day of high accomplishment compared with most of my days. This was quite a contrast to the days of prior years when I was juggling full-time work and graduate school. It felt as if life as I had known it had pretty much ended.

I started doing the sauna program in 1993, after I had done the detox diet and after having my metal fillings removed. Since I had been a chemist and had had much more than routine everyday chemical exposure, I spent seven weeks in the full sauna program, more than most people would need. I didn't feel noticeably better right away, but I remember the day that everything turned around not long after completing the sauna program. I was walking at a strip mall, not paying attention to my surroundings, when I walked right past the open door of a nail salon and I got a lungful of the chemicals that they use. I quickly passed by the door and immediately leaned against the outside wall, a strategic move that I had learned would keep me from slumping to the sidewalk.

Nothing happened, though, and I have not had a reaction to chemicals in the fifteen-plus years since. My internal level of chemicals had dropped down to a point where I was no longer reactive. My energy and mental capacity were slower to recover. However, by 1994 I was a practitioner at the Center for Advanced Medicine, working full time, and in 1996 the books I coauthored, ***Surviving the Toxic Crisis*** and ***Thriving in a Toxic World***, were published. By 1999 I was the proud owner of two doctoral degrees, one in Naturopathy (ND) and one in Nutrition (PhD). Not bad for someone for whom a shampoo was once an event that took as much energy as I could muster.

As with most such success stories, there is some complexity to mine; it wasn't a matter of just doing one thing and having my life turn right around. In my case, although I had dietary issues, mercury from my fillings, and structural (chiropractic) issues to contend with, chemicals were the major problem for me, and sauna gave me my life back.

Metal Detoxification

Safe Mercury Removal and Other Dental Considerations

The information in this book, the Metals chapter in particular, may well have convinced you to have your toxic, problem-causing metal fillings removed. The Mercury chapter in ***Surviving the Toxic Crisis***, written by the authors of this book, details the many ways in which mercury, found primarily in dental fillings, can cause harm. This chapter in ***Surviving the Toxic Crisis*** contains over 200 scientific references, a fraction of those available. Mercury poisoning can cause or contribute to a wide variety of problems that are almost too numerous to list. These may include but are not limited to:

- Light sensitivity
- Loss of smell and taste
- Asthma
- Ulcers
- Allergies
- Fatigue
- Constipation, bloating, gas
- Muscle cramps, twitches or tremors
- Mood swings, irritability, depression
- Poor circulation, cold or numb hands and feet, low body temperature
- Overall body pain (fibromyalgia)

In almost all cases it is to your advantage to have the metal fillings removed. However – and **this is very important – it is crucial that the fillings be removed properly and safely** and replaced with biocompatible materials. As mentioned in the Introduction, it is important to do the right thing, in the right way, in the right order. If filling removal is not done properly, mercury can be absorbed into the body during the removal process through breathing, swallowing, and absorption through the mouth tissues. In such a case the body burden of mercury, and the associated symptoms, may increase, and dealing with the additional load of mercury can take more time and money than having the fillings removed properly in the first place.

Dental testing for mercury vaporizing from your fillings is quick, painless and safe, and is available at some progressive clinics such as the Center for Advanced Medicine in Encinitas, CA. A number of books on the subject have been published as well. The procedure, described in ***Surviving the Toxic Crisis***, makes use of a mercury vapor tester that is also used by the EPA to monitor air quality. Ironically, the amount of mercury in the air is strictly monitored and controlled, yet there is no such monitoring or controlling of the mercury vapor in the mouth – and therefore the body – yet such levels might be many times higher than those allowed in ambient or workplace air according to EPA and OSHA standards.

Other types of testing for mercury, such as urine and hair testing, are often not reliable due to the volatile nature of mercury – it can be lost during sample collection and preparation. In addition, it can be present in a number of forms: metallic mercury, ionic mercury (mercury salt), or methylmercury, among others, which complicates testing. Provocative chelation, especially with DMSA, can give a false negative (lower) mercury result if cadmium is present. If there are symptoms of mercury poisoning along with low or negative test results, the symptoms are usually the more accurate indicator.

Aren't dentists interchangeable?
Before you run to the nearest or cheapest dentist to have your fillings removed, read on.

Although any dentist knows how to remove a filling, it is important that the dentist you choose knows how to remove mercury fillings **safely**. A dentist who simply drills out the old and puts in the new without treating the removed amalgam like the toxic material it is can do more harm than good. With unsafe removal, the patient may be exposed to as much as a year's worth of mercury in an hour, and it is not uncommon for health problems to come on or worsen soon after improper removal. These health problems may include those listed above as well as those discussed in this book, especially in the Ailments section.

In fact, proceed with caution if the dentist places new mercury fillings at all in any patient, does or even recommends root canals, or puts in stainless steel / nickel crowns, caps, bridges, or root canal posts. Such a dentist apparently does not understand the toxicity of mercury and other metals, or the dangers of electrical charges, which are explained in ***Surviving the Toxic Crisis*** and can also be tested for.

There are three types of dentists as far as mercury filling removal is concerned:

- **Toxic dentists**, the fortunately dwindling majority, who put in mercury fillings and so would probably not take proper precautions. Their technique can be described as "drill, fill and bill."
- **Non-toxic dentists**, who follow some of the procedures recommended here.
- **Excellent non-toxic biocompatible dentists**, who follow all of the procedures recommended here.

What precautions should be taken to remove mercury fillings safely?
Some recommendations for safe removal, and safe dental work in general, are:

- Use a **rubber dental dam** (latex sheet) in the mouth to keep from swallowing mercury particles.

- Use a **high speed vacuum** to remove drilled-out bits and mercury vapor.
- Use **drapes** so you don't carry mercury chips home on your clothes or absorb mercury through your exposed skin.
- Breathe **oxygen** or clean air through a nosepiece rather than mercury vapor-laden air from your mouth.
- Use a lighted **magnifying instrument** to see and remove every last bit of amalgam.
- Uses a **mercury suction pump** that goes above the body; it has a charged plate that attracts mercury that gets into the air.
- Using a special blue light, the dentist should check teeth for **cracks**, which are common with mercury fillings. These cracks should then be repaired to stabilize tooth structure before crowns are needed.
- Test **tooth voltage** from metal components before removal, removing those teeth with the highest negative charge first if possible.
- The dentist should protect him/herself with **gloves and mask**, otherwise this may be an indication that he/she does not take mercury toxicity seriously.
- **Cut up** the filling and remove it in sections rather than drilling it out, as drilling produces a fine mercury mist which can be inhaled or ingested.
- Use an **air filtering system** in the dental office.
- Have a **biocompatibility test** done for any replacement materials, adhesives, anesthetics, or other chemicals used. This can be a blood test or a muscle test.
- Use biocompatible **replacement materials** with the lowest level of toxicity possible.
- Use intravenous **chelation** with vitamin C to remove any mercury that may have gotten into the body before it enters the tissues and becomes more difficult to remove.
- Have an office that is as **chemical-free** as possible, including using air and water filters and fans venting to the outside, and having a no-cologne policy.

- **Sonicate and autoclave** (clean and sterilize) drill handpieces as well as dental drill bits to kill microorganisms from blood or saliva.

What about root canals?

Although root canals are less involved in the topic of toxicity than mercury, they still bear mentioning. With root canals, foreign materials are placed in, as well as possible infectious material left in, the mouth, and therefore in the body, so they should be dealt with.

If you have root canals, it may be in your best interest to have the teeth extracted. This is a decision to be made after discussing your health problems with your practitioner, focusing on whether your symptoms are consistent with root canal related toxicity.

If root canalled (or any) teeth are extracted, it is important to have cavitations cleaned out. This involves cleaning and smoothing out the bone around and at the bottom of the tooth socket with a low speed drill so it heals properly. If this is not done, the same jawbone infection that caused the initial health problems is still there, potentially causing continuing problems. Many if not most dentists do not take the time to do a cavitation cleaning, or don't understand its importance.

What is the cost for proper amalgam removal?

Dental work is rarely cheap, and a dentist who takes all or even most of the above precautions is likely to be more expensive than most dentists due to the additional time and equipment required. The difference in care, however, is well worth the extra cost.

What is the cost of improper amalgam removal?

Your health can be at risk when amalgam is removed improperly. Since your health is more valuable than money, this is a risk not worth taking. The bottom line is: you can pay with your wallet, or pay with your health – your choice. The problems with poor work continue long after the low price is forgotten.

Where can I find a good non-toxic dentist?

A listing of non-toxic dentists throughout the country and even the world is provided by the International Academy of Medicine and Toxicology (IAOMT), which has the website IAOMT.org. Their listings do not distinguish between non-toxic dentists and excellent biocompatible non-toxic dentists who take all precautions, but their recommendations are still a lot better than choosing a dentist at random out of the phone book.

What should be done after the dental work?

Chelation to remove heavy metals, especially mercury, is often a good idea, along with provocative chelation, a urine test for the presence of heavy metals. All mercury must be removed from the mouth before chelation is done, with the exception of vitamin C chelation during or right after each amalgam removal appointment.

Checklist for choosing a dentist

- [ ] Never places mercury fillings
- [ ] Takes mercury toxicity seriously in conversation
- [ ] Never does or recommends root canals
- [ ] Does not put in stainless steel / nickel crowns, caps, bridges, or root canal posts
- [ ] Recommended by IAOMT
- [ ] Recommended by a practitioner you trust
- [ ] Recommended by friends with your concerns and values
- [ ] Cleans cavitations after extractions
- [ ] Protects self with mask
- [ ] Uses air filtering system in the dental office
- [ ] Has chemically clean office
- [ ] Does biocompatibility test for replacement materials, and uses such materials
- [ ] Tests for voltage and uses this as guideline for order of removal, if possible
- [ ] Uses rubber dental dam
- [ ] Uses drapes
- [ ] Sonicates or autoclaves drill handpieces
- [ ] Gives patient oxygen through mask
- [ ] Uses blue light to check for cracks
- [ ] Uses high speed vacuum
- [ ] Offers chelation after mercury removal

The more check marks, the better the dentist is likely to be as far as meeting your needs.

What else can be done to detoxify the mouth?
Swish some olive oil in your mouth once a day for five minutes. This helps to pull toxins out of the mouth and parotid (salivary) glands.

Chelation

What is chelation?
Chelation is a term whose root means "claw" or "to bind." Most chelation is done by introducing an intravenous chelation solution into the veins. The chelator grabs hold of metal ions, forming a chemical compound which is water soluble and can more easily be excreted by the body. Excretion is done via urine, feces, and sweat.

Why is chelation done?
Chelation helps to remove metals from the body tissues. These metals come from a number of sources including metal dental materials and mercury amalgam fillings. Metals can cause free radical damage in the body, and this damage can lead to:

- Arteriosclerosis and atherosclerosis, blood vessel blockage
- Heart problems
- Cancer, autoimmune disease, arthritis, and other degenerative disease
- Fatigue and difficulty concentrating, particularly from mercury
- Leg cramps
- Depression and anger

Arteriosclerosis and heart problems are the #1 killer in the U.S. Cancer is #2, with 1/3 of Americans developing some form of cancer in their lifetime. Both of these can be linked in many cases to metals in the body.

Not everyone needs chelation, even if fillings have been removed. The use, amount, and type of chelation should be determined after an evaluation of your health.

What are some conditions that benefit from chelation?
Chelation can benefit nearly any condition in which metals are a contributory cause. Most research, however, has focused on the benefit to the blood vessels.

Chelation has been used to reduce calcium plaquing on the insides of arteries. This plaquing narrows the blood vessels, possibly leading to a heart attack in time if blood flow is sufficiently reduced. Chelation's action is believed to be twofold: it directly removes the excess of calcium from the arteries, and it removes heavy metals such as mercury from dental amalgam fillings, cadmium from cigarettes, and lead from gasoline from the body. These metals set up conditions conducive to inflammation, which is buffered by the calcium. Calcium coats the inflamed areas in the blood vessels like a bandage, patching up one problem but creating another. Metals can also change the blood pH (acidity), and calcium is taken from the bones to try to buffer the body fluids back to their normal pH. The removal of calcium from the bones can lead to osteoporosis, so chelation can be beneficial in that area also.

Nearly 90% of patients with peripheral vascular disease (blocked leg arteries) showed marked improvement after chelation therapy. Another study showed that all patients with peripheral vascular disease had significant improvement after only ten treatments of chelation therapy.[1] Fifty percent of cardiac arrhythmias were normalized.[2]

Plaque in the arteries can also be due to structural and other problems. It is important to identify and treat the basic problem and to use the correct chelator, if any, for the problem.

EDTA chelation can be useful in the treatment of Alzheimer's disease, most likely by removing the aluminum and other heavy metals from the brain and thus increasing the effectiveness of the body's metal chelators. There are cases of improvement in Alzheimer's symptoms with chelation in addition to a slowing or stopping of the disease progress.[3]

> **Patient profile**
> One patient, an 80-year-old man, had problems with impotence, low energy and brain fog. His wife suspected senility or early Alzheimer's disease. His problems improved markedly after 1 to 2 months of chelation therapy.[4]

What about chelation and cancer?
A documented benefit of chelation therapy is that it significantly reduced cancer mortality rates.[5]

Research has shown that there is a decrease in cancer deaths after EDTA treatment. In some forms of cancer, the use of EDTA was found to strip the tumor cells of their protective coat, allowing mechanisms such as protein-digesting enzymes to destroy the cancers.[6]

> **Patient profile**
> Jerry had a cancerous tumor of the parotid (salivary) gland. When he came to the clinic in February, it was the size of a golf ball. He had chelation done using DMSA, DMPS, and high-dose glutathione. By June the tumor was the size of a pimple; by the end of summer it was gone.

How do I know whether I need chelation?
You or your doctor may suspect that you have metals in your body. For example, you may have symptoms of metal toxicity, or you work with metals, or you have metal dental work or have recently had mercury fillings or root-canalled teeth removed. In these cases a test for metals may be wise, to be followed by treatment if indicated by the testing. Sometimes the indications of metal toxicity are so strong that a test is considered to be unnecessary.

Provocative chelation is an accurate type of urine test. The chelator, or metal-grabbing molecule, such as EDTA, DMPS, glutathione, or even vitamin C is introduced into the body intravenously (IV). The chelator binds with the metals in the blood and allows them to be excreted in the urine, which is then analyzed.

Hair analysis can also be done. A small sample of hair is sent to a laboratory for metals testing. Another advantage of hair analysis is that it can reveal levels of necessary minerals in the body.

What if a toxic level of metal is found or strongly suspected?
If a person has a problem with metal toxicity, the treatment is twofold:

- Identify and eliminate continued exposure to the metal
- Remove existing metal from the body tissues

Metal in the body may be slowly eliminated over a period of about 25 years if no more toxic metal is entering the system, even if nothing is done to speed up the process. However, the metal remaining in the body during the natural detoxification process is still doing its damage. It is therefore advantageous to intervene in order to help the body eliminate the metal faster. The usual method is through chelation, as well as through kinase modulators such as MetalloClear and DMSA.

What should be done before chelation treatments start?
It is important to stop the source of the metals, such as removing mercury fillings, or chelation will have to be done indefinitely to remove the metals that have accumulated since the last chelation. In fact, some chelators can pull mercury out of the teeth and into the body as fast as they get rid of the mercury, like leaving the faucet on and the tub drain open at the same time. For this reason metal must be removed from the teeth before beginning chelation treatment.

A complete physical and blood test should be done to assess your overall condition and to provide a baseline by which your progress toward health can be measured.

Do not take large doses of minerals, including Kona Gold, for about 8-12 hours before and after the chelation treatment. Chelation removes minerals as well as metals, so it is best if the chelator can concentrate on removing the metals. Minerals are replaced after the 12 hours has passed.

How is chelation treatment administered?
Chelation treatment is usually administered intravenously (IV), although it can also be given orally or by intramuscular injection. However, oral chelators are not usually as effective as intravenous administration. Even oral chelation is not a strictly do-it-yourself project, because the most effective chelators are prescription medications. However, there are over-the-counter oral

chelators and supporters, including Captomer, MetalloClear, Sun Chlorella, coriander, charcoal, bentonite clay, garlic, and vitamin C.

Each treatment lasts between ten minutes and three hours depending on the type of chelator used and the health problem being treated. The ten-minute DMPS IV is more often used for metals; the much longer EDTA IV is used to remove calcium plaquing. The size of your veins is also a factor, as the solution can flow more readily into larger veins. Your practitioner determines the number of treatments, taking into consideration the severity of your metal-related health problems. The usual range is three to twenty treatments, with ten being about average. The number of treatments can go as high as 40 in severe cases, but this is still safer and cheaper than heart bypass surgery.

In a professional chelation setting, skilled medical and nursing staff are available to help with any discomfort or problems that may arise.

How safe is chelation?
Chelation therapy has been used safely on more than five hundred thousand patients over the last forty years.[7] According to current drug safety standards, aspirin is about three and a half times more toxic than EDTA, one of the more common chelating agents.[8]

What can I expect after treatment?
As with all therapies, individual progress can vary. Typically, the patient may feel a bit tired and weak immediately after the treatment due to mineral depletion (chelators also grab onto and remove minerals). The appropriate mineral supplementation as recommended by your practitioner can prevent or alleviate these symptoms. Often the patient reports feeling noticeably better as soon as the day of or the day after the first treatment, with continuing improvement with successive treatments.

How do I know when chelation is done?
Knowing when you are done with chelation is an art more than a science, so a treatment more or less isn't crucial. Your practitioner can evaluate your progress and make a recommendation. In general, once your urine pH has stabilized at pH 6 and your metal-related symptoms have been mostly alleviated, your treatment is probably at an end.

Cleansing of Detox Organs

Lymphatic Massage and Exercises

What is the lymph system?

The lymphatic system, which consists of nodes and vessels, is an important part of the body's detoxification network. The nodes are located near the diaphragm in the torso and chest, and in the groin, armpits, neck, backs of the knees, and at the shoulder blades. Toxins and infectious material collect in the lymph nodes, and are released from the lymph nodes to be dealt with by the body when the nodes are squeezed by the muscles as we walk or exercise. It is not coincidental that the nodes are located where they can be massaged as we move and breathe.

Deep breathing, discussed later in this book section, squeezes the lymph glands in the chest and upper abdomen. Chewing moves the head sutures, which stimulates the lymph nodes located in that area, as well as the movement of the spinal fluid. There is wisdom in the old adage – chew each mouthful of food thirty times, which has benefits other than those related to lymph.

All of these movements push toxins out through your pores as sweat and into the bloodstream for elimination, as well as the waste products lactic and uric acid which are byproducts of exercise.

What can block the lymph system?

If you have difficulty bending and stretching, one possible cause may be lymph nodes which are full of toxins.

Dairy products can contribute to lymphatic blockages and the formation of cysts and lumps under the skin.[1] Both the detox diet, which eliminates dairy, and lymphatic exercises and massage can help to release these blockages.

Bras, especially underwire bras, constrict the lymph nodes in the breasts and prevent their drainage. There is a link between the amount of time a bra is regularly worn (per day, and number of years) and the development of breast cancer,[2-4] since the bra and underwire allows the toxins to accumulate in the lymph glands in that area without permitting them to drain.

How can one best exercise the lymph system?

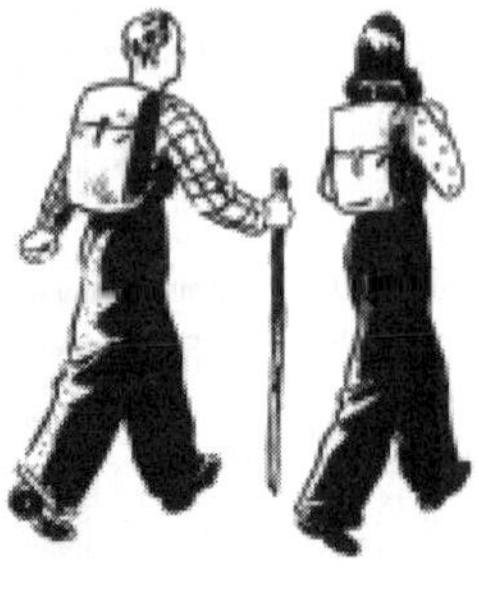

If you are reasonably active and do a fair amount of walking, your lymph system might be getting the workout it needs. However, many people are not active, and nearly anyone can benefit from exercise to increase the effectiveness of the lymphatic system. These exercises, also called tissue cleansing exercises, help to remove toxins from the lymph nodes located where movement would stimulate them – behind the knees and in the neck, groin, and armpits.

The exercises are an essential part of the sauna detox, but can benefit anyone; they can be done inside the sauna or outside during session breaks. These exercises help move toxins so that fewer chelation treatments are necessary. Doing a colonic after these exercises or lymph massage can help speed toxins out of the body more effectively.

In addition to or as part of the following specific exercises, exercising on a rebounder, a mini trampoline, can enhance the lymph workout and benefits. These exercises should be done very slowly. In most cases, for best results take 60 seconds to move to the new position, then hold it for 10 seconds, and then take another 60 seconds to move back to the original position.

Neck exercises:

- Move your head slowly from side to side as if you were shaking your head "no."
- Bend your head to try to touch your ear to your shoulder on either side.
- Nod your head forward and back.

Shoulder exercises:

- Shrug shoulders up towards ears, and then relax.
- Roll shoulders, then reverse direction.
- Cross arms in front, then try to touch them in back.
- Bring your shoulders towards the front as if trying to get them to touch, and then towards the back, again as if trying to get them to touch.

Leg exercise:

- Exaggerate steps, lifting the leg up as high as possible while bending the knee. This works the lymph nodes in both the groin and the back of the knee. If possible the exercises should be done on tiptoe to work the calf.

Torso exercise:

- Bend to either side, front, and back.

How does lymphatic massage help?

Lymphatic massage, concentrated in the node areas, works the lymph nodes, facilitating movement of toxins out of the nodes and from there out of the body. The massage is done working from the extremities to the central nodes in the breastbone area.

For further support

Red root tea helps to cleanse lymph system, and is a good adjunct to the lymphatic exercises and massage.

A lymph lamp can be used to liquefy lymph fluids so they can flow.

Colonics and Enemas

What is the difference between a colonic and an enema?
Colonics, done by a trained practitioner with special equipment, clean out the entire colon. An enema is like a "lite" version of the colonic. On the plus side, they are typically a do-it-yourself procedure; on the minus side they are not as thorough as colonics, since they only clean out the end part of the colon. Both have their uses in assisting detoxification through the bowels.

A colonic apparatus has a lighted viewing tube, which helps make this particular detoxification method unique: you actually get to see which toxins and wastes are leaving your body, which is actually pretty interesting. The visual aid also helps you and your practitioner to judge the effectiveness of your program.

Why might a colonic be needed?
Our bodies are designed to eliminate waste matter, dietary and otherwise, through the colon, which is essentially the sewer system of the body. However, sometimes elimination can use a bit of help. With a diet of complex carbohydrates, vegetables, oils, and plenty of water, along with sufficient exercise, the colon eliminates waste on its own. However, the standard American diet is full of refined starches, sugars, and dairy products, and often contains little fiber and insufficient water; in addition, many people get little or no exercise. Consequently, waste matter can build up on the colon walls, causing bloating, constipation, reduced absorption of nutrients, and toxins released into the body. A colonic can help to release this accumulated waste, which can be years or even decades old.

Another purpose for a colonic is to aid in detoxification. The colon is a major route of detoxification, because toxins accumulated and released by the liver exit via this route. A colonic can stimulate the dumping of toxins by the liver as well as the flushing out of these toxins, making it a wonderful adjunct to other detoxification methods; when done following a detox diet or liver flush, a colonic can boost the effectiveness of these.

What is colon hydrotherapy?
Colon hydrotherapy, another term for a colonic, utilizes warm water to soften any hardened fecal matter, help to evacuate it, and irrigate the colon. It is done by a trained practitioner. Colon massage during the procedure helps with this process.

The colonic experience
Unlike the case with an enema, when you have a colonic you can lie back and let the practitioner administer it. You won't be filled to bursting, nor will you have to make a mad dash for the toilet. Your only role is to provide feedback. The colonic typically lasts 45-55 minutes.

During the procedure you can wear any or all of your upper clothing, and you will be wearing a gown as well. The colonic therapist is well aware that this is a socially sensitive area and conducts herself accordingly, so there is rarely any embarrassment.

Warm water enters the colon in a series of fill-and-release sessions. The therapist explains what is happening as you go along. You are in control as you direct the therapist to stop filling or to release the water at any time.

After the colonic and while the equipment is still in place, you can have an implant of beneficial human strain bacteria including acidophilus and bifidus, herbs, or minerals. The solution is introduced through the tube and held as long as possible so the bacteria can re-colonize the intestine.

How safe is a colonic?

Everything that leads to your body is disposable, and the colonic machine is designed so there is no chance of material from a previous user entering your body.

Some people worry that a colonic will condition the body to be lazy and not work as well on its own. This rarely happens, and only in those who do a great many colonics over time without giving the body a chance to work on its own. In fact, one of the benefits of a colonic is that the digestive system tends to work better after the colonic or a series of colonics than before, as impediments to proper function are washed away and peristalsis – the natural motion of the intestinal walls – is stimulated.

What about an enema?

A number of enema kits are available commercially, with instructions for their use.

Adjuncts for intestinal cleansing

A number of supplements can help to clean out the digestive system, either as an adjunct to colonics and enemas or on their own. These include:

- Bentonite clay
- Aloe vera powder
- Charcoal
- Acidophilus and bifidus beneficial bacteria
- Diatomaceous earth

In many people, there are paths or channels through the waste in the colon, rather like the trails through the dirt in an ant farm. The waste moves through these ever-narrowing channels. Enzymes, taken orally, help to eat away at this built-up waste. Although enzymes are useful in themselves, a colonic or enema can flush away this now-loosened waste.

Liver and Gallbladder Flush

What does the liver do and why would it need cleaning?

The liver, which at three pounds is the largest organ in the body, is located on the right side of the body above the waist. The liver makes enzymes which cause the many biochemical reactions in the body, and it is assisted by the gallbladder in its digestion of fats.

The liver in its simplest form is a filter that removes toxins and sends them into the colon for elimination. The liver is actually quite an amazing organ. It filters two quarts of blood each minute of every day. This is equivalent to a backyard swimming pool filter cleaning out half of the pool's water every minute.[5]

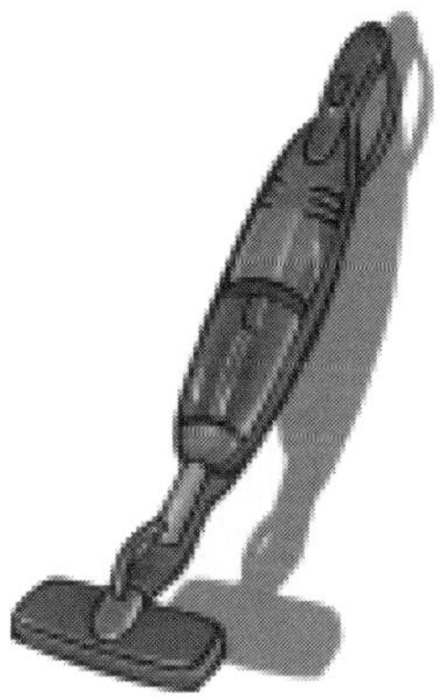

Think for a moment of one of those bagless vacuum cleaners. It vacuums okay but not great, so you take off the dirt compartment, empty it, and scrape out the dust and debris that collects in the folds of the filter. Now it works much better, picking up an amazing amount of dirt that it missed when the carpet was vacuumed with a dirty filter. The liver, unlike the vacuum cleaner filter, is self-cleaning, but only up to a point, and in today's toxin-laden lifestyle it could certainly benefit from some cleaning assistance. Once cleaned out, it will reward you with increased ability to remove toxins. A person who has done a liver cleansing often reports feeling increased energy and clarity as soon as the next day.

One way to clean out the liver is via a liver flush, which detoxifies, cleanses, and stimulates the liver and gallbladder. The liver flush also cleans out and tunes up the gallbladder, which helps in the digestion of fats and oils. In many cases, gallstones are flushed out, and a properly functioning gallbladder tends not to form as many of them. In some cases gallbladder removal surgery can be averted – don't take it out, just clean it out and reuse it.

There are many variations of the liver flush, but most of them have several things in common. They use an oil, most commonly extra virgin olive oil, as well as an acidic liquid such as lemon juice or grapefruit juice. At least one version uses apple juice or cider instead of lemon, but that version, although more pleasant to taste, introduces too much sugar into the system so it isn't recommended unless yeast overgrowth is not a problem. The simplest flush involves drinking the oil and juice combination only; more effective protocols, such as the one here, have preparatory steps for maximum cleansing on the day of the flush

What is the actual liver/gallbladder flush protocol?

The week before – This is the protocol for the seven days preceding the flush, including the day of the flush. Your diet does not need to be modified during this time.

- Take ¼ cup (4 tablespoons) of extra-virgin olive oil per day. Bertolli's brand is recommended; not Pompeii brand because it tastes too oily to many people. The oil can be taken as dressing on salad.
- Take ¼ cup of lemon juice in water twice a day, first thing in the morning and last thing at night. Use freshly juiced lemons, preferably organic, and not bottled or frozen. Do not add sugar to make lemonade.
- Add Phos-Food, 45 drops three times a day in a glass of water.

Other optional additions are:

- Boldo, an Amazon herbal preparation, ten drops three time a day after meals for these seven days.
- Lipogen for fat digestion and absorption, two tablets with each meal the night before and the two meals the day of the flush, six tablets total.
- Liv-Long contains artichoke and sarsaparilla, from the same family as silymarin, a liver cleansing herb. Take two before each meal.
- A sonogram is recommended before the flush, preferably the day of the flush or the day before. This both detects gallstones and loosens up the sludge in the gallbladder.
- A parasite protocol, if directed by your practitioner, can be done in conjunction with the flush.

The day of the flush – eat breakfast and lunch, but nothing thereafter. You may drink water with or without lemon as desired.

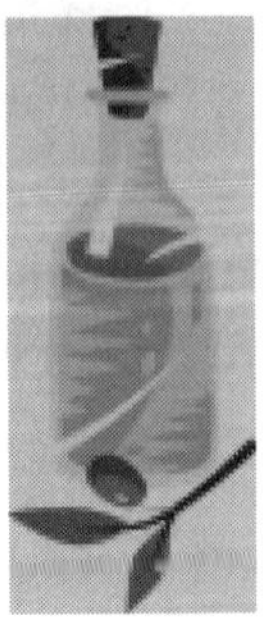

At night, mix together ½ cup extra-virgin olive oil and ½ cup fresh lemon juice. The flush should be done at night just before bed. Drink the mixture – you'll have to keep shaking it – while already in bed. Immediately lie on your right side with your right knee pulled up close to your chest for at least thirty minutes, which allows gravity to help the mixture to enter and stay in the liver and gallbladder, which are on your right side. Do not drink water after doing the flush.

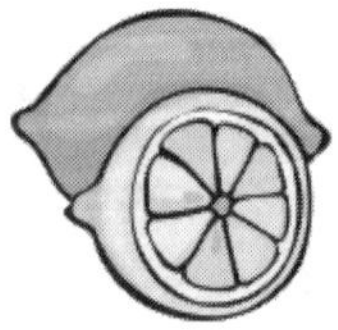

What can I expect after the flush?

Slight to moderate nausea may be experienced. Vomiting occurs rarely; drink salt water to bring your sodium level back up.

You may have some discomfort the next day, and/or an increased need to be near a toilet; because of this, plan ahead.

You may pass gallstones the day after the flush. They are in the stool, usually gray-green, and can be grape seed to cherry seed size. Small stones tend to be light in color; larger ones tend to be darker. Passing these is desirable and is a sign that the flush is doing its work.

What should be done just after the liver flush?

A great adjunctive treatment to the liver/gallbladder flush is a colonic or enema. The best timing is to schedule or do one the day after the flush, or the day after that. People who have done colonics, in which the evacuated sludge can be viewed in a viewing tube, are amazed at the stuff that comes out right after a liver flush, including visible gallstones and bright yellow bile-bound pesticides.

Make sure you get plenty of Kona Gold, and take calcium 2/1 or calcium orotate/magnesium glycinate 4:1 if you have loose stools. Calcium/magnesium supplements come in different ratios, depending on need: loose, normal, or hard stools.

Kidney Support

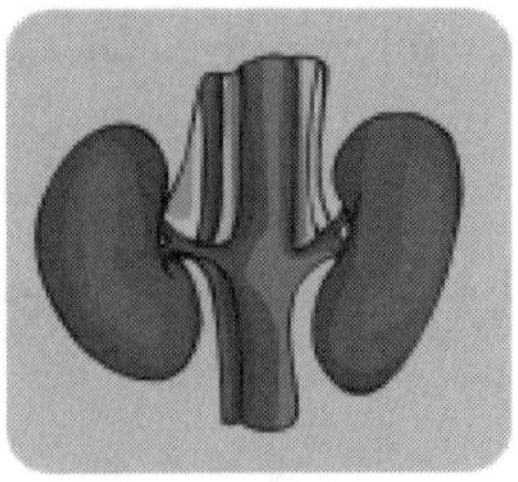

The kidneys, urinary tract, and bladder are part of the urinary system. Like the liver, the kidneys filter the blood and, in their case, send the toxins out through the urinary system. Think about it: if clear water goes in and yellow water comes out, something must be happening, right?

Like the liver, the kidneys can be overloaded with toxins and stones – calcium oxalate or urate – to the point that they don't do their job as well as they should, and they can benefit from cleaning out.

The lungs are closely aligned with the kidneys in their function; some have called the lungs "the third kidney."

The following herbs and nutrients can support the kidneys and lungs in their optimal function:

- Cranberry acidifies the urine, making it an inhospitable environment for the bacteria that can cause urinary tract infections (UTI). It coats the renal tubules of the kidneys.
- D-mannose, which is actually a type of sugar, supports urinary tract and bladder health and immune function.
- Aloe 7000 is an acidifier and antimicrobial.
- PhosFood lowers urine pH (acidifies) and breaks up kidney stones.
- Magnesium helps break up kidney stones.
- Plantain, an herb, is protective to the kidneys.
- Uva ursi is a diuretic herb that can help the urinary system flush out toxins
- Chanka piedra, also called stone-breaker herb

Breathing and Lung Cleansing

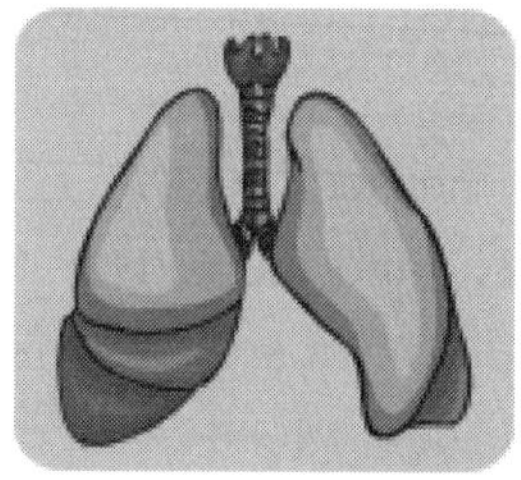

How do the lungs help with detoxification?
The lungs are major organs of detoxification, and breathing is one way that toxins find their way out of the body.

Consider for a moment what happens if you drink alcohol (Well, *you* probably wouldn't drink alcohol, being health conscious and all, but you know what we mean). You have some of your favorite alcoholic beverage, drive towards home, and on your way you are stopped and are asked to take a breathalyzer test, which, when you breathe into the little tube, gives a pretty accurate account of the amount of alcohol in your blood. Let's think about that: the alcohol has gone from your glass to your mouth to your stomach to your blood to your lungs to your breath and into that little tube, all within the space of an hour. Not only that, but your liver and kidneys have also gotten involved during that time. In addition, your brain is also feeling the effects, which is why the blood alcohol level is a pretty accurate measure of your degree of mental impairment.

In this case, and in the case with many toxins, especially volatile ones (toxins that vaporize easily), the lungs have performed their function and removed some of the toxin. Blood that is oxygenated by the lungs is sent out by the heart to the rest of the body. In the process of oxygenating the blood, however, the lungs also take on some of the volatile toxins, similar to the way a bus both discharges and then picks up passengers at the bus stop. These toxins are then breathed out. Thus the lungs perform a needed detoxification function.

I'm breathing and I'm alive, so there's obviously no problem, right?
Breathing is in some ways analogous to eating. Just because you're eating and you're alive doesn't mean there isn't plenty of room for improvement. Your diet may be anywhere from barely adequate for supporting life to optimal, and this is true of your breathing as well.

The CO_2 (carbon dioxide) level in the blood is often tested in the basic CBC blood test. If this level is low, below 24, this usually indicates that you are not breathing properly. An optimal level is 25-26. Since the body makes CO_2 out of oxygen, a too low CO_2 reading is an indicator that not enough oxygen is being taken in. A CO_2 level that is too high, over 26, can mean that there is a shortage of antioxidants in the body, and oxygen is being converted to harmful free radicals.

How can we maximize detoxification through breathing?
If you have ever watched a baby breathe, as when it is sleeping, you will notice that the baby's entire abdomen expands on the inhale. This is how we should all breathe. Try breathing normally or taking a deep breath and watch your chest and abdomen. Some people breathe shallowly and

their chest and shoulders might rise and their abdomen collapse on the inhale, which is the opposite of what should happen.

Practice breathing in a way that pushes out your abdomen. Breathing this way helps your lungs expand more fully, which in turn allows both fuller oxygenation of blood and greater capacity for detoxification through this pathway. Both functions – oxygenation and detoxification – can quickly lead to increased energy and mental clarity, always a welcome effect.

An exercise for increasing the oxygenation and detoxification capacities of the lungs is quite simple: breathe. Okay, maybe not quite that simple, since you're doing it already and things aren't optimal. First be sure you are breathing correctly, from the abdomen, not the chest. Also be sure that your shoulders are not moving upward on the inhale, or at all. Then, whenever you happen to think of it – there is no optimal schedule – breathe deliberately and deeply. First exhale all the air in the lungs by using your diaphragm muscles to push it out. This is usually much deeper than your usual exhale, and this deep exhale allows more airborne and volatile toxins to be expelled. Then inhale, deliberately deeply and slowly; again, this is typically much deeper than your usual inhalation. Sometimes, upon doing this, a sort of aching in the lungs occurs, evidence that it may have been a long time since they were expanded so much.

The diaphragm muscle lies between the lungs and the stomach, and it is the diaphragm's movement, rather than any muscular capacity of the lungs, that causes the lungs to expand and contract with inhalation and exhalation. Like any muscle, the diaphragm grows stronger with increased exercise. If you do this deep breathing when you think of it, the diaphragm grows stronger, and pretty soon you are automatically breathing more deeply and more effectively. Regular expansion of the lungs can help to develop greater lung capacity.

The deep lymph channels lie beneath the diaphragm, and the movement of the diaphragm pumps these channels and enables this detoxification route. Deeper breathing, with its greater diaphragm movement, will also help the lymph detox system.

Diaphragm movement and breathing also stimulate cranial-sacral pathways and helps to move the spinal fluid.

Is there anything else I can do to increase the lungs' detox capability?
It is important to avoid breathing anything that is toxic. The lungs' permeable surface area, which is so good at picking up toxins from the blood prior to expelling them, also makes the lungs quite efficient at picking up airborne toxins and sending them into the blood and from there around to the rest of the body. Avoiding breathing in toxins has a twofold benefit: it keeps from toxifying the rest of the body, and it keeps the lungs' capacity to detoxify existing toxins at maximum capacity. If the lungs are busy dealing with what you just inhaled, such as smoke, they

won't be available to help get rid of toxins that are already in the body. Using the bus analogy, if the bus is full it can't take on any more passengers. Airborne toxins to avoid are covered in the Part 3 of this book.

What is eucapnic breathing, and how can it help?

Eucapnic breathing (*eu* means good in Greek; *capnic* refers to carbon dioxide) was developed by K.P. Buteyko. He has found that carbon dioxide, normally considered to be a waste product exhaled by the body, has a function in maintaining the metabolism and immune system[6], and should be in balance with oxygen. One's carbon dioxide level can be too low, as measured by a blood test. Eucapnic breathing is especially effective for alleviating asthma and bronchospasm, but would be of benefit to nearly anyone who is experiencing less than optimal health.

There are coaches trained in this method, and for best results a coach should be utilized.However, the technique in its simplified form is this: On the exhale, do not inhale right away; this is called the Control Pause. When you feel the urge to breathe again, start breathing. Here's the hard part: resume breathing just as before the pause; do not take a deep breath, which is what the body will try to do. With practice, the pause should become longer and the strong desire to gasp for more air after resuming breathing should diminish. The goal here is to bring the carbon dioxide and oxygen in the blood into balance.

Wait a minute; there's a contradiction here

There seems to be a contradiction in this chapter. First we talk about getting more oxygen, which makes sense, but then we're trying to increase carbon dioxide, which sounds like the opposite. Actually, both approaches make sense. The deliberate deep breathing does bring in more oxygen, and if done often enough it can become more habitual, but it still needs to be deliberate. Eucapnic breathing increases carbon dioxide just enough to signal the body that something is wrong and needs to change, similar to the way a homeopathic remedy allows the body to become aware of an imbalance that needs to be corrected. After the carbon dioxide level is reset, deeper breathing and the intake and utilization of more oxygen should become automatic. In this way both the deep breathing and the Eucapnic breathing accomplish the same objective.

What is another breathing technique?

There is a technique in which the practitioner, typically an osteopath, holds down the diaphragm while the person breathes. A pulse develops and strengthens, which can be painful, but then it relaxes. Five gates are worked osteopathically: the cranial, thoracic, diaphragm, pubic bone, and calf. This releases diaphragmatic pressure on the lungs to allow deep breathing without pain.

Cleansing Through the Skin

Both foot baths and foot patches have become popular, although results have been mixed.

Electrical foot baths

Commercial foot baths are typically in a tub the size and shape of a dishpan. You sit with your feet immersed in plain water, into which an imperceptible current has been introduced, for about thirty minutes. Usually, but not always, the water turns a dirty color, which might be foul-smelling; this is described as toxins leaving the body through the feet. Some people who have had this done report tiredness after the treatment, followed that night by good-quality sleep and the next day by increased energy and mental clarity.

Not everyone has these results. Some have the muddy water but with no change in how they feel, and others end up with water that is barely discolored. The difference in results lies in a combination of one's initial toxicity, the particular brand and type of bath, the water that is used, and practitioner expertise. As is the case with pretty much all detox protocols, some people benefit more than others.

If you are considering buying one of these machines, it is advisable to try it out first to see what kinds of results you get from it, preferably with a knowledgeable person showing you how it is best used. In an analogous test to the placebo part of a pharmaceutical clinical trial, try out the bath with plain water – the same water source you would actually use for detox – along with the salt provided, but no feet, to be sure that any color change is a result of the actual introduction of a toxic body; if there is a color change even without feet in the water, the color change with feet is likely to be due to something other than the removal of the body's toxins.

Foot patches

Another type of product that, like the foot baths, purports to remove toxins from the body via the feet is foot patches. These are readily available at drugstores and similar stores, and are much less expensive than the foot bath. The patches are typically a mix of herbs and other ingredients in a porous bag somewhat like a teabag; a patch is adhered to the bottom of one foot and left on overnight. In theory, the toxins are pulled out of the body through the feet and into the patch. As with the foot bath, people report mixed results. A person whose feet sweat little if any is less likely to get results from the patch.

The usual results reported are of a discolored, odorous patch the next morning. Both authors of this book have tried the patch. Dr. Kellas said that his patch was discolored the next morning, and that he slept especially well that night. He also found, however, that the effect was less when the patch was used subsequently. Dr. Dworkin tried the same brand of patch, and found the patch to be discolored the next morning, with a strong odor. However, the color and odor is about what one would expect from simply dampening the patch with its strong-smelling herbs; the color change is about what one would expect from wetting a teabag. Her sleep was actually worse than usual because she kept waking up with the feeling of something large taped to the bottom of her foot, and she didn't feel any different the next day. There is no evidence that the patch can cause any harm, unless you have an allergy to one of the herbs contained in it, in which case there might be a short-lived itching where contact was made. It's safe and inexpensive and worth trying to see what kind of results you get.

Detox foot baths

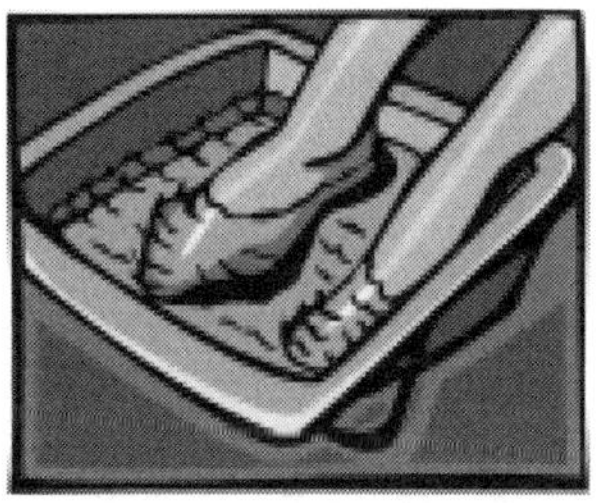

Foot baths, without the electrical component, can be useful in detoxification. Simply put warm water into a dishpan along with bentonite clay and/or the herb chaparral, and soak the feet for 20-40 minutes.

Detox bath

A good detox bath formula is as follows:

1 cup Redmond clay
16-32 oz. 3% hydrogen peroxide
1 whole large carton Epsom salts (magnesium sulfate)

Add these three ingredients to a bathtub of the warmest water you can stand. If possible use bathwater that has been treated with a filter that removes chlorine and other contaminants. Before the bath one can optionally drink a cup of ginger tea to increase detoxification. Soak for about twenty minutes. After soaking, take a brief cold shower to close the pores. This also helps to remove fluids from the joints, and stimulates the lymph and immune system.

Constitutional hydrotherapy

Alternate cold and hot wet sheets. This brings fluids containing toxins to the surface of the skin to allow the body to sweat them out.

Skin brushing

Skin brushing should be done with a soft brush. Brushing should be with the lymph, towards the heart. Skin brushing helps the lymph system remove toxins.

Parasite Cleanses

Paragon (Integris) and AP Mag are two herbal supplements that can help with parasite infestations. Take two before meals for 30-90 days.

Professional Protocols

Since most of these following protocols involve testing and prescription medications that are not available to the lay person, most of these protocols are geared towards the physician.

Roundworm and Giardia Protocol

Roundworm and giardia are often found together and the most effective protocol will go after both types of parasites. It is necessary to treat in cycles to kill the parasites as they hatch.

For roundworm: Total 18 tablets of Vermox (mebendazole)

- Chew one tablet of Vermox twice a day on an empty stomach (upon rising and before evening meal) before any nutrient intake for 3 days.
- Discontinue for 10 days.
- Then chew one tablet twice a day for 3 days as above.
- Discontinue for 10 days.
- Then chew one tablet twice a day for 3 days as above.

Wait at least 1 hour, then take 1 tsp of BifidoViden or 2 capsules of Ultra Flora, which is recommended to minimize chances of yeast infection. Finish this protocol before starting the parasite protocol.

NOTE: Do not take the Vermox along with any other protocol, anti-amoebic drug, or herbs such as AP Mag and Paragon, black walnut, Flagyl, Fasigyn, Atabrine, Quinacrine, or Yodoxin.

For giardia: Total 24 tablets of Flagyl (metronidazole), 500 mg. Alternatively, Fasigyn (tinidazole) can be used; it has fewer side effects, and is available at compounding pharmacies and outside the US.

- Day 1: 2 tablets at bedtime with food.
- Day 2: 1 tablet 3 times a day with food.
- Day 3: 1 tablet 3 times a day with food, then discontinue until day 13.
- Days 13-15: same as days 1-3, then discontinue until day 21.
- Days 21-24: same as days 1-3.

Also advised: use Clenzology Hygiene System after each bowel movement to avoid reinfection.

Helicobacter Pylori and Parasites Protocol

For helicobacter and parasites or just helicobacter, follow steps 1-7; for other parasites but not helicobacter, follow steps 2-7.

1. **For stomach protection**: Take Bismagel throughout protocol, 1 Tbsp. immediately before Flagyl/Fasigyn and tetracycline to coat the stomach. About 1½ bottles will be needed.
Per physician recommendation, take one of the following, as recommended:
   - Prilosec 20mg (prescription), 1 tablet twice a day for 14 days, then 1 tablet daily for another 14 days. Prilosec is taken before other medications to lower the HCl in the stomach.
   - 2 deglycyrrhizinated licorice (DGL) after each meal per instructions.

2. **For bacteria** that often accompany parasites: Take tetracycline, 500mg, 3 times a day or Biaxin (clarithyromycin) 500mg twice a day, for 21 days. Avoid dairy and sunlight exposure; follow strict candida diet (avoid yeasts and sugars).

3. **For amoebic/protozoal parasites**: Take Flagyl (metronidazole) or Fasigyn (tinidazole), 500mg 3 times a day for 21 days. Eat food 15 minutes after taking the dose.

4. **For fungus**: Take Nystatin, 500,000 units, 2 capsules 3 times a day, or Diflucan (fluconazole) 100mg, 1 per day, for 21 days, or Mycopril 680 three times a day with food.

5. **For fungus/yeast**: Wait at least two hours after medications, then take a probiotic such as LBC, 1 tsp. BifidoViden or LactoViden (acidophilus) or 2 capsules of Cleanzyme. Continue taking the probiotics after the rest of the protocol is complete.

6. **To avoid reinfection**: Every 5 days, put 5 droppers of Clenzology Iodine Dip into a bathtub of water. Get the solution into your nose and mucous membranes, and open and close your eyes underwater. Do not use if you are allergic to iodine. The whole family should use Clenzology to avoid reinfection

7. **For parasites** in general: Following the above 21-day treatment protocol, take 2 capsules of Paragon before each meal for 30 days.

Alinia option

Alinia (nitazoxanide) is a prescription medication that is geared primarily towards amoebic and protozoal parasites, but it is useful for worms and some bacterial parasites as well. It is a good medication to take if parasites of multiple or unknown types are suspected. If this option is used, it can replace Vermox in the Roundworm and giardia protocol, and can replace steps 2 and 3 in the helicobacter and parasites protocol.

Alinia should be taken twice a day with food; it can be chewed or swallowed whole. Sweets should be avoided on this protocol, and Nystatin, an antifungal medication, might be necessary to control yeast infection. The Clenzology iodine bath will help to avoid reinfection.

Fungus Protocol

- 1 Tbsp. Life Solubles for nutrients
- 1 Tbsp. Life Fiber to coat the intestines
- ½ tsp. Coconut oil and/or Mycopril 680, 2 before each meal
- 1-2 tsp. Intesterol; increase to 1 Tbsp. if urine pH stays above 6.5
- 1-2 tsp. Bentonite; do not use if constipated
- 1 tsp. or 2 capsules BifidoViden, Ultra Flora; rotate each meal

Combine these in a cup of water 3 times a day before meals. Follow anti-fungal diet guidelines in the Maintenance Diet.

Virus protocol

Measures to aid the body's immune system in fighting viruses are listed in the Microorganisms chapter.

Mycoplasma protocol

A protocol for mycoplasma is available at the Center for Advanced Medicine, 888-244-4420. This protocol is tailored to the individual based on body weight. Minocycline or a related antibiotic is used.

Allergy Desensitization

NAET, an allergy desensitization technique, is named for the doctor who developed it,[1,2] although others have modified it.[3] The technique works on an energy level and does not involve injections of substances, making it nearly risk-free. It is also essentially pain-free, since no needles are involved (although some practitioners, especially acupuncturists, may use acupuncture needles). Once a treatment has been completed successfully – and treatment can be for an individual substance or an entire category – the desensitization is often permanent. This technique has shown its validity many hundreds of times over.

The Theory
In a healthy person, the immune system and the body in general are able to deal with toxins and microbes appropriately, which includes the ability to identify that which is or is not dangerous.

Although many substances are inherently toxic to everyone, others are toxic or not depending on how the brain, and thus the body, perceives them and reacts to them. This selective toxicity is sometimes referred to as sensitivity or allergy. This is why so many substances (food, pollen, perfume, cat hair, etc.) cause problems for one person but not for another.

The brain-body connection has been programmed, for whatever reason, to see something more or less harmless to most people as being toxic. It follows that the brain can be reprogrammed, and if the brain is reprogrammed, it should no longer see the substance as harmful, and reactivity should improve. This is the theory behind NAET-type allergy desensitization.

Testing
Kinesiology, also called muscle testing, is used to determine what substances are problematic for the individual; electrodiagnosis, which is usually more objective, can also be used. If a substance is either toxic to everyone or a problem for that person, the muscles can grow perceptibly weak, which is the basis for muscle testing. The arm muscle is most frequently used for testing; the practitioner presses down on the arm and the person is or is not able to resist the pressure. Muscle testing is also done after a desensitization treatment to be sure the treatment has been effective.

The treatment
Physical contact with the allergen – in most cases in the form of holding a glass vial containing a solution of the allergen with its unique frequency – is a necessary part of the treatment. While holding the allergen, the patient has certain pathways stimulated, although needles are not used by most practitioners. The necessary immune mediators or antidotes are produced to that particular allergen, and these neutralize the adverse reaction to the allergen in the hand. In this way, the

brain is reprogrammed to tell the body the substance is harmless. A warning: some things are best not neutralized, for example pathogenic microorganisms or chemicals such as mercury, chlorine, or arsenic, unless one has autoimmune problems. A strong immune response is appropriate and desirable for these.

24 hours are needed for information on an energy level to circulate through the entire body and reset its twelve major systems (liver, lymph etc.), because it requires two hours to travel through each one of the systems. Therefore as many as 24 hours must pass for the new information to complete the cycle throughout the body, and for the allergy treatment to be effective. To be on the safe side, 25 hours rather than 24 are allotted for the aftermath of each treatment. During this time, exposure to the substance treated for should be avoided.

Treatment should go from the general to the specific. Combinations such as grain mix, sugar mix, mineral mix, B vitamin complex mix and others can clear allergies to all grains, sugars, and so forth in some people, although others may require some separation of substances for best results.

Even though you might be sensitive to a large number of things, it is often not necessary to clear them all. A more effective strategy might be to clear only that which is needed for detoxification, such as supplements, as well as using parasite protocols to clear out parasites and supporting the liver. After this is done, many if not most sensitivities often clear up on their own, one of the many benefits of detoxification. After the detox, any remaining allergies can be cleared if they are still a problem.

Other types of detoxification

Earthing is a term meaning to let your bare feet touch the earth. This is said to pull free electrons from our bodies into the ground. Free electrons (free radicals) are oxidants that can build up in the body. With earthing, they are grounded and pulled into the earth.

Sneezing, hiccupping, and swallowing can help to reset the central nervous system. This can release muscle tension, which allows the lymph glands to detoxify.

Wear a **copper wire** wrapped around your wrist in the shower. The water sets a flow of electrons going down the wire, as is the case with electricity. This can help to detoxify from radiation as from radon or uranium.

Avoid sleeping on **earth energy lines**, also called Hartman-Curry and ley lines. These are regular lines of radiation in the earth, which can be picked up with a dowsing rod.

Avoid sources of electromagnetic frequencies (**EMF**), such as high-tension power lines, motors and transformers, cell phones (unless a wired headset or speaker is used), or portable landline phones.

Part 5
Nutritional and Other Supporters

General Discussion of Supporters

There are any number of books on general nutrition, including a major section of ***Thriving in a Toxic World***, written by the authors of this book. This is not to minimize the importance of general nutrition. The healthier and stronger your body is in general, the better able it is to detoxify and to keep you healthy, and the better able it is to heal toxin damage after detoxification. However, this chapter focuses on those nutrients and supplements that are specific to the supporting of detoxification.

Why is nutritional support so important in detoxification?
In addition to strengthening your body in general, specific nutrients, whether they come from food or supplements, help in various aspects of detoxification. Trying to detoxify without them is like driving a car with only a bare minimum of gas in the tank – you probably won't get very far. You can't detox faster than you remineralize.

> You can only detoxify as fast as you can remineralize.

What does detoxification-related nutritional support do?
Detoxification is actually quite a complex process, involving a number of organs, elimination pathways, and quite a few biochemical pathways as toxins are broken down. Some nutrients specifically support the liver or kidneys. Some nutrients are, or help produce, antioxidants, which work against free radical damage. Some, like water and oil, help to carry toxins out of the body.

A number of nutritional supporters have been discussed throughout the book where relevant. Others are discussed in the chapters in this section.

Specific Supporters

Water

Water helps to dilute and carry toxins out of the body. It is necessary for all of the functions of the cells and body, including detoxification. The recommended amount is ½ ounce for every pound of body weight per day; if, for example, you weigh 128 pounds, that comes to 64 ounces, or a half gallon, per day. Be sure that the water you are drinking is filtered or spring water, not municipal tap water that can contain chlorine and other toxins. Although water from vegetables, fruits, and soups counts, it is a good idea to drink plenty in the form of water itself to be sure you are getting enough. As long as minerals are taken in sufficient quantity, including from food sources and from Kona Gold, it is nearly impossible to get too much, so drink up.

For people who don't breathe properly, such as those with illnesses, alkaline water can help to balance the body's pH, alkalinizing the cell and increasing nutrient absorption.

How do you know whether you are drinking enough water?
If you need to urinate approximately once every waking hour, you are taking in enough water from whatever source. If you are urinating less, you should increase your water intake.

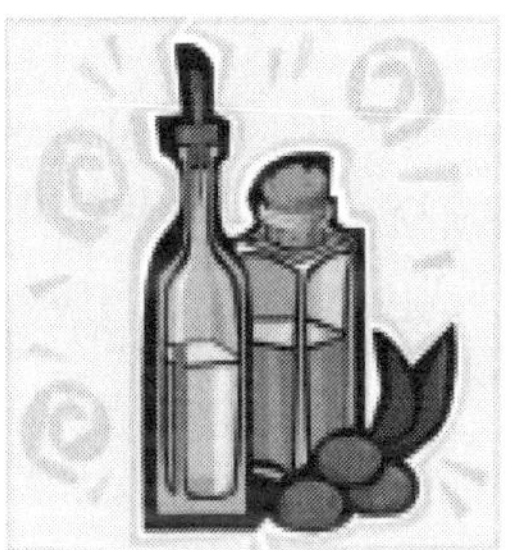

Oils

Beneficial oils, especially fish oils, cod liver oil, olive oil, and flaxseed oil, help to carry out oil-soluble toxins such as solvents and pesticides. In addition, since the cell wall has a lipid bilayer (fatty double layer) as protection from toxins outside the cell, taking in good oils can strengthen that selective barrier.

Minerals

Just as the lungs take in essential oxygen and expel the waste product carbon dioxide as well as some toxins, cells also have a cycle of intake and excretion. They take in water and nutrients and expel waste products. Minerals, especially sodium, potassium, calcium, and magnesium, are necessary for the cells to take in through the cell wall and utilize water. They are also necessary for the passage of waste products in the other direction. Minerals are essential in a number of ways, in this way they directly help to detoxify on a cellular level. They also control detoxification speed – you can't detox faster than you can replace the minerals. Sodium is one of the most crucial in this regard, but a good supply and balance of necessary minerals all play a part.

The minerals **zinc, copper, and manganese** together form the powerful antioxidant enzyme superoxide dismutase.[1] Magnesium is a cofactor in and activator of hundreds of enzymes.

Selenium is part of the enzyme glutathione peroxidase, which acts as an antioxidant.[1] It has antioxidant properties, especially in combination with vitamin E, and works with detoxifying sulfur-based amino acids such as glutathione. It is an immune system booster.

Magnesium is a cofactor in over 300 different enzyme reactions, and also helps in the removal of toxic substances.[1]

Sulfur is part of a number of amino acids such as methionine, cysteine, and glutathione, which are potent detoxifiers of chemicals and metals. Certain foods contain sulfur: garlic onions, beans, and eggs.

Zinc is required for the body's natural chelation processes. It is part of superoxide dismutase (SOD), which controls some free radicals. It also helps to boost the immune system, which is why zinc lozenges are useful for colds.

Copper, in combination with vitamin C and with the amino acid lysine, is needed for immune system function.

Molybdenum is necessary to utilize sulfur based amino acids such as glutathione, methionine and cysteine, which help clear the body of metals and toxins. Aldehyde oxidase is a molybdenum dependent enzyme that helps detoxify acetaldehyde from beverage alcohol as well as formaldehyde.

Vitamins

Vitamins can be:

- Fat soluble, with the carotenoids inside the cell; these include vitamins A and E
- Transitional: alpha-lipoic acid and glutathione
- Water soluble, such as vitamin C, with bioflavonoids outside the cell

Vitamin A is an antioxidant and immune system stimulant, especially in the form of its precursor beta-carotene as well as other carotenoids.

Vitamin C helps to raise the levels of glutathione, one of the body's natural detoxifiers. In high doses of one gram or more, either oral or intravenously, it acts as a chelator to remove toxic heavy metals. It also supports the immune system and acts as an antiviral, especially in high doses, either oral or IV, and as an antihistamine, helping to relieve cold symptoms. It can help relieve allergic symptoms. It counteracts formation of nitrosamines, which are carcinogens, from nitrates and nitrites in processed and preserved foods. It can help to reduce the toxic effects of alcohol.

Vitamin E, a fat-soluble vitamin, is incorporated into the fatty parts of cells to protect against free radicals, drugs, and radiation.[1] It works with vitamin A to protect lungs from ozone and air pollution, including damage from smoking. It is also an immune system stimulant.

PABA, in the B vitamin family, helps to prevent sun damage to skin and ozone damage to lungs.

Antioxidants

Coenzyme Q10, or CoQ10, is an antioxidant that protects cells, especially of the heart, from free radical damage. Most heart disease patients respond positively to CoQ10, and it is also of value in lowering high blood pressure. CoQ10 also protects nerves and may slow the onset of diseases such as Alzheimer's and Parkinson's. It can reduce fatigue in some CFS patients.

CoQ10 has been shown to have anticancer properties and has been implicated in improvements of some cancer patients.[2] It can also help to mitigate damage from anticancer drugs.

Pine bark extract and grape seed extract are powerful bioflavonoid antioxidants that act as free radical scavengers.[1] Pycnogenol, quercetin, rutin, resveratrol, turmeric, boswellia, and others, are also bioflavonoid antioxidants.

Amino acids

NAC, or N-acetylcysteine, is a stable form of the amino acid L-cysteine. It is converted to glutathione, a detoxifier, in the body, and is more easily absorbed and utilized than taking glutathione itself.[1] These work together to form the glutathione complex. The mineral molybdenum, the vitamins B2, B6, vitamin C, and folic acid, and the amino acids glutamine, methionine, glycine, and n-acetylcysteine (NAC), as well as cordyceps, milk thistle (silymarin), n-acetyl d-glucosamine, and quercetin, are also helpful in forming glutathione.

Cystine and **cysteine** convert from one to the other as needed. They are potent free radical destroyers and help protect the body from radiation damage, making it a good adjunctive therapy with chemotherapy and radiation treatments for cancer.[3] They promote resistance to free radical damage, chemicals, and heavy metals, and help to protect against cancer, which is often caused by free radicals.

Glycine is an amino acid produced by the body, and it is important in some of the liver functions. Since the liver is crucial in chemical detoxification, glycine is recommended as a supplement when one has had a significant chemical or drug exposure.[1]

Glutamine is also important for liver detox, and is recommended especially for those who are detoxing from alcohol, as well as for those who are taking anti-inflammatory medications or who have food sensitivities or yeast overgrowth.[1] It can help reduce alcohol and sugar cravings by feeding the brain. Supplementation with glutamine decreases the side effects of cancer chemotherapy[4] by healing the intestines.

Lysine fights viral and herpes infections, including cold sores and shingles, especially when combined with copper as copper lysinate. Lysine and arginine are shown to enhance immune function by increasing the number of lymphocytes and IgG levels.[5]

Taurine and **methionine** are two other amino acids with a role in detoxification.

Enzymes

Nothing in the body happens until the enzymes say so. The 4000-plus metabolic enzyme types are the catalysts for all of the body's reactions, rather like the spark plugs in a car's engine. Enzymes help with digestive and other bodily functions, including detoxification. In general, enzymes taken with meals help in the digestion of the food eaten, and enzymes taken away from meals help with the body's processes. The enzyme supplementation in the Detoxification diet addresses both. Food sensitivity can be a sign of low enzymes in the body, which can be addressed by enzyme supplementation.

Enzymes facilitate the breakdown of toxins to be eliminated from the body.

Protease, one type of enzyme, can dissolve the protein coatings of microorganisms so the immune system can finish them off. It is not coincidental that the tropical countries most known for intestinal microorganisms – Mexico, India, Thailand – also provide high-enzyme fruits such as pineapple, papayas and mangoes that help reduce intestinal infections in the locals.

Enzymes help to treat or prevent cancer in a number of ways, from destroying the fibrin coating that protects abnormal cells, to strengthening the immune system, to decreasing metastasis, to preventing abnormal cell formation in the first place. Enzymes can also help prevent cancer by being involved in DNA repair.

Herbs

Eleuthero, or Siberian Ginseng, enhances immune system function and increases T-cell counts, and helps the liver to detoxify chemicals and drugs.[6] Ashwaganda, an herb from India, has a similar function, and it also help to protect against radiation damage.[6]

Garlic, a good source of the minerals selenium and sulfur, enhances the immune system and helps to kill some parasites.

Herbs are discussed in greater detail in the chapter on Herbs, later in the book.

Fiber

Fiber helps to maintain digestive system health and bowel regularity, By normalizing bowel transit time, it decreases the amount of time that toxins in the bowel can contact the intestinal walls and be reabsorbed into the bloodstream. Low fiber and increased colon cancer incidence go together, likely because toxins in the fecal matter stay in contact with the colon walls longer without enough fiber.

Fiber also acts as a kind of broom to sweep toxins out of the digestive system. In addition, it encourages more water to enter the digestive tract, and water carries toxins out of the body; fiber can enhance the elimination of toxins in this way. Fiber acts as a sponge, not only for water-soluble toxins, but also for harmful fatty acids and oil-soluble toxins.

Rice bran is a beneficial type of fiber, both for its cleansing action and its nutritional content. Oryzanol is a substance found in the oil of rice bran. Even small doses of oryzanol enable certain cholesterol-controlling enzymes in the liver to function more effectively.

Other nutrients

Curcumin is a bioflavonoid compound that gives the spice turmeric, or Indian curry, its characteristic yellow color. It has been used in China and India for millennia to protect the liver and enhance bile flow.[1] It also acts as an anti-inflammatory agent.

Lecithin and choline are lipotropics. Lecithin thins the bile to allow chemicals and other toxins to flow out of the liver more readily. It also helps to break down fats[1], which can carry oil-soluble toxins out of the body.

Choline is used to make phosphatidyl choline, a key ingredient in cell membranes; cell membranes help to protect cells against toxins. It is also used for gallbladder and liver function.

Tocotrienols are members of the vitamin E family. They are potent antioxidants against lipid peroxidation, the damaging of fats by oxidation.[7] Tocotrienol is 40 to 6000 times stronger as an antioxidant than vitamin E, depending on the tocopherol fraction.[8] Tocotrienols help prevent the oxidation of LDL cholesterol to a more harmful form. They may also protect against cancer.

Octacosanol helps to reduce lipid peroxidation; that is, it lessens the formation of more damaging compounds from cholesterol and triglycerides.[9] It also helps to protect epithelial (skin) cells.[9]

Indole-3-carbinol (I3C) occurs naturally in cruciferous vegetables such as broccoli, cauliflower, Brussels sprouts and cabbage. I3C protects against dioxin, an environmental toxin. In general, it provides antioxidant protection.[10] It is especially protective against hormonal cancers such as breast, ovarian, and prostate.

Whey protein is an immune system enhancer that boosts the body's ability to fight infection and in some studies has been shown to inhibit the growth of cancer cells. Whey is a first-line immune system defense as it inhibits the growth of iron-dependent bacteria, scavenges free iron, can block the growth of pathogenic bacteria and yeast, can stimulate the beneficial intestinal microflora and has antibacterial properties. It also builds up the body's own antioxidants by raising glutathione levels; glutathione is an antioxidant that protects cells and neutralizes toxins.[11]

Probiotics – Regular use of probiotics may improve immune function[12] and increase resistance to infection.[13,14]

For more information
Minerals and herbs are discussed in greater detail in the next two chapters.

Mineral Balancing for Symptom Relief

Why is mineral balancing so important?

Minerals can become unbalanced or deficient during any detox, especially the detox diet and the sauna.

Mineral imbalances can cause unpleasant symptoms that can rapidly be remedied by taking the appropriate supplements. There are four minerals whose deficiency is common. These are needed in larger amounts than most other minerals, which are often called trace minerals. The following minerals and supplements can help relieve the following symptoms.

We recommend that you have potassium, calcium, and magnesium (citrate or malate) supplements, as well as a good quality salt such as Real Salt, on hand before beginning the detoxification diet or, for that matter, any type of detox. Symptoms to watch out for are listed in this chapter.

If you don't know which mineral to take, Kona Gold would be a good choice since it contains most minerals in balance.

Take the mineral every two hours until symptoms subside (once is usually sufficient) up to a maximum of 6 tablets/capsules unless directed otherwise by your practitioner. A symptom that is caused by a mineral deficiency will often respond dramatically, sometimes within twenty minutes or so of taking the mineral.

Potassium and sodium must be in balance, and their deficiency symptoms can be opposites. Too much of one, for example in a high-salt meal, can cause a relative deficiency of potassium. The same holds true for the calcium / magnesium pairing, which is why they are often placed together in supplements; taking calcium supplements by themselves can bring on magnesium deficiency symptoms. An example is the way magnesium deficiency can cause constipation, while either an excess of magnesium or a deficiency of calcium can cause diarrhea.

How can I identify what mineral is needed?

Potassium

Symptoms of low potassium include:

- Insomnia with mind racing, tossing and turning; typically a person with low potassium will get up to urinate during the night, and having urinated out potassium, can have trouble getting back to sleep.
- Mind racing, obsessive thinking, repetitive thinking, even getting songs stuck in your head

- Anxiety; in the case of the sauna program, low potassium can cause a feeling of "I've got to get out of here right now!"
- Fatigue, especially mid-afternoon fatigue
- Rapid or pounding heartbeat
- High pulse rate
- Kidney pain in lower back area
- Irritability
- Shallow breathing
- Twitching
- Muscle cramps, tightness or pain

Any of these can be a sign of potassium deficiency; several or all of them together are a sure sign. Take potassium on an empty stomach if possible; if you are experiencing symptoms and you have eaten recently, try the potassium anyway. Try potassium before magnesium if you are not sure which to take, since some of the same symptoms are indicative of a deficiency of either one. Potassium usually comes in 99mg capsules; you can try one or two. Caution: do not take more than this at one time, since it can throw off the sodium/potassium pump in the body and can cause an effective lowering of the sodium level, with low sodium symptoms as listed in the next paragraph.

Sodium

Symptoms of low sodium include:

- Cold hands and feet
- Heavy fatigue that may come on suddenly
- Thirst even after drinking water, or no thirst at all
- Low blood pressure
- Dizziness
- Nausea
- Loss of appetite

A typical low-sodium scenario is this: You have taken a long soak in a hot tub, and now you are feeling dizzy, nauseated, and so tired that you just want to lie down. Part of this may be due to lowered blood pressure from the heat, but usually these symptoms come on from low sodium. While you have been soaking in the hot water, you have been sweating, which, of course, would not be evident, and which would deplete your body of salt. If this has happened to you, you will have some idea of the kinds of feelings to watch out for during detox. Take sodium by taking a capsule of Kona Gold or dissolving a half to one teaspoon of mineral salt or Real Salt in water. Generally people need 1½ tsp of salt per day from all sources; people who exercise a lot or are prone to night sweats might need more since they would be sweating out some of the salt.

Magnesium

Magnesium is responsible for muscle contracting smoothly. Magnesium deficiency, therefore, can cause tightness and cramping overall. Symptoms of low magnesium include:

- Constipation
- Heart palpitations, fibrillation, or a feeling of skipped or irregular beats
- Severe menstrual cramps
- Muscle cramps
- High blood pressure: arterial walls, being muscular, contract, narrowing the arterial opening and raising the blood pressure
- Headache, which can be related to tightening muscles in the neck and scalp
- Potassium deficiency symptoms (see above) that are not relieved by potassium

Take magnesium on an empty stomach. Be aware that too much magnesium can cause diarrhea, which depletes calcium and potassium. If you do not desire the stool softening effect, take magnesium glycinate, or take the magnesium intravenously. If the stool softening effect is desired, take a different form of magnesium such as magnesium citrate.

Calcium

Symptoms of low calcium include:

- Fatigue
- Diarrhea
- Inability to stay asleep
- Lack of stamina
- Low strength
- Tooth pain
- Pain in the long bones, elbow, knee, shoulder, or hip
- Loose stools, like those caused by taking magnesium supplements; remember that low calcium and high magnesium are a pair in that they work as antagonists, and too much magnesium can cause a functional deficiency of calcium.

Take calcium on an empty stomach for best absorption. Fish oils, vitamin D, and the mineral boron also help in the absorption of calcium.

Calcium and magnesium are often found together in supplements in varying ratios. The best ratio for you can be determined by your stool. The usual ratio is 2:1 calcium to magnesium, typically 1000mg of calcium to 500mg magnesium. If you tend to have loose stools, take 3:1 (more calcium); if you tend to be constipated, take 1:1 or even 1:2 (more magnesium).

Herbs

How can herbs be useful in detoxification?

There are a number of herbs that can support detoxification in several ways:

- General detoxifier
- Blood cleansing
- Colon cleansing – strong cathartics are not included here or recommended
- Liver cleansing and support
- Kidney support, diuretic (increase urination)
- Skin cleanser, promotes sweating
- Antimicrobial

Some of the herbs used for detoxification include the following.[1] The usual dosage is 1-2 before meals.

Herb	Blood cleanser	Colon cleanser	Liver cleanser, support	Diuretic, kidney cleanser	Skin cleanser/ sweating	Anti-micro-bial	Additional properties
Artichoke			x				
Black walnut	x					x	
Buckthorn		x					
Burdock root	x		x		x	x	
Cayenne	x				x		
Chaparral	Strong				x	x	
Dandelion root	x	x	x	x			Filters toxins
Echinacea	x					x	
Garlic	x	x				x	
Ginger root			x		x		Helps nausea
Goldenseal root	x	x	x	x	x	x	
Horsetail				x			
Juniper berries				x			
Licorice root		Mild laxative					Detoxifies, soothes stomach
Milk thistle, silymarin			x				
Oregon grape root	x	x	Liver stimulant		x		
Parsley leaf				x			Freshens breath

Herb	Blood cleanser	Colon cleanser	Liver cleanser, support	Diuretic, kidney cleanser	Skin cleanser/ sweating	Anti-micro-bial	Additional properties
Plantain				x			
Purslane	x					x	
Red clover	x						
Rhubarb root		x					
Sarsaparilla root	x		x			x	Cleans lymph
Senna leaf		x					
Uva ursi				x			
Yarrow				x			
Yellow dock root	x	x	x		x		

Recommended Supplements

These supplements are recommended for almost everyone on the detox diet, or undergoing other detox protocols described in this book. Dosage should be as indicated on the container in most cases, or take as directed by your practitioner.

Supplement	Manufacturer	Purpose	Dosage and Instructions
Essential 7 (E7), Life Solubles,	Integris	Provides seven essential food groups	1-3 scoops daily up to 10 scoops if on detox diet; take with food
Goatein		Provides protein from goat source, less allergenic than cow products	1-3 scoops daily with E7 if hypoglycemic
UltraBalance, UltraClear, Ultra Clear Renew, Ultra Meal rice protein	Metagenics	Nutrition	1-3 scoops daily
Cleanzyme (or Biozyme, Fibrozyme)	Integris (Cleanzyme)	Enzyme for food digestion and bodily processes, can "digest" some microorganisms	One capsule every waking hour
Aloe 7000	Integris	Reduces sugar and bread cravings and fungus growth	Mix one part aloe to two parts water after meals, swish in mouth for 2 minutes and swallow
Kona Gold	Integris	Mineral supplement	2-8 per day before meals
SoZo capsules	Integris	Alkalizes system; puts ATP (power plants) into cells; helps bone, sleep, memory; anti-inflammatory	Take 1-3 capsules per day away from food and supplements (2 hours after or 1 hour before food)
SoZo beverage	SoZo	Increases cell regulators such as antioxidants, enzymes, glyconutrients/kinases, endorphins, and hormones	About three ounces of liquid per day
AdvaClear	Metagenics	Increases cytochrome P450 for chemical detoxification	1-2 before meals
Life Fiber	Professional Preference	Improves bowel elimination	1-2 tsp. per day
Cardio-Health	Integris	Ayurvedic herb blend to normalize heart function and blood pressure	2 pills twice a day before meals

In addition to the detox diet supplements on the previous page, these supplements are mentioned in various places throughout the book. Generic (not brand name) supplements are not covered here, nor are prescription medications. Dosages vary depending on condition being addressed.

Supplement	Manufacturer	Purpose	Dosage and Instructions
Paragon	Integris	Helps to eliminate parasites	2 before meals
MetalloClear	Metagenics	Increases metal detoxification	1 before meals
Super Aloe 450	Ortho Molecular Products	Helps with constipation	As needed, one at night
Kyo Dophilus	Kyolic	Probiotics	1-2 per day
Ultra Flora	Metagenics	Probiotics	1-2 per day
BifidoViden	Metagenics	Probiotics	1-2 per day
AgriSept	Essentially Yours	Antifungal citrus seed	4 drops in water
Dioxychlor	American Biologics	Antimicrobial	3-10 drops
Kyolic garlic	Wakunaga	Stimulates immune system	5-30 drops
Mycopril 680	TE Neesby	Caprylic acid for fungus	2 before meals
Only Whey	Integris	Hydrolyzed predigested whey	1-3 scoops per day
Real Salt	Redmond	Salt with minerals	1½ tsp per day
Aloe 7000	Integris	Digestive health, fungus	1 capful to 1 oz water, swish and swallow
MetalloClear	Metagenics	Detoxifies metals	1 before meals
Sun Chlorella	Sun Chlorella Corp.	Green superfood	5-15 per day
Phosfood	Standard Process	Digestion, pulls free calcium out of kidneys and gallbladder	3-10 drops per day
Lipo-Gen	Metagenics	For digesting oils	1-2 per meal
Liv Long	Integris	Liver cleansing	1-2 per meal
AP Mag	Ayush Herbs	Antiparasitic	1-2 per meal
BifidoViden LactoViden	Metagenics	Probiotics	1-2 per day
WBC	Dragon River	Increases white blood cells	1 dropper per day
Primal Defense	Garden of Life	Probiotics	1-2 per day
Pycnogenol	Horphag Research	Bioflavonoids	1-2 per day
pH testing tape	Micro Essentials	To test urine pH	Per instructions to test 1st AM urine
Clenzology	Garden of Life	External cleansing	Per instructions

All supplements listed on the previous two pages can be ordered from the Center for Advanced Medicine, 760-632-9042 or toll-free 888-244-4420, and from the websites www.camhealthtalk.com or www.solvingtherootcause.com. They can also be ordered from the indicated manufacturer in some cases. In addition, the Toxic Twins books, ***Surviving the Toxic Crisis*** and ***Thriving in a Toxic World***, and the ***Toxic Immune Syndrome Cookbook***, by the authors of this book, Dr. William R. Kellas and Dr. Andrea S. Dworkin, are also available if still in print. Other books by these authors may be available as well.

Saliva tests for adrenal function can be ordered from Diagnos-techs (diagnostechs.com).

Glossary and Abbreviations

Acetaldehyde – neurotoxic breakdown product of alcohol and found in cigarette smoke
ADA – American Dental Association
ADHD – attention deficit hyperactivity disorder
Aflatoxin – nervous system toxin from mold sometimes found on peanuts
Agoraphobia – fear of leaving the home
Aldehydes – toxic breakdown products
Allopathic – Western, or mainstream, medicine
ALS – amyotrophic lateral sclerosis, a nervous system disease; Lou Gehrig's disease
AMA – American Medical Association
Anaerobic – without oxygen
Ankylosing spondylitis – severe hereditary form of arthritis
Anorexia – appetite loss
Arteriosclerosis – hardening of arteries
Aspartame – neurotoxic artificial sweetener
BHT – a food preservative
Biopsy – tissue testing
BUN – blood urea nitrogen, a test of kidney function
Candida – yeast in the body
Carcinoma, carcinogen, carcinogenic – pertaining to cancer
Cardiac – referring to the heart
Cathartic – herb or drug that forcefully eliminates bowel waste
CBC – standard blood test
CDC – Centers for Disease Control, a federal agency
Celiac disease – intolerance of grain gluten
Cellulase – enzyme that breaks down fiber
CFS – chronic fatigue syndrome
Chelation – removal of metals from the body
CNS – central nervous system, brain and spinal cord
Cognitive – referring to thinking, awareness, and memory
Cytochrome P450 – the body's chemical detoxification system
Dermatitis – skin rash
Diuretic – drug or herb that increases excretion of fluid
DIY – do it yourself
DMPS, DMSA – chelators
DNA, RNA – components for cell duplication
Dolomite – natural, but not recommended, source of calcium
EBV – Epstein-Barr virus
EI – environmental illness, the same as multiple chemical sensitivity

EKG – electrocardiogram test for the heart
EMF – Electro-magnetic frequencies; types of harmful radiation
EPA – Environmental Protection Agency
ERT – estrogen replacement therapy
FDA – Food and Drug Association
FD&C – Food, Drug, and Cosmetic
Fibromyalgia – overall pain
Fluorosis – improper mineralization of bones and teeth caused by fluoride
FMS – fibromyalgia syndrome
Free radical – reactive, and harmful, form of an element
GERD – gastro-esophageal reflux disease, severe heartburn
GI – gastrointestinal
Gluten – allergenic component of most grains
HCl – hydrochloric acid in stomach
HDL – beneficial cholesterol
Helicobacter pylori – bacteria that cause ulcers
Hemoglobin – blood component that transports oxygen
Hepatitis – liver inflammation
HRT – hormone replacement therapy
Hypertension – high blood pressure
Hyperthermia – sauna, high temperature
Hypoglycemia – low blood sugar
IBS – irritable bowel syndrome
IDDM – insulin dependent diabetes mellitus, type 1 diabetes
Immunodeficient, immunocompromised – having poor immune system function
Insulin – hormone produced by the pancreas to regulate blood sugar
Ischemia – blockage
Kinesiology testing – muscle weakness testing for allergy or toxicity
LBA – live blood analysis
LDL – so-called "bad" cholesterol
Lipids – fats
MCS – multiple chemical sensitivity
Meningeal system, meninges – covering of brain and spinal cord
Metabolites – breakdown products of drugs
Metallothionein – the body's metal detoxification system
Methylmercury – a more harmful form of mercury
MRI – magnetic resonance imaging, a testing technique
MS – Multiple sclerosis
Mycoplasma – small microbe
Myelin – fatty sheath around nerve fibers

NAET – allergy desensitization technique
Neurotoxic – poisonous to the nervous system
Nightshade – category of vegetables that can contribute to arthritis in sensitive people
NSAIDs – non-steroidal anti-inflammatory drugs (painkillers)
Opiates – class of strong painkilling drugs
Organochlorines – harmful chemicals formed from organic chemicals and chlorine
OSA – oxidative stress analysis, a blood test
OSHA – Occupational Safety and Health Agency
Osteomalacia – softening of bones, may precede osteoporosis
Osteoporosis – porous and fragile bone
OTC – over the counter drug
Pathogenic – harmful, relating to microbes
Peristalsis – the normal downward propelling motion of the intestine
pH – acidity or alkalinity of a liquid
ppm – parts per million, a measure of concentration
Probiotics – beneficial bacteria such as acidophilus and bifidus
Renal – referring to the kidneys
Solanine – toxin in potatoes
Specific gravity – density of a liquid such as urine
Statins – drugs to lower cholesterol
Structure – skeleton, bones, joints, and their relationship to each other
Sublingual – under the tongue
Sulfites – food preservatives, often allergenic
Tartrazine – allergenic yellow food dye
Tbsp – tablespoon
Trans fatty acids – harmful oils
Triglycerides – blood fats, usually undesirable
tsp – teaspoon
Vegan – diet with no animal products at all
Villi – projections in the intestine for food absorption
Xenoestrogens – estrogen-like chemicals, like pesticides, that come from outside the body

References

Part 1

Assessment

1. Kellas, William, and Andrea S. Dworkin, ***Thriving in a Toxic World***, Professional Preference, Olivenhain CA, 1996.

Part 2

Neurological

1. Carper, Jean, ***Your Miracle Brain***, HarperCollins, NY, 2000.
2. Petty, CS, "Organic phosphate insecticide poisoning," ***American Journal of Medicine***, Vol. 24, 1958, pp. 467-470.
3. Kellas, William, and Andrea S. Dworkin, ***Surviving the Toxic Crisis***, Professional Preference, Olivenhain CA, 1996.
4. Feldman, ***American Journal of Industrial Medicine***, 1980.
5. ***Neurotoxins: At Home and the Workplace***, Report by the Committee on Science and Technology, U.S. House of Representatives, Sept. 16, 1986, Report 99-827.
6. Hatherill, J Robert, ***The Brain Gate***, LifeLine Press, Washington DC, 2003.
7. Vroom, FQ and M Greer, "Mercury vapor intoxication," ***Brain***, Vol. 95, 1972, pp. 305- 318.
8. Echevarria, D et al, "Neurobehavioral effects from exposure to dental amalgam Hg," ***FASEB Journal***, Vol. 12, 1998, pp. 971-980.
9. Cutler, Andrew Hall, ***Amalgam Illness: Diagnosis and Treatment***, Sammamish WA, 1999.
10. Moen B, Hollund B, Riise T, "Neurological symptoms among dental assistants: A cross-sectional study," ***Journal of Occupational Medicine and Toxicology***, May 18, 2008, Vol. 3, p. 10.
11. Colino, Stacey, "Why you've got that headache," ***Redbook***, Feb. 2004, Vol. 202, No. 2, pp. 46-54.
12. "Don't feed your headache," ***Reader's Digest***, Sept. 2003, p. 196.
13. Shirlow, MJ and CD Mathers, "A study of caffeine consumption and symptoms: Indigestion, palpitations, tremor, headache and insomnia," ***International Journal of Epidemiology***, Vol. 14, No. 2, 1985, pp. 239-248.
14. Rao, Linda, "Headache in a can," ***Prevention***, Dec. 2003, Vol. 55, No. 12, p. 42.
15. Batmanghelidj, Fereydoon, ***Your Body's Many Cries for Water***, Global Health Solutions, Inc., Vienna VA, 3rd edition, 1997.
16. Kane, LE and T Alaria, "Sensory irritation to formaldehyde and acrolein during single and repeated exposures in mice," ***American Industrial Hyg. Assoc. Journal***, Vol. 38, 1977, p. 509.
17. Klotter, Jule, "Toluene," ***Townsend Letter for Doctors***, No. 118, May 1993, p. 518.
18. Jetter, Alexis, "How safe is your food?" ***Reader's Digest***, Aug. 2003, pp. 64-71.
19. Till, T and K Maaly, "Mercury in tooth roots and in jaw bones," ***ZRW***, Vol. 87, Issue 6, 1978, pp. 288-90.
20. Harrison, DP, "Copper as a factor in the dietary precipitation of migraine," ***Headache***, Vol. 26, No. 5, 1986, pp. 248-250.
21. Mindell, Earl, ***Earl Mindell's Secret Remedies***, Fireside (Simon & Schuster), NY, 1997.
22. Manning, Betsy Russell (editor), ***Candida, Silver Mercury Fillings and the Immune System***, Greensward Press, San Francisco CA, 1985.
23. Siblerud, Robert, "Evidence that mercury from silver dental fillings may be an etiological factor in multiple sclerosis," ***The Science of the Total Environment***, Vol. 142, 1994, pp. 191-205.
24. Giraudon, P, and A Bernard, "Chronic viral infections of the central nervous system: Aspects specific to multiple sclerosis," ***Rev. Neurol.*** (Paris), Aug. 3, 2009, pubmed.gov.
25. Sullivan, Kip, "The evidence linking silver-mercury fillings to Alzheimer's disease: A literature review," ***Townsend Letter for Doctors and Patients***, Aug./Sept., 1997, Vol. 169/170, pp. 74-83.
26. Redhe, R and J Pleva, "Recovery from Amyotrophic Lateral Sclerosis and from allergy after removal of dental amalgam fillings," ***International Journal of Risk Safety Medicine***, 1994, Vol. 4, pp. 229-236.
27. Qureshi M, Brown RH Jr, Rogers JT, Cudkowicz ME, "Serum ferritin and metal levels as risk factors for amyotrophic lateral sclerosis," ***Open Neurology Journal***, Sept. 12, 2008, Vol. 2, pp. 51-54.
28. Kreisher, Otto, "Survey links Lou Gehrig's disease, Gulf War service," ***The San Diego Union-Tribune***, Dec. 11, 2001, p. A13.
29. Kellas, William, and Andrea S. Dworkin, ***Thriving in a Toxic World***, Professional Preference, Olivenhain CA, 1996.
30. Kane, LE, and T Alaria, "Sensory irritation to formaldehyde and acrolein during single and repeated exposures in mice," ***American Industrial Hyg. Assoc. Journal***, Vol. 38, 1977, p. 509.
31. "Fluoridation death," ***Townsend Letter for Doctors***, No. 112, Nov. 1992, p. 988.
32. Ritz, B, and F. Yu, "Parkinson's disease mortality and pesticide exposure in California 1984-1994," ***International Journal of Epidemiology***, 2000, Vol. 29, pp. 323-329.
33. Fleming, L, JB Mann et al, "Parkinson's disease and brain levels of organochlorine pesticides," ***Annals of Neurology***, Vol. 36, No. 1, July 1994, pp. 100-3.
34. Butterfield, PG, BG Valanis et al, "Environmental antecedents of young-onset Parkinson's disease," ***Neurology***, Vol. 43, No. 6, June 1993, pp. 1150-8.

35. Tonkonogy J, Geller J., "A neuropsychiatry service in a state hospital: Adolf Meyer's approach revisited," ***Psychiatry Quarterly***, Sept. 2007, Vol. 78, No. 3, pp. 219-235.

36. Lipscomb, JW, JE Kramer and JB Leikin, "Seizure following brief exposure to the insect repellent N,N-diethyl-m-toluamide," ***Annals of Emergency Medicine***, Vol. 21, No. 3, March 1992, pp. 3115-7.

Cancer

1. Servan-Schreiber, David, "The anticancer lifestyle," ***AARP The Magazine***, March/April 2009, Vol. 52, No. 2C, pp. 20-23.
2. Grossman, Michael J, and Jodi L Jones, ***The Vitality Connection***, Vitality Press Publications, Rancho Santa Margarita CA, 2003.
3. Lichtenstein, P et al, ***New England Journal of Medicine***, 2000, Vol. 343, No. 2, pp. 78-85.
4. Dragani TA, Zocchetti C., "Occupational exposure to vinyl chloride and risk of hepatocellular carcinoma," ***Cancer Causes Control***. Dec. 2008, Vol. 19, No. 10, pp. 1193-1200.
5. Besaratinia, A and GP Pfeiffer, "Weak yet distinct mutagenicitiy of acrylamide in mammalian cells," ***Journal of the National Cancer Institute***, June 2003, Vol. 95, No. 12, pp. 889-896.
6. Kellas, William, and Andrea S. Dworkin, ***Surviving the Toxic Crisis***, Professional Preference, Olivenhain CA, 1996.
7. Forasteire F, A Quercia et al, "Cancer among farmers in central Italy," ***Scand. Journal of Work and Environmental Health***, Vol. 19, No. 6, Dec. 1993, pp. 382-9.
8. McDuffie, HH, "Women at work: Agriculture and pesticides," ***Journal of Occupational Medicine***, Vol. 36, No. 11, Nov. 1994, pp. 1240-6.
9. Goldberg, Burton (ed.), ***Alternative Medicine: The Definitive Guide***, Future Medicine Publishing Inc., Tiburon CA, 2nd ed., 1999.
10. ***Neurotoxins: At Home and the Workplace***, Report by the Committee on Science and Technology, U.S. House of Representatives, Sept. 16, 1986, Report 99-827.
11. Arnold, Kathryn, "Is your hair dye safe?" ***Delicious***, July/Aug. 1993, pp. 50+.
12. Casarett and Doull, ***Toxicology***, Macmillan Publishing Company, New York, 1986, 3rd edition.
13. Eyre R, Feltbower RG, Mubwandarikwa E, Eden TO, McNally RJ, "Epidemiology of bone tumours in children and young adults," ***Pediatric Blood Cancer.*** Jul 17, 2009, pubmed.gov.
14. "Re: Fluoridation," ***Townsend Letter for Doctors***, No. 115/116, Feb./Mar. 1993, p. 206.
15. Taylor, Alfred and Nell Carmichael Taylor, "Effect of sodium fluoride on tumor growth," ***Proceedings of the Society for Experimental Biology and Medicine***, Vol. 119, 1965, pp. 252-5.
16. http://www.jurak.com/include/healthststats.htm, accessed 3/24/04.
17. Balch, James F. and Mark Stengler, ***Prescription for Natural Cures***, John Wiley and Sons, Hoboken NJ, 2004.
18. Quillin, Patrick, "Using nutrition to augment medical therapies in cancer patients," ***ACAM Nutrition and Cancer***, Nov. 2001, pp. 1-11.
19. Yam, D, A Fink, I Nir, and P Budowski, "Insulin-tumor interrelationships in thymoma bearing mice: Effects of dietary glucose and fructose," ***British Journal of Cancer***, Vol. 64, No. 6, 1991, pp. 1043-6.
20. Marietta C, Thompson LH, Lamerdin JE, Brooks PJ., "Acetaldehyde stimulates FANCD2 monoubiquitination, H2AX phosphorylation, and BRCA1 phosphorylation in human cells in vitro: implications for alcohol-related carcinogenesis," ***Mutation Research,*** .May 12, 2009, Vol. 664(1-2), pp. 77-83
21. Potter, JD and AJ McMichael, "Alcohol, beer and lung cancer: A meaningful relationship?" ***International Journal of Epidemiology***, Vol. 13, No. 2, June 1984, pp. 240-2.
22. Lueth NA, Anderson KE, Harnack LJ, Fulkerson JA, Robien K, "Coffee and caffeine intake and the risk of ovarian cancer: the Iowa Women's Health Study," ***Cancer Causes Control.*** Dec. 2008, Vol.19, No.10, pp.1365-72.
23. Joseph, P, "Mechanisms of cadmium carcinogenesis," ***Toxicol Appl Pharmacol***. Aug 1, 2009, Vol. 238, No. 3, pp. 272-9
24. ***American Journal of Epidemiology***, 2002, Vol. 156, pp. 1002-10, cited in "Vitamin E fights bladder cancer," GreatLife, June 2003, Vol. 6, No. 6, p. 12.
25. Maugh, TH, "Experts downplay cancer risk of chlorinated water," ***Los Angeles Times***, July 2, 1992.
26. Levy, Stephen J, ***Managing the Drugs in Your Life***, McGraw-Hill Publishing Co., New York, 1983.
27. Pearson, Durk, and Sandy Shaw, ***Life Extension***, Warner Books, New York, 1982.
28. Bosetti C, McLaughlin JK, Tarone RE, Pira E, La Vecchia C, "Formaldehyde and cancer risk: a quantitative review of cohort studies through 2006," ***Annals of Oncology***, Jan. 2008;19(1), pp. 29-43.
29. ***Journal of Occupational Environmental Medicine***, April 1998, Vol. 40, pp. 332-9.
30. Kellas, William, and Andrea S. Dworkin, ***Thriving in a Toxic World***, Professional Preference, Olivenhain CA, 1996.
31. Roswit, Bernard, and Herbert Edlis, "Carcinoma of the male breast: A thirty year experience and literature review, Current concepts in cancer," ***Radiation Oncology Biology Physics***, 1978, Vol. 4, pp. 711-6
32. Clorfene-Casten, Liane, "Breast cancer: Poisons, profits and prevention," ***Townsend Letter for Doctors and Patients***, May 1998, Vol. 178, pp. 24-31.
33. Longnecker, MP, PA Newcomb et al, "Risk of breast cancer in relation to lifetime alcohol consumption," ***Journal of the National Cancer Institute***, Vol. 87, No. 12, June 21, 1995, pp. 923-9.
34. Balch, James F. and Phyllis A. Balch, ***Prescription for Nutritional Healing***, Avery Publishing Group, Garden City Park, NY, 2nd ed., 1997.

35. Snyderman, Nancy, "Good question," ***Health***, June 2000, Vol. 14, No. 5, p. 160.

36. Rudel RA, Brody JG, Spengler JD, et al. "Identification of selected hormonally active agents and animal mammary carcinogens in commercial and residential air and dust samples," ***Journal of Air Waste Management Association***, 2001;51(4):499-513.

37. Dadd, Debra Lynn, ***Nontoxic and Natural***, Jeremy P. Tarcher Inc., Los Angeles CA, 1984.

38. www.webmd.com/content/article/123/115255.htm

39. www.new-cancer-treatments.org/articles/rootcanals.html.

40. "Breast cancer and PCBs: A possible link," ***Business Week***, April 6, 1992, p. 36.

41. Tsubura A, Yuri T, Yoshizawa K, Uehara N, Takada H, "Role of fatty acids in malignancy and visual impairment: epidemiological evidence and experimental studies," ***Histol Histopathol.*** Feb. 2009, Vol. 24(2), pp. 223-34.

42. Andrews, Dominique, "Body briefs," ***Ladies' Home Journal***, Jan. 2002, Vol. 119, No. 1, p. 34.

43. Maugh, TH, "Experts downplay cancer risk of chlorinated water," ***Los Angeles Times***, July 2, 1992.

44. ***American Journal of Public Health***, 1997, Vol.87, pp. 1168-76.

45, Werbach, Melvyn R, "Nutrients to protect against colon cancer," ***Townsend Letter for Doctors and Patients***, Nov. 1998, Vol. 184, p. 156.

46. Rosenfeld, Isadore, ***Doctor, What Should I Eat?*** Warner Books, NY, 1995.

47. Vaughn, TL, DS Strader, S Davis and JR Daling, "Formaldehyde and cancers of the pharynx, sinus and nasal cavity, II. residential exposures," ***International Journal of Cancer***, Vol. 38, 1986, p. 685.

48. Kaye, JA, MW Myers, and H Jick, "Acetaminophen and the risk of renal and bladder cancer in the general practice research database," ***Epidemiology***, Nov. 2001, Vol. 12, No. 6, pp. 690-4.

49. Faloon, William, "Acetaminophen risks understated," ***Life Extension***, May 2004, Vol. 10, No. 5, pp. 11-12.

50. Shroeder, Henry A, ***The Poisons Around Us***, Indiana University Press, Bloomington IN, 1974.

51. Lowengart, RA et al, "Childhood leukemia and parents' occupational and home exposures," ***Journal of the National Cancer Institute***, Vol. 79, No. 1, July 1987, pp. 39-46.

52. Huggins, Hal A, "Proposed role of dental amalgam toxicity in leukemia and hematopoietic dyscrasias," ***International Journal of Biosocial and Medical Research***, Vol. 11, No. 1, 1989, pp. 84-93.

53. Wynder, Ernest et al, "Tobacco smoking as possible etiologic factor in bronchogenic carcinoma," ***Journal of the American Medical Association***, May 1950, pp 329-338.

54. "Nickel may pose health hazard," ***Dentistry Today***, April 1985, p. 8.

55. Prasher, D, "Heavy metals and noise exposure: Health effects," ***Noise Health***, July-Sept. 2009, Vol. 11, No. 44, pp. 141-4.

56. Schechter, Steven R, ***Fighting Radiation with Foods, Herbs, and Vitamins***, East West Health Books, Brookline MA, 1988.

57. Handler, Sheldon Saul, ***The Oxygen Breakthrough***, William Morris and Co., NY, 1989.

58. Lovelady, Sara, "100% natural way to detoxify," ***Healthy Living***, Vol. 9, No. 6, pp. 19-21.

59. ***Journal of Epidemiology and Community Health***, 1998, Vol. 52, pp. 651-6.

60. Ursin, G et al, "Milk consumption and cancer incidence: A Norwegian prospective study," ***British Journal of Cancer***, Vol. 61, No. 3, March 1990, pp. 456-9.

61. Nahas, G, and C Latour, "The human toxicity of marijuana," ***Med. Journal Aust.***, Vol. 156, No. 7, April 6, 1992, pp. 495-7.

62. Holmes, GKT et al, "Malignancy in coeliac disease – Effect of a gluten free diet," ***Gut***, Vol. 30, 1989, pp. 333-8.

63. Elkins, Rita, "Prostate Disorders and Natural Medicine," Woodland Health Series, Woodland Publishing Inc., Pleasant Grove UT, 1995.

64. FC&A Medical Publishing editors, ***The Folk Remedy Encyclopedia***, FC&A, Peachtree City GA, 2001.

65. Kohout J, Ouda Z, Hora M [Risk factors in carcinoma of the prostate]. ***Cas. Lek. Cesk.***, 134: 679-680, 1995.

66. Soraham T, Waterhouse JA, "Cancer of prostate among nickel-cadmium battery workers," ***Lancet***, 1: 459, 1985.

67. Lee JD, Wu SM, Lu LY, Yang YT, Jeng SY, "Cadmium concentration and metallothionein expression in prostate cancer and benign prostatic hyperplasia of humans," ***Journal of the Formosa Medical Association***, July 2009, Vol. 108, No. 7, pp. 554-9.

68. Sahl, WJ, S Glore, P Garrison, K Oakleaf and SD Johnson, "Basal cell carcinoma and lifestyle characteristics," ***Int. Journal of Dermatology***, Vol. 34, No. 6, June 1995, pp. 398-402.

69. FC&A editors, ***Inner Cleansing Cures***, FC&A Publishing, Peachtree City GA, 1998.

Cardiovascular problems

1. Dahhan, SS and H Orfaly, "Electrocardiographic changes in mercury poisoning," ***American Journal of Cardiology***, Vol. 14, 1964, pp. 178-183.

2. Ellis, RW and SC Fang, "Elimination, tissue accumulation and cellular incorporation of mercury in rats receiving an oral dose of 203Hg-labeled phenylmercuric acetate and mercuric acetate," ***Toxicology and Applied Pharmacology***, Vol. 11, 1967, pp. 104-113.

3. Stortebecker, Patrick, "Mercury poisoning from dental amalgam – A hazard to the human brain," Karolinska Institute, Stockholm, Sweden.

4. Ziff, Michael, "The missing link? A persuasive new look at heart disease as it relates to mercury," BioProbe Inc., 1991.

5. Wertheim, Alfred H, "Trans fats," ***Townsend Letter for Doctors and Patients***, No. 150, Jan. 1996, pp. 106-7.

6. Mago, L, "The effects of industrial chemicals on the heart," ***Cardiac Toxicology***, T. Balazo (ed.), CRC Press, Boca Raton FL, 1981.

7. Thompson, Betty J, "Going cold turkey," ***Natural Health***, May/June 2003, Vol. 33, No. 4, p. 10.
8. Werbach, Melvyn R, "How to reduce arrhythmias through diet," ***Townsend Letter for Doctors and Patients***, Vol. 197, Dec. 1999, p. 144.
9. Weed, Susun S, ***Menopausal Years the Wise Woman Way***, Ash Tree Publishing, Woodstock NY, 1992.
10. Rosenfeld, Isadore, ***Doctor, What Should I Eat?*** Warner Books, NY, 1995.
11. Casarett and Doull, ***Toxicology***, Macmillan Publishing Company, New York, 3rd edition, 1986.
12. Palmer, JR, L Rosenberg, RS Rao and S Shapiro, "Coffee consumption and myocardial infarction in women," ***American Journal of Epidemiology***, Vol. 141, No. 8, April 15, 1995, pp. 724-31.
13. Klatz, Ronald M, "Food and Drug Administration Report 69 Viagra-Related Deaths in the US," ***Townsend Letter for Doctors and Patients***, February / March 1999, Vol. 187/188, p. 64.
14. "Bad at any age," ***Time***, Sept. 6, 2004, Vol. 164, No. 10, p. 102.
15. Cool, Lisa Collier, "A silent killer," ***Ladies' Home Journal***, Feb. 2004, Vol. 121, No. 2, pp. 158-170.
16. Turk, Michele, "Cutting heart attack risk," ***American Health***, March 1993, pp. 12-14.
17. "Ban butts, save hearts," ***Prevention***, Dec. 2003, Vol. 55, No. 12, p. 38.
18. Mercola, Joseph M, "Too much iron ups heart risk," ***Townsend Letter for Doctors and Patients***, May 1998, Vol. 178, p. 37.
19. National Vital Statistics Reports, Vol. 50, No. 15, in http://www.jurak.com/include/healthststats.htm, accessed 3/24/04.
20. Stelfox HT et al, "Conflict of interest in the debate over calcium-channel antagonists," ***New England Journal of Medicine***, 1998, Vol. 338, pp. 101-6.
21. Nygard, O et al, "Coffee consumption and plasma total homocysteine: The Hordaland Homocysteine Study," ***American Journal of Clinical Nutrition***, Vol. 65, 1997, pp. 136-143.
22. Gajilan, A. Chris, "Up in smoke," ***Time***, May 10, 2004, Vol. 163, No. 19, p. 82.
23. Grant, William B, "The role of sugars in ischemic heart disease," ***Townsend Letter for Doctors and Patients***, February / March 1999, Vol. 187/188, pp. 80-85.
24. Challem, Jack, Burton Berkson, and Melissa Diane Smith, ***Syndrome X***, John Wiley & Sons, NY, 2000.
25. Atkins, Robert C, ***Dr. Atkins' Age-Defying*** Diet, St. Martin's Press, NY, 2001.
26. Rosick, Edward R, "Arginine can improve your blood pressure," ***Life Enhancement***, Jan. 2003, pp. 9-12.
27. Brown, Jody, "Battling the silent killer," ***Healthy Living***, Vol. 9, No. 6, pp. 22-23.
28. Carper, Jean, ***The Miracle Heart***, Harper Paperbacks, NY, 2000.
29. Glauser, SC, CT Bello and EM Gauser, "Blood cadmium levels in normotensive and untreated hypertensive humans," ***Lancet***, Vol. 1, April 1976, pp. 717-8.
30. Kellas, William, and Andrea S. Dworkin, ***Surviving the Toxic Crisis***, Professional Preference, Olivenhain CA, 1996
31. Mercola, Joseph, M, "Viagra, male impotence pill, will have complications," ***Townsend Letter for Doctors and Patients***, July 1998, Vol. 180, p. 25.
32. Casarett and Doull, ***Toxicology***, Macmillan Publishing Company, New York, 3rd edition, 1986.
33. Sanchez-Delgado, E, and H Liechti, "Lifetime risk of developing coronary heart disease," ***Lancet***, 1999, Vol. 353, p. 934.
34. FC&A Medical Publishing editors, ***The Folk Remedy Encyclopedia***, FC&A, Peachtree City GA, 2001.
35. Rogers, Sherry A, ***Tired or Toxic?*** Prestige Publishing, Syracuse NY, 1990.
36. Spreen, Allan N, ***Nutritionally Incorrect***, Woodland Publishing, Pleasant Grove UT, 2nd ed., 2002.
37. Brophy, Christine, "Lower your stroke risk," ***Family Circle***, March 9, 2004, Vol. 117, No. 3, p. 108.
38. Andrews, Dominique, "Easy on the aspirin," ***Ladies Home Journal***, Dec. 2001, p. 58.
39. Airola, Paavo, ***Every Woman's Book***, Health Plus Publishers, Phoenix AZ, 1979.
40. Cutler, Andrew Hall, ***Amalgam Illness: Diagnosis and Treatment***, Sammamish WA, 1999.
41. Siblerud, Robert, "Evidence that mercury from silver dental fillings may be an etiological factor in multiple sclerosis," ***The Science of the Total Environment***, Vol. 142, 1994, pp. 191-205.
42. Huggins, Hal, "Observations From the Metabolic Fringe," ICBM Conference, Colorado, 1988.
43. Lorscheider and Vimy, ***The Lancet***, Vol. 337, May 4, 1991.
44. Granato, Heather, "Building up, not breaking down," in www.enzymeuniversity.com/artandexc.html.
45. Cousins, Norman, ***Anatomy of an Illness***, WW Norton & Co., NY, 1979.
46. ***New England Journal of Medicine***, Dec. 23, 1999, Vol. 341, pp. 1986-95.
47. "Microwave your prostate," ***Men's Health Newsletter***, June 1991, p. 7.
48. Kellas, William, and Andrea S. Dworkin, ***Thriving in a Toxic World***, Professional Preference, Olivenhain CA, 1996.

Bone and joint problems

1. Kellas, William, and Andrea S. Dworkin, ***Surviving the Toxic Crisis***, Professional Preference, Olivenhain CA, 1996.

2. Dreher R, Buttgereit F, Demary W, Görtz B, Hein G, Kern P, Schulz A, "Insufficiency fractures in rheumatology: Case report and overview," ***Z Rheumatol***. Sep. 2006, vol.65(5), pp. 417-23.

3. Waldbott, George et al, ***Fluoridation: The Great Dilemma***, Coronado Press, Lawrence KS, 1978.

4. Balch, James F and Phyllis A Balch, ***Prescription for Nutritional Healing***, Avery Publishing Group, Garden City Park, NY, 2nd ed., 1997.

5. Goldberg, Burton (ed.), ***Alternative Medicine: The Definitive Guide***, Future Medicine Publishing Inc., Tiburon CA, 2nd ed., 1999.

6. Gaby, Alan R, "Do non-steroidal anti-inflammatory drugs damage cells?" ***Townsend Letter for Doctors***, Vol. 126, Jan. 1994, p. 13.

7. Murray, Michael T, ***Seven Valuable Tips for Managing Osteoarthritis***, Vital Communications Inc., Issaquah WA.

8. Bridges, AJ, "Rheumatic disorders in patients with silicone implants: A critical review," ***Journal of Biomater. Sci. Polym. Ed.***, 1995, Vol. 7, No. 2, pp. 147-57.

9. Freundlich, B, C Altman, et al, "A profile of symptomatic patients with silicone breast implants: A Sjogrens-like syndrome," ***Semin. Arthritis and Rheumatism***, Aug. 1994, Vol. 24, pp. 44-53.

10. Asakawa J, Kobayashi S, Kaneda K, Ogasawara H, Sugawara M, Yasuda M, Hashimoto H, "Reactive arthritis after influenza vaccination: report of a case," 2005, Vol. 15(4), pp. 283-5

11. Mercola, Joseph M, "Hepatitis B vaccine linked to autoimmune rheumatoid diseases," ***Townsend Letter for Doctors and Patients***, February / March 1999, Vol. 187/188, p. 54.

12. Thiel, Robert J, "Musculoskeletal pain relief for people with arthritis, lupus and fibromyalgia," ***Townsend Letter for Doctors and Patients***, Nov. 1997, Vol. 172, pp. 91-92.

13. D'Adamo, Peter, ***Eat Right 4 Your Type***, GP Putnam's Sons, NY, 1996.

14. Stackel, Leslie, "Are naturopaths the family docs for the 21st century?" ***Healthy Living***, May 1998.

15. FC&A editors, ***Inner Cleansing Cures***, FC&A Publishing, Peachtree City GA, 1998.

16. Peltonen, R, Nenonen M, Helve T et al, "Faecal microbial flora and disease activity in rheumatoid arthritis during a vegan diet," ***British Journal of Rheumatology***, 1997, Vol. 36, pp. 64-68.

17. ***American Journal of Clinical Nutrition***, 1999, Vol. 70, pp. 1077-82.

18. Appelboom, T, and P. Durez, "Effects of milk product deprivation on spondyloarthropathy," ***Annals of Rheumatic Disease***, 1994, Vol. 53, pp. 481-2.

19. Gaby, Alan R, "Milk and ankylosing spondylitis," ***Townsend Letter for Doctors and Patients***, August/September 1999, Vol. 193-4, p. 31.

20. Sutherland, Caroline M, ***The Body Knows***, Hay House, Carlsbad CA, 2001.

21. FC&A Medical Publishing editors, ***The Folk Remedy Encyclopedia***, FC&A, Peachtree City GA, 2001.

22. Sahud, MS and RJ Cohen, ***Lancet***, May 8, 1971.

23. Cousins, Norman, ***Anatomy of an Illness***, WW Norton & Co., NY, 1979.

24. Cooper, Cyrus et al, "Water fluoridation and hip fracture," ***Journal of the American Medical Association***, Vol. 266, July 1991, pp. 513-4.

25. Danielson, C et al, "Hip fractures and fluoridation in Utah's elderly population," ***Journal of the American Medical Association***, Vol. 268, 1992, pp. 746-8.

26. Riggs, B. Lawrence, "Effect of fluoride treatment on the fracture rate in postmenopausal women with osteoporosis," ***New England Journal of Medicine***, Vol. 322, 1990, pp. 802-9.

27. Schnitzler, CM et al, "Bone fragility of the peripheral skeleton during fluoride therapy for osteoporosis," ***Clin. Orthop.***, Vol. 261, 1990, pp. 268-275.

28. Rico, H, "Alcohol and bone disease," ***Alcohol and Alcoholism***, Vol. 25, No. 4, 1990, pp. 345-352.

29. Casagrande, G, and F Michot, "A randomized bone marrow study in alcohol-dependent individuals," ***Blut.***, Vol. 59, No. 3, Sept. 1989, pp. 231-6.

30. Muraki S, Yamamoto S, Ishibashi H, Oka H, Yoshimura N, Kawaguchi H, Nakamura K, "Diet and lifestyle associated with increased bone mineral density: cross-sectional study of Japanese elderly women at an osteoporosis outpatient clinic," ***Journal of Orthopedic Science***, July 2007, Vol. 12(4), pp. 317-20.

31. Kiel, DP et al, "Caffeine and the risks of hip fracture. The Framingham study," ***American Journal of Epidemiology***, vol. 132, No. 4, Oct. 1990, pp. 675-684.

32. Huston, James E and L Darlene Lanka, ***Perimenopause***, New Harbinger Publications Inc., Oakland CA, 1997.

33. Schaaf, Rachelle Vander, "I thought I was too young for osteoporosis," ***Redbook***, Feb. 2003, Vol. 200, No. 2, pp. 30-38.

34. ***Journal of Clinical Investigation***, 1998, Vol. 102.

35. Andrews, Dominique, "Body briefs," ***Ladies' Home Journal***, Jan. 2002, Vol. 119, No. 1, p. 34.

36. Robbins, John, ***Reclaiming Our Health***, HJ Kramer, Tiburon,CA, 1996.

37. "Understanding Osteoporosis," American Medical Association pamphlet, 2000

38. Gaby, Alan R, "Drinking milk does not prevent fractures," ***Townsend Letter for Doctors and Patients***, Oct. 1998, Vol. 183, p. 36.

39. Rude KK, M. Olerich, "Magnesium deficiency: Possible role in osteoporosis associated with gluten-sensitive enteropathy," ***Osteoporosis Int.***, 1996, Vol. 6, pp. 453-461.

40. Field, Stan, "The curse of the soft drink," ***Townsend Letter for Doctors and Patients***, Dec. 1998, Vol. 185, pp. 119-121.

41. Mazariegos-Ramos, E. et al, "Consumption of soft drinks with phosphoric acid as a risk factor for the development of hypocalcemia in children: A case-control study," ***Journal of Pediatrics***, Vol. 126, 1995, pp. 940-2.

42. Barnard, Neal, ***Turn Off the Fat Genes***, Harmony Books, NY, 2001.

43. Nordin, BEC, AG Need, HA Morris, and M Horowitz, "The nature and significance of the relationship between urinary sodium and urinary calcium in women," ***Journal of Nutrition***, 1993, Vol. 123, pp. 1615-22.

44. Coats, C, "Negative effects of a high-protein diet," ***Family Practice Recertification***, Vol. 12, No. 12, Dec. 1990, pp. 80-94.

45. ***American Journal of Clinical Nutrition***, March 1983.

46. ***American Journal of Clinical Nutrition***, Vol. 73, 2001, pp. 118-122.

47. Kennedy, David, ***How To Save Your Teeth***, Health Action Press, Delaware OH, 1993.

48. Muha, Laura, "Advice from Dr. Paul Lachance: Eat better, stay younger," ***Biography***, Oct. 2000, pp. 79-82+.

49. Feskanich, D, et al, "Milk, dietary calcium, and bone fractures in women: A 12 year prospective study," ***American Journal of Public Health***, 1997, Vol. 87, pp. 992-7.

Gastrointestinal problems

1. Summers, AO, J Wireman, MJ Vimy et al, "Mercury released from dental 'silver' fillings provokes an increase in mercury and antibiotic resistant bacteria in primates' oral and intestinal flora," ***Antimicrobial Agents and Chemotherapy***, Vol. 37, 1993, pp. pp. 825-834.

2. Casarett and Doull, ***Toxicology***, Macmillan Publishing Company, New York, 3rd edition, 1986.

3. Kellas, William, and Andrea S. Dworkin, ***Surviving the Toxic Crisis***, Professional Preference, Olivenhain CA, 1996

4. Friend, WG, "The cause and treatment of idiopathic pruritis ani," ***Diseases of the Colon and Rectum***, Vol. 20, 1977, pp. 40-42.

5. Hales, Dianne, "The doctors' guide to bloating," ***Ladies' Home Journal***, July 1996, Vol. 113, No. 7, pp. 126-9.

6. Kellas, William, and Andrea S. Dworkin, ***Thriving in a Toxic World***, Professional Preference, Olivenhain CA, 1996

7. Gordon, Sandra, "Gut advice," ***New Age's Body & Soul***, 2001, pp. 34-39.

8. Pizzorno, Joseph E. and Michael T. Murray, ***A Textbook of Natural Medicine***, John Bastyr College Publications, Seattle WA, 1989.

9. Allbritton, Jen, "Conquering constipation," Vitamin Cottage ***Health Hotline***, March 2005, pp. 6-7.

10. Iacono, G et al, "Intolerance of cow's milk and chronic constipation in children," ***New England Journal of Medicine***, 1998, Vol. 339, pp. 1100-4.

11. Spreen, Allan N, ***Nutritionally Incorrect***, Woodland Publishing, Pleasant Grove UT, 2nd ed., 2002.

12. Mettler, Molly, and Donald W. Kemper, ***Healthwise for Life***, Healthwise Inc., Boise ID, 2nd ed., 1996.

13. Michaud, Ellen and Lila L. Anastas, ***Listen to Your Body***, Rodale Press, Emmaus PA, 1988.

14. Dean, Carolyn, "Ask the experts: Horrible heartburn," ***Natural Health***, Sept. 2000, Vol. 30, No. 7, pp. 47-8.

15. Snyderman, Nancy, "Good question," ***Health***, Oct. 2001, p. 164.

16. Grumman, Rachel, "The perils of pain pills," ***Ladies' Home Journal***, July 2003, Vol. 120, No. 7, p. 140.

16. Halstead, Bruce W, ***Fossil Stony Coral Minerals and Their Nutritional Application***, Health Digest Publishing Company, Cannon Beach OR, 1999.

17. "Acute pancreatitis following continuous exposure to organophosphate insecticide," ***Internal Medicine World Report***, March 1-14, 1989.

Mental and behavioral problems

1. Larson, Joan Mathews, ***Depression-Free, Naturally***, Ballantine Publishing Group, NY, 1999.

2. Null, Gary, "Mercury dental amalgams – Analyzing the debate," ***Townsend Letter for Doctors***, No. 109/110, Aug./Sept. 1992, pp. 760-9.

3. Echevarria, D, et al, "Neurobehavioral effects from exposure to dental amalgam Hg," ***FASEB Journal***, Vol. 12, 1998, pp. 971-980.

4. Cutler, Andrew Hall, ***Amalgam Illness: Diagnosis and Treatment***, Sammamish WA, 1999.

5. Siblerud, Robert, "The relationship between mercury from dental amalgam and mental health," ***American Journal of Psychiatry***, Vol. 43, No. 4, Oct. 1989.

6. Siblerud, Robert, "Psychometric evidence that mercury from silver dental fillings may be an etiological factor in depression, excessive anger and anxiety," ***Psychological Reports***, Vol. 74, 1994, pp. 67-80.

7. "Yeast-related mental disturbances: An interview with Richard G. Jaeckle," ***Mastering Food Allergies***, Jan./Feb. 1995.

8. ***Candida Yeast Answer, The***, Candida Wellness Center, Provo UT, rev. Jan. 2004.

9. Tenney, Louise, "Allergies," Woodland Health Series, Woodland Publishing Inc., Pleasant Grove UT, 1996.

10. Carper, Jean, ***Your Miracle Brain***, HarperCollins, NY, 2000.

11. Dager, SR et al, "Panic disorder precipitated by exposure to organic solvents in the workplace," ***American Journal of Psychiatry***, Vol. 144, No. 8, August 1987, pp. 1056-8.

12. Klotter, Jule, "Toluene," ***Townsend Letter for Doctors***, No. 118, May 1993, p. 518.

13. webmd.com/drugs/drug-6816-Halcion+Oral.aspx?drugid=6816&...+Oral

14. Pfeiffer, Carl C, ***Nutrition and Mental Illness: An Orthomolecular Approach to Balancing Body Chemistry***, Healing Arts Press, Rochester VT, 1987.

15. Carlton, Richard M, "Food and our moods / Food and our bodies," in ***Unpublicized Health Breakthroughs, Warnings, Secrets***, Boardroom Inc., 2001.

16. Bjerklie, David, "Do implants trigger suicide?" ***Time***, March 17, 2003, Vol. 161, No. 11.

17. "Causes and Effects," ***Newsweek***, Oct. 13, 2003, Vol. 147, No. 15, p. 23 (advertising section).

18. Balch, James F and Phyllis A Balch, ***Prescription for Nutritional Healing***, Avery Publishing Group, Garden City Park, NY, 2nd ed., 1997.

19. Bjerklie, David, "Pills, teens and suicide," ***Time***, June 23, 2003, Vol. 161, No. 25, p. 79.

20. Till, T, and K Maaly, "Mercury in tooth roots and in jaw bones," ***ZRW***, Vol. 87, Issue 6, 1978, pp. 288-90.

21. Casarett and Doull, ***Toxicology***, Macmillan Publishing Company, New York, 3rd edition, 1986.

22. "Synthetic food coloring and behavior: a dose response effect in a double-blind, placebo-controlled, repeated-measures study," ***Journal of Pediatrics***, 1994 Nov;125(5 Pt 1):691-8.

23. Hatherill, J Robert, ***The Brain Gate***, LifeLine Press, Washington DC, 2003.

24. Metcalf and Holmes, ***Annals of the New York Academy of Science***, Vol. 160.

25. Regenstein, Lewis, ***America the Poisoned***, Acropolis, 1982.

26. Kellas, William, and Andrea S. Dworkin, ***Surviving the Toxic Crisis***, Professional Preference, Olivenhain CA, 1996.

27. Rosenfeld, Isadore, "What you need to know now," ***Parade Magazine***, Jan. 15, 2006, pp. 6-8.

28. Shumaker, Sally A et al, "Estrogen plus progestin and the incidence of dementia and mild cognitive impairment in postmenopausal women," ***JAMA***, 5-28-03.

29. ***Physician's Desk Reference***, Medical Economics Co., Oradell NJ, 1993.

30. Mettler, Molly, and Donald W Kemper, ***Healthwise for Life***, Healthwise Inc., Boise ID, 2nd ed., 1996.

31. FC&A Medical Publishing editors, ***The Folk Remedy Encyclopedia***, FC&A, Peachtree City GA, 2001.

32. Solowij, N, PT Michie and AM Fox, "Differential impairments of selective attention due to frequency and duration of cannabis use," ***Biol. Psychiatry***, Vol. 37, No. 10, May 15, 1995, pp. 731-9.

33. Godfrey, ME and Hal Huggins, "The pathophysiology of long-term exposure to dental amalgam: A potential hazard for senile dementia," ***Clinical Practice of Alternative Medicine***, Vol. 1, No. 2, Summer 2000, pp. 107-112.

34. Sullivan, Kip, "The evidence linking silver-mercury fillings to Alzheimer's disease: A literature review," ***Townsend Letter for Doctors and Patients***, Aug./Sept., 1997, Vol. 169/170, pp. 74-83.

35. ***NeuroToxicology***, 18:2, 1997, pp. 315-324.

36. Jetter, Alexis, "How safe is your food?" ***Reader's Digest***, Aug. 2003, pp. 64-71.

37. Casdorph, HR, "EDTA Chelation Therapy: Efficacy in Brain Disorders," in ***A Textbook on EDTA Chelation Therapy***, Elmer M. Cranton (ed.), ***Journal of Advancement in Medicine***, Vol. 2, Nos. 1-2, Human Sciences Press, NY, 1989, pp. 131-153.

38. Neri, LC and D Hewitt, "Aluminum, Alzheimer's disease and drinking water," ***Lancet***, Vol. 338, 1991, p. 390.

39. McLachlan, DRC et al, "Intramuscular desferrioxamine in patients with Alzheimer's disease," ***Lancet***, Vol. 337, 1991, pp. 1304-8.

40. Kellas, William, and Andrea S. Dworkin, ***Thriving in a Toxic World***, Professional Preference, Olivenhain CA, 1996.

41. FC&A editors, ***Inner Cleansing Cures***, FC&A Publishing, Peachtree City GA, 1998.

42. Verner, Judith A, Karl F Jensen, William Horvath and Robert L Isaacson, "Chronic administration of aluminum-fluoride or sodium-fluoride to rats in drinking water: Alterations in neuronal and cerebrovascular integrity," ***Brain Research***, Vol. 784, 1998, Elsevier Science.

43. Mullenix, Phyllis and Jack Hein, ***Neurotoxicology and Teratology***, Vol. 17, 1995, pp. 169-177.

44. Roberts, HJ, ***Aspartame (NutraSweet): Is It Safe?***, The Charles Press, 1990, cited in Balch, James F. and Phyllis A. Balch, ***Prescription for Nutritional Healing***, Avery Publishing Group, Garden City Park, NY, 2nd ed., 1997, p. 9.

45. "Survey shows link between antibiotics and developmental delays in children," ***Townsend Letter for Doctors and Patients***, No. 147, Oct. 1995, p. 9.

46. Aesoph, Lauri, "The Poisonous Legacy of Pesticides," ***Delicious***, April 1994, pp. 32-4.

47. Hotton, Donald, "Roaring water: Fluoride toxicity and ADHD," ***Townsend Letter for Doctors and Patients***, April 1998, Vol. 177, p. 76.

48. Klotter, Jule, "Lead poisoning," ***Townsend Letter for Doctors***, No. 107, June 1992, p. 533.

49. Berlin, M., "Prenatal exposure to mercury vapor: Effects on brain development," ***Fundamentals of Applied Toxicology***, Vol. 19, 1992, pp. 319-329.

50. Lombardi, Raymond M., "ADHD: Bringing it into focus," ***Delicious Living***, Nov. 2000, pp. 40-46.

51. Boris, M and FS Mandel, "Foods and additives are common causes of the attention deficit hyperactive disorder in children," ***Annals of Allergy***, 1994, Vol. 72, pp. 462-7.

52. Brody, Jane E, "Kids really do get a sugar buzz, new study shows," ***The Seattle Post-Intelligencer***, March 15, 1995.

53. Pelsser, L et al, "Favorable effect of a standard elimination diet on the behavior of young children with attention deficit hyperactivity disorder (ADHD): A pilot study," ***Ned Tijdschr Geneeskd***, Dec. 2002, Vol. 146, No. 52, pp. 2543-7.

54. Egger, J et al, "Controlled trial of oligoantigenic treatment in the hyperkinetic syndrome," ***Lancet***, 1985, pp. 540-5.

55. Feingold, BF, ***Why Your Child Is Hyperactive***, Random House, NY, 1975.

56. Hunt, Douglas, ***No More Cravings***, Warner Books, 1987.

57. Vojdani, Aristo, N. Brautbar and A.W. Campbell, "Antibody to silicone and native macromolecules in women with silicone breast implants," ***Immunopharmacology and Immunotoxicology***, Nov. 1994, Vol. 16, No. 4, pp. 497-523.

58. Prevention editors, ***The Complete Book of Vitamin Cures***, Rodale Press, Emmaus PA, 1998.

59. Crenshaw, Mary Ann, ***End of the Rainbow***, Macmillan Publishing Co., NY, 1981.

60. Tanzer, Peter P, ***The Doctor's Guide to Sleep Without Pills***, Tresco Publishers, Canton OH, 1994.

61. "Excessive sunlight exposure, skin melanoma, linked to vitamin D," ***International Journal of Biosocial and Medical Research***, Vol 13, No. 1, 1991, pp. 13-14.

62. ***Science***, 1998, Vol. 279, pp. 333+.

63. Schwarzbein, Diana and Nancy Neville, ***The Schwarzbein Principle***, Health Communications Inc., Deerfield Beach FL, 1999.

Skin problems

1. Balch, James F, and Phyllis A Balch, ***Prescription for Nutritional Healing***, Avery Publishing Group, Garden City Park, NY, 2nd ed., 1997.
2. Gottleib, Bill (editor), ***New Choices in Natural Healing***, Rodale Press Inc., Emmaus PA, 1995.
3. Von Boehmer, Harald, and Pawel Kisielow, "How the immune system learns about self," ***Scientific American***, Oct. 1991, pp. 74-81.
4. ***Folk Remedy Encyclopedia, The***, editors of FC&A Medical Publishing, Peachtree City GA, 2001.
5. Kellas, William, and Andrea S. Dworkin, ***Thriving in a Toxic World***, Professional Preference, Olivenhain CA, 1996.
6. Kellas, William, and Andrea S. Dworkin, ***Surviving the Toxic Crisis***, Professional Preference, Olivenhain CA, 1996.
7. Cutler, Ellen, ***Winning the War Against Asthma and Allergies***, Delmar Publishers, Albany NY, 1998.
8. Sutherland, Caroline M., ***The Body Knows***, Hay House, Carlsbad CA, 2001.
9. Manning, Betsy Russell (editor), "Benefits of Electroacupuncture by Voll," ***Candida, Silver Mercury Fillings, and the Immune System***, Greensward Press, San Francisco CA, 1985, pp. 69-71.
10. Howard, Beth, "Too embarrassed to ask?" ***Ladies' Home Journal***, July 2001, Vol. 18, No. 7, pp. 56-60.
11. Mellette, J Ramsey et al, "Fluoride toothpaste: A cause of perioral dermatitis," ***Archives of Dermatology***, Vol. 112, 1976, pp. 730-1.
12. Airola, Paavo, ***Every Woman's Book***, Health Plus Publishers, Phoenix AZ, 1979.
13. Rosenberg, EW et al, "Response to Crohn's disease and psoriasis," ***New England Journal of Medicine***, 1983, Vol. 308, p. 101.
14. Grossman, Michael J, and Jodi L Jones, ***The Vitality Connection***, Vitality Press Publications, Rancho Santa Margarita CA, 2003.

Endocrine problems

1. Diamanti-Kandarakis E, Bourguignon JP, Giudice LC, Hauser R, Prins GS, Soto AM, Zoeller RT, Gore AC, "Endocrine-disrupting chemicals: an Endocrine Society scientific statement," ***Endocrine Reviews***, June 2009, Vol. 30(4), pp. 293-342.
2. Colborn, Theo and Coralie Clement (editors), ***Chemically Induced Alterations in Sexual and Functional Development***, Princeton Scientific Publishing Co., Princeton NJ, 1992.
3. "Mercury in fish," ***Bulletin of W.H.O.***, Vol. 64, No. 5, 1986, p. 634.
4. Ziff, Sam, ***Silver Dental Fillings - The Toxic Time Bomb***, Aurora Press, Santa Fe NM, 1986. Chapter 5, "Do We Really Have Electricity In Our Mouths?" pp. 65-70.
5. "Hormone hub: Thyroid," ***Body & Soul***, Nov./Dec. 2003, pp. 16-18.
6. Boas M, Main KM, Feldt-Rasmussen U, "Environmental chemicals and thyroid function: an update," ***Current Opinion Endocrinology Diabetes and Obesity***, Jul 21, 2009, pubmed.gov.
7. www.naturalhealthconsult.com/wilsons.html.
8. ***Merck Index***, Merck and Co. Inc, Rahway NJ, 1968, p. 959.
9. FitzGerald, Frances, "Slowing down?" ***Taste for Life***, Aug. 2003, pp. 30-32.
10. Shomon, Mary J, ***Living Well With Hypothyroidism***, Quill (HarperCollins), NY, 2000.
11. Huggins, Hal A, ***Position Papers: The Amalgam Issue, Root Canals, Cavitations***, Huggins Diagnostic Center, Colorado Springs CO, 1991.
12. Sutherland, Caroline M, ***The Body Knows***, Hay House, Carlsbad CA, 2001.
13. Gaby, Alan R, "Soy interferes with thyroid therapy," ***Townsend Letter for Doctors and Patients***, April 1998, Vol. 177, p. 33.
14. "Acute pancreatitis following continuous exposure to organophosphate insecticide," ***Internal Medicine World Report***, March 1-14, 1989.
15. McGinnis, Marianne, "Cigarettes raise diabetes risk," ***Prevention***, Feb. 2004, Vol. 56, No. 2, p. 40.
16. Madsbad, S, P McNair, CD. Christensen et al, "Influence of smoking on insulin requirement and metabolic status in diabetes mellitus," ***Diabetes Care***, 1980, Vol. 3, pp. 41-43.
17. ***New England Journal of Medicine***, 1998, Vol. 338, pp. 645+.
18. www.medicineforthedefense.com/Main/articles/newspubs-a-29.aspx, accessed 7/16/09.
19. Foster, Harold D, "Aluminum buildup implicated in diabetes," ***Townsend Letter for Doctors and Patients***, Vol. 197, Dec. 1999, p. 113.

20. Jiang, R, JE Manson, JB Meigs, J Ma, N Rifai, FB Hu, "Body iron stores in relation to risk of type 2 diabetes in apparently healthy women," ***JAMA***, Feb. 11, 2004, Vol. 291, No. 6, pp. 711-7.

21. Fettner, Ann Giudici, ***Viruses: Agents of Change***, McGraw-Hill Publishing Co., New York, 1990.

22. Balch, James F, and Mark Stengler, ***Prescription for Natural Cures***, John Wiley and Sons, Hoboken NJ, 2004.

Overweight

1. Shomon, Mary J, ***Living Well With Hypothyroidism***, Quill (HarperCollins), NY, 2000.
2. Dworkin, Norine, "Can't lose weight?" ***Family Circle***, March 9, 2004, Vol. 117, No. 3, pp. 110-115.
3. Whitman, Stacy, "The truth about metabolism," ***Shape***, Sept. 2003, pp. 110-114.
4. Atkins, Robert C, ***Dr. Atkins' New Diet Revolution***, Avon Books Inc., NY, 1992, 1999.
5. Heller, Richard F, and Rachael F. Heller, ***The Carbohydrate Addict's Lifespan Program***, Plume (Penguin Putnam), NY, 1997.
6. Kellas, William, and Andrea S. Dworkin, ***Thriving in a Toxic World***, Professional Preference, Olivenhain CA, 1996.
7. Hatherill, J Robert, ***The Brain Gate***, LifeLine Press, Washington DC, 2003.
8. Hunt, Douglas, ***No More Cravings***, Warner Books, 1987.
9. Barnard, Neal, ***Turn Off the Fat Genes***, Harmony Books, NY, 2001.
10. Dancey, Elisabeth, ***The Cellulite Solution***, St. Martin's Paperbacks, NY, 1996.

Chronic fatigue, fibromyalgia, MCS

1. Metcalf and Holmes, ***Annals of the New York Academy of Science***, Vol. 160.
2. Vojdani, Aristo, N Brautbar and AW Campbell, "Antibody to silicone and native macromolecules in women with silicone breast implants," ***Immunopharmacology and Immunotoxicology***, Nov. 1994, Vol. 16, No. 4, pp. 497-523.
3. Goldberg, Burton, ***Alternative Medicine Guide to Chronic Fatigue, Fibromyalgia and Environmental Illness***, Future Medicine Publishing, Tiburon CA, 1998.
4. Crook, William G, ***Chronic Fatigue Syndrome and The Yeast Connection***, Professional Books, Jackson TN, 1992.
5. Buttram, Harold E, "Routine childhood vaccinations –A probable contributory cause of the chronic fatigue syndrome in young adults," ***Townsend Letter for Doctors***, Jan. 1994, p. 60.
6. Till, T, and K Maaly, "Mercury in tooth roots and in jaw bones," ***ZRW***, Vol. 87, Issue 6, 1978, pp. 288-90.
7. Casarett and Doull, ***Toxicology***, Macmillan Publishing Company, New York, 3rd edition, 1986.
8. Tanzer, Peter P, ***The Doctor's Guide to Sleep Without Pills***, Tresco Publishers, Canton OH, 1994.
9. Rosenbaum, Michael, and Murray Susser, ***Solving the Puzzle of Chronic Fatigue Syndrome***, Life Sciences Press, Tacoma WA, 1992.
10. "When fatigue isn't just fatigue," ***Family Circle***, Mar. 9, 1999, Vol. 112, No. 4, p. 52.
11. Price, Weston A, ***Nutrition and Physical Degeneration***, Harper & Brothers, NY, 1939.
12. www.fibromyalgia-resource.org, accessed 5/28/06.
13. Weisshaar, Rachel, "Silicone Breast Implant Victims to See Settlement Dollars," June 1, 2004, http://www.now.org/issues/health/060104settlement.html.
14. FDA – "Fibromyalgia and ruptured silicone gel breast implants – Updates," FDA Consumer, Nov-Dec. 2001, http://www.findarticles.com/p/articles/ mi_m1370/is_6_35/ai_80681267.
15. Shomon, Mary J, ***Living Well With Hypothyroidism***, Quill (HarperCollins), NY, 2000.
16. Ashford, Nicholas A, and Claudia S Miller, ***Chemical Exposures: Low Levels and High Stakes***, Van Nostrand Reinhold, NY, 1990.
17. Rea, William J, ***Chemical Sensitivity***, Volume I, Lewis Publishers, Boca Raton FL, 1992.
18. Weil, Andrew, "Frustrated by fibromyalgia?" 7/1/03, http://www.drweil.com/u/QA/QA269355/
19. ***Townsend Letter for Doctors***, 11/96, #160, p. 16
20. Miller CS, Mitzel HC. "Chemical sensitivity attributed to pesticide exposure versus remodeling," ***Archives of Environmental Health***, 1995, Vol.50, pp. 119-29.
21. Ross, Gerald H, Rea, WJ, & Johnson, AR (1989, Feb. 23-26), "A prospective cross sectional study comparing environmentally-sensitive patients and controls, measuring biochemical, hematological, immunological and toxicological parameters," ***Proceedings of the 7th Annual International Symposium on Man and his Environment in Health and Disease***, Dallas, TX.
22. Ross, Gerald H, "Treatment Options in Multiple Chemical Sensitivity," ***Toxicology and Industrial Health***, 1992, 8(4), 87-94.
23. "Detox," Thorne Research, Inc., Dover ID, May 2000.

<u>Part 3</u>

Pesticides

1. "Acute Pancreatitis Following Continuous Exposure to Organophosphate Insecticide," ***Internal Medicine World Report***, March 1-14, 1989.

2. Colborn, Theo and Coralie Clement (editors), ***Chemically Induced Alterations in Sexual and Functional Development***, Princeton Scientific Publishing Co., Princeton NJ, 1992.
3. Petty, CS, "Organic Phosphate Insecticide Poisoning," ***American Journal of Medicine***, Vol. 24, 1958, pp. 467-470.
4. Aesoph, Lauri, "The Poisonous Legacy of Pesticides," ***Delicious***, April 1994, pp. 32-4.
5. Raloff, Janet, "That Feminine Touch," ***Science News***, Vol. 145, Jan. 22, 1994, pp. 56-8.
6. Dadd, Debra Lynn, ***Nontoxic and Natural***, Jeremy P. Tarcher Inc., Los Angeles CA, 1984.

Solvents

1. Rogers, Sherry A, ***The E.I. Syndrome***, Prestige Publishing, Syracuse NY, 1986.
2. Dadd, Debra Lynn, ***Nontoxic and Natural***, Jeremy P. Tarcher Inc., Los Angeles CA, 1984.
3. Kaura, SR, ***Understanding and Preventing Cancer***, Health Press, Santa Fe NM, 1991.
4. Rogers, Sherry A, ***Tired or Toxic?*** Prestige Publishing, Syracuse NY, 1990.
5. Vaughn, TL, DS Strader, S Davis and JR Daling, "Formaldehyde and Cancers of the Pharynx, Sinus and Nasal Cavity, II: Residential Exposures," ***International Journal of Cancer***, Vol. 38, 1986, p. 685.
6. Aschwanden, Christie, "Problems with plastic," ***Oprah Magazine***, April 2009, Vol. 10, No. 4, p. 104.

Air pollution

1. Dadd, Debra Lynn, ***Nontoxic and Natural***, Jeremy P. Tarcher Inc., Los Angeles CA, 1984.

Water pollution

1. Yiamouyiannis, John, ***Fluoride: The Aging Factor***, Health Action Press, Delaware OH, 1986.
2. Dadd, Debra Lynn, ***Nontoxic and Natural***, Jeremy P. Tarcher Inc., Los Angeles CA, 1984.

Personal care products

1. Ashford, Nicholas A. and Claudia S. Miller, ***Chemical Exposures: Low Levels, High Stakes***, 1991.
2. ***Neurotoxins: At Home and the Workplace***, Report by the Committee on Science and Technology, U.S. House of Representatives, Sept. 16, 1986, Report 99-827.
3. "Making Sense of Scents," ***Townsend Letter for Doctors***, No. 132, July 1994, pp. 765-7.
4. Arnold, Kathryn, "Is Your Hair Dye Safe?" ***Delicious***, July/Aug. 1993, pp. 50+.
5. www. pharmsolutions.com/docs/NationalOrganicProgramReportonSodiumLaurylSulfate...

Drugs

1. ***Webster's II New Riverside University Dictionary***, Houghton Mifflin Co., Boston MA, 1994, p. 880.
2. Roe, DA, "Nutrient and Drug Interactions," ***Nutrition Reviews***, Vol. 42, No. 4, April 1984, pp. 141-154.
3. Beardsley, Tim, "Cannabis Comprehended," ***Scientific American***, Vol. 263, Oct. 1990, p. 38.
4. Levy, Stephen J., ***Managing the Drugs in Your Life***, McGraw-Hill Publishing Co., New York, 1983.
5. Krogh, David, ***Smoking: The Artificial Passion***, W.H. Freeman and Co., New York, 1991.
6. Abramson, R, "EPA Officially Links Passive Smoke, Cancer," ***Los Angeles Times***, Vol. 112, June 8, 1993, p. A27.
7. Roberts, Marjory, "Mouth Cancer from a Morning Gargle?" ***U.S. News and World Report***, Vol. 111, July 1, 1991, p. 63.
8. Gloeckner, Carolyn, "From Drinking to Disease," ***Current Health***, Vol. 17, Oct. 1990, pp. 23-5.
9. Thompson, WG, "Coffee: Brew or Bane?" ***American Journal of Medical Science***, Vol. 3308, No. 1, July 1994, pp. 49-57.
10. Simon, D, S Yen and P Cole, "Coffee Drinking and Cancer of the Lower Urinary Tract," ***Journal of the National Cancer Institute***, Vol. 54, No. 3, March 1975, pp. 587-591.

Food additives

1. Steinman, David, ***Diet For A Poisoned Planet***, Ballantine Books, NY, 1990.
2. Kellas, William R. and Andrea S. Dworkin, ***Surviving The Toxic Crisis***, Professional Preference, Olivenhain CA, 1996.
3. Rinzler, Carol Ann, ***Nutrition For Dummies***, IDG Books, Foster City CA, 1997.
4. Winter, Ruth, ***A Consumer's Dictionary of Food Additives***, Crown Publishing, NY, 1984.

Metals

Mercury

1. Huggins, Hal, and Sharon Huggins, ***It's All in Your Head***, Life Sciences Press, Colorado Springs CO, 1986.
2. Heintz, Edwardson, Derand and Birkhed, "Methylation of Mercury From Dental Amalgam and Mercuric Chloride by Oral Streptococci," ***Scandinavian Journal of Dental Research***, Vol. 91, 1983, pp. 150-2.
3. Begley, Sharon, and Patricia King, "Drilling for Danger," ***Newsweek***, Oct. 15, 1990.
4. Taylor, Joyal, ***The Complete Guide to Mercury Toxicity from Dental Fillings***, Scripps Publishing, San Diego CA, 1988.
5. Hahn et al, ***The FASEB Journal***, Vol. 3, Dec. 1989, pp. 2643+.
6. Till, T, and K Maaly, "Mercury in Tooth Roots and in Jaw Bones," ***ZRW***, Vol. 87, Issue 6, 1978, pp. 288-90.

7. Casarett and Doull, ***Toxicology***, Macmillan Publishing Company, New York, 3rd edition, 1986.
8. Balch, James F, and Phyllis A. Balch, ***Prescription for Nutritional Healing***, Avery Publishing Group, Garden City Park, NY, 1990.
9. Balch, James F, and Phyllis A Balch, ***Prescription for Nutritional Healing***, Avery Publishing Group, Garden City Park, NY, 2nd ed., 1997.
10. Ward, NI and JA Mason, "Neutron Activation Analysis Techniques for Identifying Elemental Status in Alzheimer's Disease," ***Journal of Radioanalytical Nuclear Chemistry***, Vol. 113, No. 2, 1987, pp. 515-526.
11. Wenk, GL and KL Stemmer, "Suboptimal Dietary Zinc Intake Increases Aluminum Accumulation Into the Rat Brain," ***Brain Research***, Vol. 288, 1983, pp. 393-5.

Microorganisms

1. Graham, Barbara, "A New Bug in Town," ***Health***, Oct. 1990, pp. 38-40.
2. Shepherd, RW, and PFL Boreham, "Recent Advances in the Diagnosis and Management of Giardiasis," ***Scand. J. Gastroenterology***, 1989, Vol. 24, pp. 60-64.
3. Diaczok, BJ, J Rival, "Diarrhea Due to Blastocystis Hominis: An Old Organism Revisited," ***Southern Medical Journal***, July 1987, Vol. 80, No. 7, pp. 931-2.
4. Schmidt, Gerald D, and Larry S. Roberts, ***Foundations of Parasitology***, Times Mirror / Mosby College Publishing, St. Louis MO, 3rd ed., 1985.
5. ***McGraw-Hill Encyclopedia of Science and Technology***, McGraw-Hill Book Co., 1992, 7th ed.
6. Rodolsky, Doug M, "Kill the Bug and You Kill the Ulcer," ***U.S. News and World Report***, Vol. 110, May 13, 1991, p. 94.
7. Whitman, Sylvia, "Hepatitis," ***Current Health***, Vol. 18, Sept. 1991, pp. 12-13.
8. Fettner, Ann Giudici, ***Viruses: Agents of Change***, McGraw-Hill Publishing Co., New York, 1990.
9. Eisenberg, Steve, "From One Lover to Another: The Infection That Can Lead to Cancer," ***Health***, Vol. 20, Sept. 1988, pp. 62-64+.
10. Shoemaker, Ritchie C, with Patti Schmidt, ***Mold Warriors***, Gateway Press, Baltimore MD, 2005.
11. Smith, Alice Lorraine, ***Principles of Microbiology***, C.V. Mosby Co., St. Louis MO, 9th ed., 1981.

Part 4

Detox diet

1. Haas, Elson, and Daniella Chace, ***The New Detox Diet***, Celestial Arts, Berkeley CA, 2004.

Sauna detoxification

1. Schnare, DW et al, "Evaluation of a Detoxification Regimen for Fat Stored Xenobiotics", ***Medical Hypotheses***, Vol. 9, no. 3, 1982, pp. 265-282.
2. Gard, Zane R. and Erma J. Brown, "Literature review and comparison studies of sauna / hyperthermia in detoxification", ***Townsend Letter for Doctors and Patients***, August/September 1999, Vol. 193-4, pp. 76-86.
3. Thrash, A and CL Thrash Jr, ***Home Remedies: Hydrotherapy, Massage, Charcoal, and Other Simple Treatments***, New Life Books, Grovel-and CA, 1981.
4. Goldberg, Burton (ed.), "Hyperthermia", ***Alternative Medicine: The Definitive Guide***, Future Medicine Publishing, Inc., Puyallup WA, 1999, 2nd ed., pp. 299-305.

Metal detoxification

1. Olszewer, E, and JP Carter, "EDTA Chelation Therapy: A Retrospective Study of 2,870 Patients," in ***A Textbook on EDTA Chelation Therapy***, Elmer M. Cranton (ed.), ***Journal of Advancement in Medicine***, Vol. 2, No. 1-2, Human Sciences Press, NY, 1989, pp. 197-211.
2. Alsleben, HR, and WE Shute, ***How to Survive The New Health Catastrophes***, Survival Publications Inc., Anaheim CA, 1973.

3. Hoffer, Abram, "Alzheimer's – An anecdote," ***Townsend Letter for Doctors and Patients***, June 1998, Vol. 179, pp. 107-9.

4. Kellas, William, and Andrea S. Dworkin, ***Surviving the Toxic Crisis***, Professional Preference, Olivenhain CA, 1996.

5. Blumer, W, and EM Cranton, "Ninety percent reduction in cancer mortality after chelation therapy with EDTA," in ***A Textbook on EDTA Chelation Therapy***, Cranton EM ed., Special issue, Journal of Advancement in Medicine, 1989, Vol. 2, No. 1-2, Human Sciences Press, NY, p. 183.

6. www.holistic-online.com/Chelation/chel_ben_cancer.htm, accessed 3/24/04.

7. Olszewer, E, and Carter, JP, "EDTA Therapy in Chronic Degenerative Disease," Medical Hypotheses, Vol. 27, No. 1, Sept. 1988, pp. 41-49.

8. Strohecker, James (ed.), "Chelation Therapy," ***Alternative Medicine: The Definitive Guide***, Future Medicine Publishing, Inc., Puyallup WA, 1994, pp. 126-133.

Cleansing of detox organs

1. Sutherland, Caroline M., ***The Body Knows***, Hay House, Carlsbad CA, 2001.

2. Hill, TL, "The Link Between Breast Cancer and Bras," ***Nude and Natural***, Vol. 15, No. 2, 1996, pp. 40-42.

3. Gaby, Alan R, "Does Wearing a Bra Cause Breast Cancer?" ***Townsend Letter for Doctors and Patients***, No. 154, May 1996, p. 29.

4. Singer, Sydney Ross and Soma Grismaijer, "Dressed to Kill: The Link Between Breast Cancer and Bras," ***Townsend Letter for Doctors and Patients***, No. 151/152, Feb./Mar. 1996, p. 42.

5. Colbert, Don, ***Toxic Relief***, Siloam Press, Lake Mary FL, 2001.

6. Novozhilov, A, ***Buteyko Method***, 2003.

Allergy

1. Nambudripad, Devi, ***Say Goodbye To Illness***, Delta Publishing Company, Buena Park, CA, 1993.

2. Nambudripad, Devi, ***The NAET Guidebook***, Delta Publishing Company, Buena Park, CA, 1994.

3. Cutler, Ellen, ***The Food Allergy Cure***, Harmony Books, 2001.

Part 5

Supporters

1. Colbert, Don, ***Toxic Relief***, Siloam Press, Lake Mary FL, 2001.

2. Carper, Jean, ***Miracle Cures***, HarperCollins Publishers, NY, 1997.

3. "Amino acids," www.healingwith nutrition.com/aminoacid.html.

4. Muscaritoli, M et al, "Oral glutamine in the prevention of chemotherapy-induced gastrointestinal toxicity," ***European Journal of Cancer***, 1997, Vol. 33, pp. 319-320.

5. Azzara, A et al, "Effects of Lysine-Arginine Association on Immune Functions in Patients with Recurrent Infections," ***Drugs Experimental Clinical Research***, Vol. 21, 1995, pp. 71-78.

6. www.virtualhealthinfo.com/herb/Siberian_ginseng.htm.

7. Kamal-Eldin, A, and L Appelqvist, "The chemistry and antioxidant properties of tocopherols and tocotrienols," ***Lipids***, 1996, Vol. 31, pp. 671-80.

8. www.naturalhealthconsult.com/monographs/tocotrienol.html.

9. www.1stplace-supplements.com/energe-5000.phtml.

10. www.lef.org/newshop/items/item00456.html.

11. Draper, Dave, "Whey protein," www.davedraper.com/whey-protein.html.

12. Meydani, SN and WK Ha, "Immunologic effects of yogurt," ***American Journal of Clinical Nutrition***, 2000, Vol. 71, p. 861.

13. Smirnov, VV, SR Reznic et al, "The current concepts of the mechanisms of the therapeutic-prophylactic action of probiotics from bacteria in the genus bacillus," ***Mikrobiolohichnyi Zhurnal***, 1993, Vol. 55, No. 4, pp. 92-112.

14. Melnikova, VM, NM Gracheva, GPBelikov et al, "The chemoprophylaxis and chemotherapy of opportunistic infections," ***Antibiotiki i Khimioterapiia***, 1993, Vol. 38, pp. 44-48.

Herbs

1. Haas, Elson, and Daniella Chace, ***The New Detox Diet***, Celestial Arts, Berkeley CA, 2004.

Index

(Also see Glossary for definitions)

F

N

O

P